CADRE

For updated information on
insulin and oral agents,
please visit the "What's New" section of
the CADRE website at
www.cadre-diabetes.org

D1509080

# Insulin Therapy

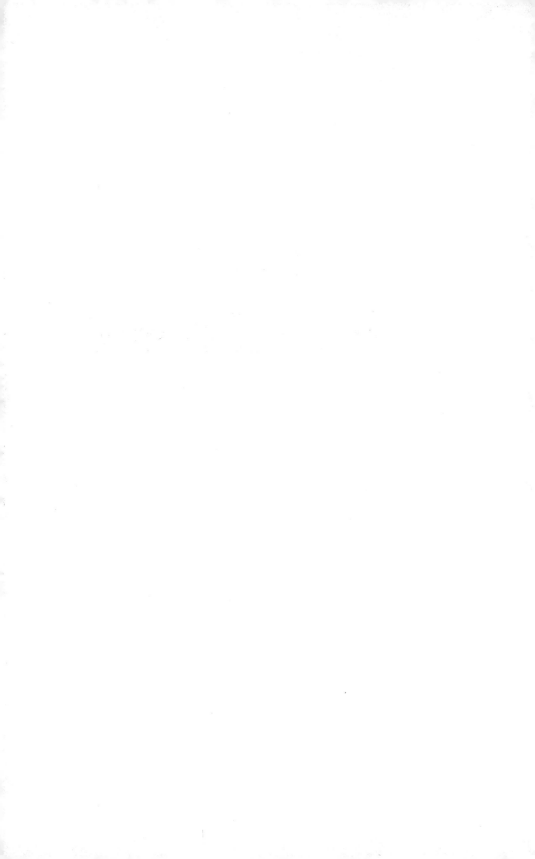

# Insulin Therapy

edited by

## Jack L. Leahy
## William T. Cefalu

*University of Vermont College of Medicine*
*Burlington, Vermont*

MARCEL DEKKER, INC.          NEW YORK · BASEL

**ISBN: 0-8247-0711-7**

This book is printed on acid-free paper.

**Headquarters**
Marcel Dekker, Inc.
270 Madison Avenue, New York, NY 10016
tel: 212-696-9000; fax: 212-685-4540

**Eastern Hemisphere Distribution**
Marcel Dekker AG
Hutgasse 4, Postfach 812, CH-4001 Basel, Switzerland
tel: 41-61-261-8482; fax: 41-61-261-8896

**World Wide Web**
http://www.dekker.com

The publisher offers discounts on this book when ordered in bulk quantities. For more information, write to Special Sales/Professional Marketing at the headquarters address above.

**PRINTED IN THE UNITED STATES OF AMERICA**

# Preface

During the 1990s, diabetes mellitus emerged as an international health crisis. Much of the attention has focused on type 2 diabetes, reflecting the skyrocketing incidence of obesity and associated illness around the world. Many oral therapies are available for type 2 diabetes, and practicing physicians are generally knowledgeable about their use. However, given the progressive nature of type 2 diabetes, more than one oral antidiabetic agent is often required, and combination oral therapy is now considered the standard of care for most patients. Continued progression of the disease causes oral therapy to eventually fail in many patients, requiring exogenous insulin either as monotherapy or in combination with oral agents. Thus, when glycemic control is not achievable in the type 2 diabetic patient as determined by failure to achieve the target $HbA_{1c}$ level with traditional oral therapies, it is appropriate to consider insulin.

Insulin therapy has undergone major changes over the last few years. Insulin analogs (often referred to as *designer insulins*) are now available that closely approximate the delivery of insulin from a healthy pancreas. Injection equipment is easy to use, and for most patients injections are painless. Further, in a few years we will likely have inhaled insulin or some other noninvasive approach for insulin delivery. However, these advances have not been easily integrated into clinical practice. Insulin therapy of both type 1 and type 2 diabetes remains a difficult, frustrating experience for physicians and patients, reflecting most patients' wish to avoid self-injection therapy, plus the concerns of many physicians about hypoglycemia, weight gain, or worsening cardiovascular risk. Contributing to this is a dearth of educational material regarding insulin therapy; many caregivers do not feel knowledgeable about how to use insulin optimally.

The current volume is intended to be a comprehensive, up-to-date, clinically based resource for practicing providers and those in training regarding insulin therapy. Contributors were charged to use a "how to" format, but also to include physiological and pharmacological concepts to make understandable the design and troubleshooting of inpatient and outpatient insulin programs.

The book is divided into three sections. Part I (Chapters 1–6) provides a general background: a rationale for optimal glycemia control in diabetes and standards of care, injection and glucose-monitoring equipment, dietary practices, physiology of insulin secretion and blood glucose regulation, and pharmacokinetics of the available insulin preparations. Part II (Chapters 7–12) applies these principles to specific patient populations: those with type 1 and type 2 diabetes, children, inpatients, pregnant women, and patients experiencing hyperglycemic emergencies. Part III (Chapters 13–15) addresses prevention and therapy of hypoglycemia, insulin pumps, and noninvasive approaches for insulin delivery.

There is one style issue. The term "analog" is used throughout the text: prior medical literature mostly used "analogue," but this alternative spelling is now increasingly used.

We would like to thank the many contributors to this volume. Without their diligence, patience, and humor, this project would have remained simply a fantasy of the editors.

**Jack L. Leahy**
**William T. Cefalu**

# Contents

*Preface*                                                                    *iii*

*Contributors*                                                                *vii*

## Part I: BACKGROUND

1. **Rationale for and Strategies to Achieve Glycemic Control**        **1**
   *William T. Cefalu*

2. **Goals of Treatment**                                             **13**
   *Nathaniel G. Clark*

3. **Insulin Syringes, Pens, and Glucose-Monitoring Equipment
   and Techniques**                                                   **21**
   *Margaret Costello*

4. **Nutrition Assessment and Therapy**                               **47**
   *Linda Tilton*

5. **Physiology of Glucose Homeostasis and Insulin Secretion**        **61**
   *Robert A. Ritzel and Peter C. Butler*

6. **Insulin Pharmacokinetics**                                       **73**
   *Steven D. Wittlin, Hans J. Woehrle, and John E. Gerich*

## Part II: PATIENT POPULATIONS

7. **Intensive Insulin Therapy in Type 1 Diabetes Mellitus**     87
   *Jack L. Leahy*

8. **Insulin Therapy in Type 2 Diabetes Mellitus**     113
   *Andrew J. Ahmann and Matthew C. Riddle*

9. **Insulin Therapy in Children**     127
   *William V. Tamborlane and JoAnn Ahern*

10. **Insulin Therapy in Pregnancy**     139
    *Lois Jovanovic*

11. **Insulin Management of Hospitalized Diabetic Patients**     153
    *Muriel H. Nathan and Jack L. Leahy*

12. **Hyperglycemic Emergencies: Diabetic Ketoacidosis and
    Nonketotic Hyperosmolar Syndrome**     173
    *Muriel H. Nathan*

## Part III: PREVENTION AND THERAPY

13. **Insulin Therapy and Hypoglycemia**     193
    *Anthony L. McCall*

14. **The Art and Science of Insulin-Pump Therapy**     223
    *Alan O. Marcus*

15. **Noninvasive Insulin-Delivery Systems: Options and Progress
    to Date**     245
    *William T. Cefalu*

*Index*     *261*

# Contributors

**JoAnn Ahern, M.S.N., A.P.R.N., C.D.E.**   Department of Pediatrics, Yale School of Medicine, New Haven, Connecticut

**Andrew J. Ahmann, M.D.**   Division of Endocrinology, Diabetes and Clinical Nutrition, Department of Medicine, Oregon Health and Science University, Portland, Oregon

**Peter C. Butler, M.D.**   Division of Endocrinology and Diabetes, Department of Medicine, Keck School of Medicine, University of Southern California, Los Angeles, California

**William T. Cefalu, M.D.**   Division of Endocrinology, Diabetes, and Metabolism, Department of Medicine, University of Vermont College of Medicine, Burlington, Vermont

**Nathaniel G. Clark, M.S., R.D., M.D.**   American Diabetes Association, Alexandria, Virginia

**Margaret Costello, R.N, M.S., C.D.E.**   Vermont Regional Diabetes Center, Fletcher Allen Health Care, University of Vermont College of Medicine, Burlington, Vermont

**John E. Gerich, M.D.**   University of Rochester School of Medicine and Dentistry, Rochester, New York

**Lois Jovanovic, M.D.**   Sansum Medical Research Institute, Santa Barbara, California

**Jack L. Leahy, M.D.**   Division of Endocrinology, Diabetes, and Metabolism, Department of Medicine, University of Vermont College of Medicine, Burlington, Vermont

**Alan O. Marcus, M.D.**   University of Southern California Medical School, Los Angeles, and Saddleback Memorial Medical Center, Laguna Hills, California

**Anthony L. McCall, M.D., Ph.D., F.A.C.P.**   Division of Endocrinology and Metabolism, Department of Internal Medicine, University of Virginia Health System, Charlottesville, Virginia

**Muriel H. Nathan, M.D., Ph.D**   Division of Endocrinology, Diabetes, and Metabolism, Department of Medicine, University of Vermont College of Medicine, Burlington, Vermont

**Matthew C. Riddle, M.D.**   Division of Endocrinology, Diabetes and Clinical Nutrition, Department of Medicine, Oregon Health and Science University, Portland, Oregon

**Robert A. Ritzel, M.D.**   Division of Endocrinology and Diabetes, Department of Medicine, Keck School of Medicine, University of Southern California, Los Angeles, California

**William V. Tamborlane, M.D.**   Pediatric Pharmacology Research Unit and Children's Clinical Research Center, Department of Pediatrics, Yale School of Medicine, New Haven, Connecticut

**Linda Tilton, M.S, R.D., C.D.E.**   Vermont Regional Diabetes Center, Fletcher Allen Health Care, University of Vermont College of Medicine, Burlington, Vermont

**Steven D. Wittlin, M.D.**   University of Rochester School of Medicine and Dentistry, Rochester, New York

**Hans J. Woehrle, M.D.**   University of Rochester School of Medicine and Dentistry, Rochester, New York

# Insulin
# Therapy

# 1

## Rationale for and Strategies to Achieve Glycemic Control

**William T. Cefalu**

University of Vermont College of Medicine, Burlington, Vermont

### INTRODUCTION

The prevalence of diabetes is increasing in epidemic proportions on a worldwide basis. In the United States alone, it has been estimated that there are approximately 16 million patients with diabetes, representing about 6% of the population. In addition, an estimated 5.4 million people are undiagnosed. On a more alarming note, it has been estimated that approximately 20 million people have impaired glucose tolerance, a clinical state felt to be representative of pre-diabetes. The projected increase in new cases of diabetes is also expected to increase the prevalence of complications associated with the disease, i.e., retinopathy, neuropathy, nephropathy, and cardiovascular disease. In addition to the morbidity and mortality resulting from these complications, the financial cost is staggering. It has been estimated that the total cost to care for diabetes and its related complications in the United States alone was over $98 billion for the year 1997. Thus, the current and evolving emphasis in diabetes management is to 1) evaluate strategies for the prevention of the disease and 2) implement clinical treatment regimens, as outlined in subsequent chapters, with the goal of reducing or delaying the progression of these devastating complications.

There have been significant advances in the understanding of the etiology and pathogenesis of both type 1 and type 2 diabetes. Whereas type 1 diabetes has been established to be an autoimmune process associated with pancreatic destruction, resulting in an absolute insulin-deficient state, type 2 diabetes is associated with insulin resistance, increased hepatic glucose production, and, in all cases, a "relative" deficiency of insulin. As such, despite laboratory studies suggesting a normal or elevated insulin level in subjects with type 2 diabetes compared with nondiabetic subjects, the insulin level is not sufficient to completely compensate for the increased insulin resistance of the peripheral tissues—i.e., muscle and fat—required to maintain glycemia. The failure of adequate insulin secretory compensation ultimately results in hyperglycemia and the diagnosis of type 2 diabetes.

Despite differences in the etiology of type 1 and type 2 diabetes, the common biochemical manifestation is hyperglycemia. Chronic hyperglycemia is considered a major factor in the development of microvascular complications in both type 1 and type 2 diabetes and contributes greatly to the pathogenesis of macrovascular disease. As such, diabetes remains a major cause of premature death and disability in the United States: It remains the leading cause of new cases of blindness in adults, and it is responsible for over 50% of nontraumatic lower-extremity amputations and approximately 50% of new cases of end-stage renal disease. It has also been established that the presence of diabetes causes a two- to fourfold increase in cardiovascular risk. Because of the accelerated cardiovascular risk, the most recent National Cholesterol Education Program (NCEP) guidelines suggest that diabetes represents a "risk equivalent" for cardiovascular disease and warrants treatment to lipid goals comparable to that for patients with pre-existing cardiovascular disease. It is hard to imagine that at one time the contribution of hyperglycemia to development of these complications was questioned. Yet the studies reported over the past 10 years leave little doubt that hyperglycemia is indeed a major causative factor in the development of complications. The precise mechanism(s) by which chronic hyperglycemia promotes tissue complications, however, is still an area of great debate and research interest.

## ROLE OF HYPERGLYCEMIA IN THE DEVELOPMENT OF COMPLICATIONS: EVIDENCE TO DATE

Clinical evidence supporting glycemic control as a primary goal of management exists for both type 1 and type 2 diabetes (Table 1). The landmark study, the Diabetes Control and Complications Trial (DCCT), was reported in 1993. This trial evaluated a total of 1441 subjects with type 1 diabetes and included 726 subjects with no retinopathy at baseline (primary-prevention cohort) and 715 with mild retinopathy (secondary-intervention cohort). The subjects were randomly assigned to intensive treatment (administered either with an external insulin pump

TABLE 1  Clinical Evidence for Benefits of Glycemic Control

| | Study (subject type) | | | |
| --- | --- | --- | --- | --- |
| | DCCT (type 1) | Kumamoto (type 2) | UKPDS (type 2) | SDIS (type 1) |
| Retinopathy | 63% | 69% | 17–21% | 63 vs. 33%[b] |
| Nephropathy | 54% | 70% | 24–33% | 26 vs. 7[b] |
| Neuropathy | 60% | — | — | 32 vs. 14[b] |
| Macrovascular Dx | 41%[a] | — | 16%[a] | — |
| HbA$_{1c}\Delta$ | 9–7% | 9–7% | 8–7% | 9.5–7.2% |

[a] Not statistically significant.
[b] Compared with standard treatment.

or by three or more insulin injections) or to conventional therapy (one or two daily insulin injections). The subjects were followed for a mean of 6.5 years, and the appearance and progression of retinopathy and other complications were assessed regularly. The trial demonstrated conclusively that control of clinical hyperglycemia, as evidenced by a reduction in HbA$_{1c}$, reduced retinopathy by 75%, nephropathy by 54%, and neuropathy by 60%. There was also a 41% reduction in macrovascular disease, but this was not statistically significant because of the low number of events.

The Stockholm Diabetes Intervention Study (SDIS) also evaluated the benefit of glycemic control in type 1 subjects. In this trial, 43 subjects were randomized to intensified conventional treatment (ICT) and 48 subjects randomized to standard treatment (ST). Subjects were followed for 10 years while vascular complications, treatment side effects, well-being, and risk factors for complications were studied. HbA$_{1c}$ (normal range 3.9–5.7%) was reduced from 9.5 $\pm$ 1.4% (mean $\pm$ SD) in the ICT group and 9.4 $\pm$ 1.2% in the ST group to a mean (during 10 years) to 7.2 $\pm$ 0.6% and 8.3 $\pm$ 1.0%, respectively ($p < 0.001$). Serious retinopathy (63 vs. 33%; $p = 0.003$), nephropathy (26 vs. 7%; $p = 0.012$), and symptoms of neuropathy (32 vs. 14%; $p = 0.041$) were more common in the ST group after 10 years.

Several landmark studies have been reported for type 2 diabetic subjects. The Kumamoto Study examined whether intensive glycemic control could decrease the frequency and severity of diabetic complications. This prospective study of Japanese subjects with non-insulin-dependent diabetes (NIDDM) included 110 subjects with NIDDM who were randomly assigned to either the multiple insulin injection treatment (MIT) group or the conventional insulin injection treatment (CIT) group. Fifty-five subjects who showed no retinopathy and urinary albumin excretions <30 mg/24 hours at baseline were evaluated in the primary prevention cohort, and the other 55 NIDDM subjects (who showed simple retinopathy and urinary albumin excretions <300 mg/24 hours) were evaluated in the secondary intervention cohort. The appearance and progression of retinopathy, nephropathy, and neuropathy were evaluated every 6 months over a 6-year period. A significant difference in glycemic control was demonstrated between groups as assessed by a 2.3% difference in $HbA_{1c}$ levels. The progression in retinopathy and nephropathy after 6 years was significantly less for the MIT group than for the CIT group, for both the primary and secondary intervention cohorts. In neurological tests, the MIT group showed significant improvement in the nerve conduction velocities, while the CIT group showed significant deterioration in the median nerve conduction velocities and vibration threshold. From this study, a $HbA_{1c}$ of <6.5% was indicated as the glycemic threshold to prevent the onset and progression of diabetic microangiopathy.

The United Kingdom Prospective Diabetes Study (UKPDS) was a multicenter, randomized, controlled trial in over 4000 type 2 diabetic subjects conducted between 1977 and 1997. Subjects were followed every 3 months for 3, 6, or 9 years. The study objectives were to determine whether intensive therapy of type 2 diabetic subjects reduces the risk for complications and to compare intensive pharmacological therapy with conventional therapy. Subjects were first placed on a low-fat, high-carbohydrate, high-fiber diet for 3 months and then randomized to diet alone, insulin, sulfonylurea, or metformin. Over 10 years, $HbA_{1c}$ was 7.0% (6.2–8.2) in the intensive group versus 7.9% (6.9–8.8) in the conventional group—an 11% reduction. There was no difference in $HbA_{1c}$ among agents in the intensive group. Compared with the conventional group, the risk in the intensive group was 12% lower (95% CI 1–21; $p = 0.029$) for any diabetes-related endpoint, 10% lower (−11 to 27; $p = 0.34$) for any diabetes-related death, and 6% lower (−10 to 20; $p = 0.44$) for all-cause mortality. Most of the risk reduction in the any-diabetes-related aggregate endpoint was due to a 25% risk reduction (7–40; $p = 0.0099$) in microvascular endpoints, including the need for retinal photocoagulation. There was no difference for any of the three aggregate endpoints between the three intensive agents (chlorpropamide, glibenclamide, or insulin).

In addition, 753 overweight subjects were included in a randomized controlled trial comparing conventional policy, primarily with diet alone ($n = 411$), with intensive blood glucose control policy with metformin, aiming for fasting plasma glucose <6 mmol/L ($n = 342$). A secondary analysis compared the 342 subjects allocated metformin with 951 overweight subjects allocated intensive blood glucose control with chlorpropamide ($n = 265$), glibenclamide ($n = 277$), or insulin ($n = 409$). Median $HbA_{1c}$ was 7.4% in the metformin group versus 8.0% in the conventional group. Subjects allocated metformin, compared with the conventional group, had risk reductions of 32% (95% CI 13–47; $p = 0.002$) for any diabetes-related endpoint, 42% for diabetes-related death (9–63; $p = 0.017$), and 35% for all-cause mortality (9–55; $p = 0.011$).

**TABLE 2** Epidemiological Analysis of the UKPDS

|  | Risk reduction relative to $HbA_{1c}$ (%) | |
| --- | --- | --- |
|  | $-1$ | $-1.5$ |
| Mortality |  |  |
| All causes | 14 | 17–21 |
| Related to diabetes | 21 | 24–33 |
| Events |  |  |
| Any diabetes-related endpoint | 21 | 32 |
| Microvascular disease | 37 | 56 |
| Amputation/death PVD | 43 | 65 |
| MI | 14 | 21 |
| CVA | 12 | 18 |
| CHF | 16 | 24 |

*Source*: Stratton et al., 2000.

Further analysis of the UKPDS suggests risk reduction for several endpoints; Table 2 demonstrates the risk reduction relative to specific decreases in $HbA_{1c}$.

The findings of the clinical trials demonstrate conclusively that intensive therapy, by significantly improving clinical glycemia, reduces the risk of microvascular and neurological complications. It is also seen from these trials that exogenous insulin therapy did not increase the risk of complications, in particular, macrovascular disease. This concept is well demonstrated by the UKPDS results, in which insulin therapy appeared to control glycemia as well as the pharmacological therapies, but there appeared to be no difference in macrovascular events between those treated with insulin and those taking the other oral therapies. The UKPDS study also suggested that type 2 diabetes, the most common form of the disease, is indeed a progressive disease that will require additional therapies (i.e., combination oral therapies and/or addition of insulin) in order to control glycemia over time.

Finally, clinical trials to date have also provided the data required to suggest target levels for glycemic control, as assessed with the $HbA_{1c}$. Current ADA guidelines suggest a target of $<7\%$. However, in the epidemiologic data from the UKPDS, there appears to be no lower threshold for $HbA_{1c}$ levels for which complications are not reduced (Figure 1). A number of small cohort trials, preceding and during the large interventional trials, further corroborate the significance of $HbA_{1c}$ elevations greater than 6.5%. These findings are also consistent with a number of epidemiological studies implicating the association of hyperglycemia

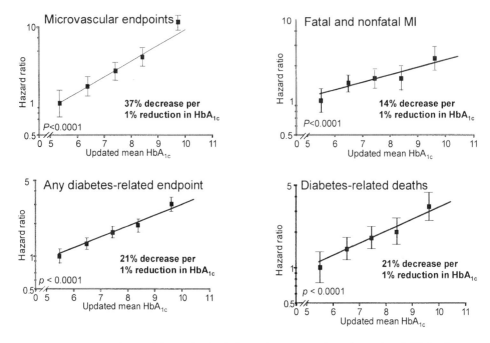

FIGURE 1 UKPDS epidemiological data demonstrating the role of HbA₁c in the hazard ratio for microvascular and macrovascular complications. (From Stratton et al., 2000.)

with the development of diabetic complications. A more recent study also pointed to the observation that a lowered HbA₁c may be favorable for cardiovascular events. This had been suggested by the EPIC-Norfolk Study, in which the relative risk for cardiovascular disease was much less, with recorded HbA₁c levels of <5%. Based on the evidence, a Consensus Conference of the American College of Endocrinology was recently convened; this conference suggested that the primary target for obtaining glycemic control should be <6.5%.

## ASSESSMENT OF CLINICAL GLYCEMIC CONTROL

The clinical trials to date have objectively assessed glycemic control by measuring the glycated hemoglobin level, a readily available clinical test and a mainstay for diabetes management for many years. This test relies on the nonenzymatic attachment of glucose to amino groups on proteins; since this reaction is nonenzymatic, the major factors contributing to the degree of protein "glycation," i.e., attachment of glucose to the protein, are the magnitude of the clinical hyperglycemia and the duration of exposure of the protein to clinical hyperglycemia. Numerous techniques are used in laboratories to assess glycated hemoglobin levels. The "total glycated hemoglobin" is a measure of the percentage of glycation of all hemoglobin species and traditionally has been assessed with an affinity chromatography technique. The most common assay, however, $HbA_{1c}$, has traditionally employed ion-exchange methodology and specifically measures the glycation of the major glycated hemoglobin species. It is important to recognize which test is offered in your clinic, because a measure of total glycated hemoglobin would be reported as a higher level than that of $HbA_{1c}$. Because the hemoglobin in the red blood cell has a half-life of approximately 60–90 days, measurement of glycated hemoglobin gives an overall objective index of glycemic control for the preceding 2–3 months.

Recently there has been interest in measuring glycation of other proteins, primarily albumin, that have shorter circulating half-lives (days or weeks instead of months). This would offer the clinician an objective measure of more recent glycemic control. These tests, which are commercially available, are performed by obtaining a plasma or serum fructosamine level. Assessment of serum fructosamine will provide an objective index over the past 1–2 weeks. These tests may be ideal in situations in which more frequent objective tests are needed, such as in pregnancy. Research also suggests that glucose may nonenzymatically attach to long-lived tissue protein, such as myelin in nerves and collagen in kidneys and arteries. It has been postulated that the glucose attached to these proteins may result in cross-linkage of proteins and lead to products referred to as advanced glycated end-products, or AGE proteins. The presence of these AGE proteins on long-lived tissue proteins has been postulated to alter protein structure and characteristics and therefore provide a mechanism by which hyperglycemia may contribute to the development of diabetic complications.

Clinical glycemia can be described as consisting of two components: 1) basal or fasting glucose levels, and 2) meal-related glycemic, or postprandial, elevations (Figure 2). The fasting glucose level is influenced by hepatic glucose production and hepatic sensitivity to insulin. Postprandial glucose levels are influenced by: 1) the preprandial glucose level, 2) meal-related insulin secretion, 3) the glucose load from the meal, and 4) peripheral tissue sensitivity to insulin. As demonstrated in Figure 2, the preprandial glucose is normally maintained in a narrow range. However, in subjects with diabetes, in which alterations occur in the factors controlling these parameters, both the fasting and postprandial levels are elevated. Thus, an elevated $HbA_{1c}$ level in diabetic states is reflective of contributions from the elevated fasting or preprandial glucose level and the postprandial glycemic rise. This concept is very important on clinical grounds, as it suggests that control of both fasting/preprandial and postprandial glucose levels is required to normalize the $HbA_{1c}$ level.

Traditionally, it has been the targeting of preprandial levels that has

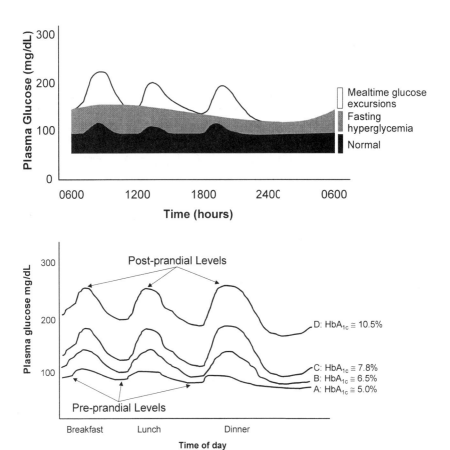

**Figure 2** (Top) Relative contributions of FPG and mealtime glucose excursions to 24-hour glycemic control. (From Riddle MC. Evening insulin strategy. Diabetes Care 13:676–686, 1990.) (Bottom) 24-hour glucose profiles for representative patients at various levels of glycemic control.

guided changes in insulin therapy. However, recent observations suggest that targeting postprandial levels may be an alternative clinical strategy. First, one could argue that targeting postprandial glucose levels is important based on the observations that postprandial glucose abnormalities are the earliest detectable glycemic change in diabetes. Second, it is postulated that postprandial glucose levels may correlate better to the $HbA_{1c}$ level; supporting this concept are studies in outpatient trials demonstrating that targeting treatment to control postprandial, as compared with preprandial, glucose levels in outpatient trials results in a more significant drop in HbA$_{1c}$. Third, evidence is mounting on the importance of postprandial glucose in the development of complications, particularly vascular complications. Specifically, the importance of postprandial glucose levels was demonstrated in the Honolulu Heart Study, which suggested that a significant increase in both fatal and total coronary heart disease was observed with increasing postprandial glucose. However, the most convincing data on postprandial glucose and cardiovascular disease have been compiled in the Diabetes Epidemiology: Collaborative Analysis of Diagnostic Criteria in Europe (DECODE) study. This study involved 13 centers in Europe and 25,364 patients with unknown glucose tolerance at baseline. Included were 13 studies of men (132,785 patient-years) and six studies of women (48,900 patient-years). The average follow-up was 10 years, with a median follow-up of 7.3 years. This study showed a highly significant increase in the hazard ratio for death in those with increased postprandial glucose >200 mg/dl (Figure 3) and strongly supports the concept of postprandial glycemia as an important marker of cardiovascular disease.

The emergence of postprandial glycemia as a contributor to diabetic complications provides an additional clinical target, as it is understood that both the fasting/preprandial glucose and postprandial glycemic excursion contribute to the HbA$_{1c}$ level. Figure 1B outlines four 24-hour glucose profiles representing

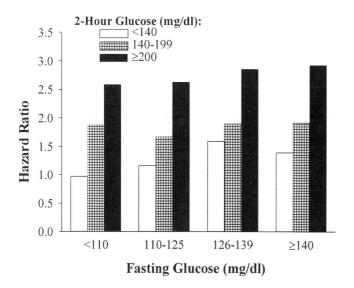

**FIGURE 3** Hazard ratios (95% CI) for death according to the fasting glucose and 2-hour glucose in individuals not known as diabetic. (From DECODE, 1999.)

"normal" and various levels of glycemic control. As demonstrated, profile A represents glucose levels for a nondiabetic individual with control of both pre- and postprandial excursions; one could suggest an approximate $HbA_{1c}$ of 5% for this individual based on the lowered glycemic profile. In contrast is a patient with uncontrolled hyperglycemia, as represented by profile D, with both elevated fasting and preprandial glucose levels, along with postprandial glycemic excursions. This profile may be representative of a patient with an $HbA_{1c}$ of approximately 10.5%. With improved control and improvement in both pre- and postprandial glucose levels, 24-hour glucose may be further improved, resulting in an $HbA_{1c}$ of approximately 7.8%, as suggested by profile C. This represents a very common clinical profile in that preprandial glucoses are controlled, yet the $HbA_{1c}$ is still not at target. This is a situation in which checking postprandial glycemia may be indicated, and adjusting therapy as needed to control these postprandial spikes. By improving postprandial hyperglycemia in the patient represented by profile C, a further reduction in $HbA_{1c}$ can be obtained, as outlined in the patient profile labeled B.

In summary, there is now definitive clinical evidence that hyperglycemia is related to the progression and development of diabetic complications. Although several mechanisms have been postulated, the precise mechanism(s) by which hyperglycemia contributes is not specifically known. Based on the clinical trials to date, we now have defined clinical goals for which to target levels of glycemic control. Further evolving concepts in the management of diabetes would suggest that understanding postprandial control may benefit our patients greatly by improving $HbA_{1c}$ and possibly by improving cardiovascular outcomes. However, the latter observation has not been clinically tested in prospective intervention trials.

## BIBLIOGRAPHY

ACE Consensus Conference on Guidelines for Glycemic Control [article online], 2001. Available from http://www.aace.com/pub/press/releases/diabetesconsensuswhite paper.php. Accessed Aug 24, 2001.

Adler AI, Stratton IM, Neil HA, Yudkin JS, Matthews DR, Cull CA, Wright AD, Turner RC, Holman RR. Association of systolic blood pressure with macrovascular and microvascular complications of type 2 diabetes (UKPDS 36): prospective observational study. Br Med J 321:412–419, 2000.

Cefalu WT, Wang ZQ, Bell-Farrow AD, McBride D, King T. Clinical validity of a self-test fructosamine in outpatient diabetic management. Diabetes Technol Ther 1:435–441, 1999.

DECODE Study Group. European Diabetes Epidemiology Group. Glucose tolerance and mortality: comparison of WHO and American Diabetes Association diagnostic criteria. Diabetes Epidemiology: Collaborative Analysis of Diagnostic Criteria in Europe. Lancet 354:617–621, 1999.

Diabetes Control and Complications Trial Research Group. The effect of intensive treatment of diabetes on the development and progression of long-term complications in insulin-dependent diabetes mellitus. N Engl J Med 329:977–986, 1993.

NCEP. Executive Summary of the Third Report of the National Cholesterol Education Program (NCEP) Expert Panel on Detection, Evaluation, and Treatment of High Blood Cholesterol in Adults (Adult Treatment Panel III). JAMA 285:2486–2497, 2001.

Ohkubo Y, Kishikawa H, Araki E, Miyata T, Isami S, Motoyoshi S, Kojima Y, Furuyoshi N, Shichiri M. Intensive insulin therapy prevents the progression of diabetic microvascular complications in Japanese patients with non-insulin-dependent diabetes mellitus: a randomized prospective 6-year study. Diabetes Res Clin Pract 28:103–117, 1995.

Reichard P, Berglund B, Britz A, Cars I, Nilsson BY, Rosenqvist U. Intensified conventional insulin treatment retards the microvascular complications of insulin-dependent diabetes mellitus (IDDM): the Stockholm Diabetes Intervention Study (SDIS) after 5 years. J Intern Med 230:101–108, 1991.

Reichard P, Pihl M, Rosenqvist U, Sule J. Complications in IDDM are caused by elevated blood glucose level: the Stockholm Diabetes Intervention Study (SDIS) at 10-year follow up. Diabetologia 39:1483–1488, 1996.

Shichiri M, Kishikawa H, Ohkubo Y, Wake N. Long-term results of the Kumamoto Study on optimal diabetes control in type 2 diabetic patients. Diabetes Care 23(suppl 2): B21–B29, 2000.

Singh R, Barden A, Mori T, Beilin L. Advanced glycation end-products: a review. Diabetologia 44:129–146, 2001.

Stratton IM, Adler AI, Neil HA, Matthews DR, Manley SE, Cull CA, Hadden D, Turner RC, Holman RR. Association of glycaemia with macrovascular and microvascular complications of type 2 diabetes (UKPDS 35): prospective observational study. Br Med J 321:405–412, 2000.

Turner RC, Cull CA, Frighi V, Holman RR. UK Prospective Diabetes Study (UKPDS) Group. Glycemic control with diet, sulfonylurea, metformin, or insulin in patients with type 2 diabetes mellitus: progressive requirement for multiple therapies (UKPDS 49). JAMA 281:2005–2012, 1999.

UK Prospective Diabetes Study (UKPDS) Group. Effect of intensive blood-glucose control with metformin on complications in overweight patients with type 2 diabetes (UKPDS 34). Lancet 352:854–865, 1998.

UK Prospective Diabetes Study (UKPDS) Group. Intensive blood-glucose control with sulphonylureas or insulin compared with conventional treatment and risk of complications in patients with type 2 diabetes (UKPDS 33). Lancet 352:837–853, 1998.

Ulrich P, Cerami A. Protein glycation, diabetes, and aging. Recent Prog Horm Res 56: 1–21, 2001.

# 2

## Goals of Treatment

**Nathaniel G. Clark**

American Diabetes Association, Alexandria, Virginia

### INTRODUCTION

The aim of this chapter is to describe the current treatment guidelines and goals of therapy for patients with diabetes mellitus as outlined by the American Diabetes Association (ADA) (1–3; Table 1). Each year the ADA publishes "Clinical Practice Recommendations," which are standards that have been shown to minimize the risk of both short-term (i.e., hypoglycemia) and long-term complications of diabetes. Such standards also allow objective assessment of the care provided by practitioners in managing patients with diabetes.

Over the past few years, the federal government has indicated great interest in improving diabetes care in the United States. The Diabetes Quality Improvement Project (DQIP), a collaborative effort of many groups involved with diabetes care, resulted in the development of a set of diabetes-specific performance and outcome measures—the first nationwide performance measures widely adopted by the health-care community. The National Committee for Quality Assurance (NCQA) included the DQIP measures in HEDIS 2000 (Health Employment Data Information Set), its evaluation program for accrediting health-care plans. In addition, the Heath Care Financing Administration (HCFA) now requires all health plans contracting with Medicare to report their DQIP data.

TABLE 1   American Diabetes Association Standards of Care

| Measure | Standard |
| --- | --- |
| Diagnosis of diabetes | |
| Fasting blood glucose (FBG) | >126 mg/dl |
| Casual (random) BG | >200 mg/dl (with symptoms) |
| 2-hour OGTT value | >200 mg/dl |
| Blood glucose goals | |
| Preprandial | 80–120 mg/dl |
| Bedtime | 100–140 mg/dl |
| Hemoglobin $A_{1c}$ | <7.0% |
| Lipids | |
| LDL | <100 mg/dl (children: <110 mg/dl) |
| HDL | >45 mg/dl (men), >55 mg/dl (women) |
| Triglycerides | <200 mg/dl |
| Blood pressure | <130/80 (children: <90th percentile for age) |
| Urinary microalbumin/creatinine ratio | <30 mg/g creatinine |
| Dilated eye exam | Yearly |
| Aspirin | Encouraged unless contraindicated |
| Foot exam | Each visit (high-risk patients); yearly complete exam in all patients |
| Smoking | Document status, encourage cessation |
| Immunizations | |
| Influenza | Yearly |
| Pneumococcal | Once. Revaccination of those >64 years of age (see text) |

## DIAGNOSTIC CRITERIA FOR DIABETES

In 1997, in collaboration with the World Health Organization, the ADA revised the guidelines for the diagnosis of diabetes mellitus into three criteria. If any single criterion is met, the diagnosis of diabetes is made.

1. The presence of the typical symptoms of ongoing hyperglycemia such as polyuria, polydipsia, and weight loss *and* a casual (random) plasma glucose concentration ≥200 mg/dl (11.1 mmol/L) *or*
2. A fasting plasma glucose ≥126 mg/dl (7.0 mmol/L). Fasting is defined as no caloric intake for at least 8 hours prior to the test *or*
3. A blood glucose level ≥200 mg/dl (11.1 mmol/L) at the 2-hour point of a 75-g oral glucose tolerance test (OGTT).

It is recommended that these criteria be confirmed by repeat testing on a different day before the diagnosis is firmly established.

Defining blood glucose levels for the diagnosis of diabetes also provided an opportunity to define blood glucose levels that, while not consistent with diabetes, did not fall within the normal range. Impaired fasting glucose (IFG) is defined as 110 to 125 mg/dl (6.1–7.0 mmol/L) and impaired glucose tolerance (IGT) is a 2-hour value on the OGTT of 140 to 199 mg/dl (7.8–11.1 mmol/L).

*Comment*: The need to obtain a confirmatory positive test on a different day needs to be considered in the context of the individual patient. A fasting blood glucose (FBG) of 135 mg/dl (7.5 mmol/L) in the absence of any symptoms of hyperglycemia warrants repeating, whereas an FBG of 300 mg/dl (27.7 mmol/L) in the setting of polyuria, polydipsia, and weight loss clearly indicates clinical diabetes and need not be repeated prior to beginning treatment. The hemoglobin $A_{1c}$ ($HbA_{1c}$) was not recommended as a diagnostic test for diabetes because it is not rigorously standardized around the world and the normal range can vary based on the assay used. Nonetheless, while a normal $HbA_{1c}$ does not rule out diabetes, an elevated value is highly significant and supports the diagnosis of diabetes or at least indicates a need for further testing.

## GLYCEMIC CONTROL

### Blood Glucose

The average preprandial blood glucose level should be 80–120 mg/dl (4.4–6.7 mmol/L). Action, i.e., changing the treatment plan, would be appropriate if this value were consistently below 80 mg/dl (4.4 mmol/L) or more than 140 mg/dl (7.8 mmol/L). It is recommended that the average bedtime glucose level be 100–140 mg/dl (5.6–7.8 mmol/L). Action is suggested if this value is consistently less than 100 or more than 160 mg/dl (8.8 mmol/L).

### Hemoglobin $A_{1c}$ ($HbA_{1c}$)

Although blood glucose levels obtained by self-monitoring using a blood glucose meter are extremely important in the day-to-day management of diabetes, hemoglobin $A_{1c}$ is accepted as the best measure of overall blood glucose control. This test has been used in all the major research studies that examined the relationship between glycemic control and complications. $HbA_{1c}$ provides a measure of average blood glucose level over the preceding 2–3 months (Table 2).

It is recommended that $HbA_{1c}$ be checked every 6 months in patients who are currently achieving blood glucose treatment goals and if the therapeutic regimen is stable. More frequent monitoring is recommended in those individuals who do not meet these criteria. For the majority of patients, checking $HbA_{1c}$ every 3 months would be prudent. In most laboratories in the United States, the

TABLE 2  Relationship Between Hemoglobin
$A_{1c}$ (HbA$_{1c}$) and Mean Blood Glucose Level

| Hemoglobin A$_{1c}$ (%) | Mean blood glucose level (mg/dl) |
|---|---|
| 5.0 | 90 |
| 6.0 | 120 |
| 7.0 | 150 |
| 8.0 | 180 |
| 9.0 | 210 |
| 10.0 | 240 |
| 11.0 | 300 |
| 12.0 | 330 |

normal range for individuals who do not have diabetes is approximately 4–6%. The goal for patients with diabetes is an HbA$_{1c}$ level less than 7%, with action suggested if the value is more than 8%.

*Comment*: The standards for HbA$_{1c}$ and blood glucose levels are the same for patients with type 1 and type 2 diabetes. It is well known, however, that the risk of hypoglycemia that accompanies very tight blood glucose control is much greater in patients with type 1 than in those with type 2 diabetes. With this in mind, the standards need to be individualized for each patient. A prior history of significant hypoglycemia is an important factor in setting the goal for blood glucose control. In addition, the goal should be *achievable* to prevent patient discouragement. A reduction of HbA$_{1c}$ from 10 to 8% is very significant clinically and should be positively reinforced even though the stated goal of less than 7% has not yet been achieved.

## LIPID CONTROL

The ADA has defined "low-risk" (<100 mg/dl, 2.60 mmol/L), "borderline" (100–129 mg/dl, 2.60–3.35 mmol/L), and "high-risk" (≥130 mg/dl, ≥3.38 mmol/L) LDL levels for adults. The goal for LDL in adults with diabetes is less than 100 mg/dl (<2.60 mmol/L). Similarly, levels of risk have been defined for HDL cholesterol. In men, "high-risk" is less than 35 mg/dl (<0.90 mmol/L), "borderline risk" 35–45 mg/dl (0.90–1.15 mmol/L), and "low-risk" more than 45 mg/dl (>1.15 mmol/L). For women, these values are increased by 10 mg/dl. The HDL goal is more than 45 mg/dl (>1.15 mmol/L) for men with diabetes and more than 55 mg/dl (>1.40 mmol/L) for women. In regard to plasma triglycerides, "high-risk" is greater than or equal to 400 mg/dl (≥4.50 mmol/L), "borderline risk" 200–399 mg/dl (2.30–4.50 mmol/L), and "low-risk" less than 200 mg/dl (<2.30 mmol/L). The goal for triglycerides in individuals with diabetes is less than 200 mg/dl (<2.30 mmol/L).

In children with risk factors for cardiovascular disease (e.g., diabetes), the goal for total cholesterol is less than 170 (4.4 mmol/L) and for LDL less than 110 mg/dl (<2.80 mmol/L). There are no stated guidelines for HDL or triglycerides in this population (4).

*Comment*: Recently published guidelines from the National Cholesterol Education Program (NCEP) state that the goal for LDL should be based on the patient's prior history of a significant cardiovascular event or the presence of defined risk factors for coronary disease (5). Previously, diabetes was simply considered a risk factor with the same relative weight as such other factors as family history of heart disease, smoking, hypertension, and gender. Recent studies have suggested that having diabetes confers a risk of cardiovascular disease equal to that of having had a previous cardiovascular event (6). In the 2001 NCEP guidelines, diabetes is considered a ''CHD risk equivalent,'' and the LDL goal when diabetes is present is less than 100 mg/dl.

## BLOOD-PRESSURE CONTROL

Hypertension should be treated aggressively in patients with diabetes. The goal for blood pressure is less than 130/80 in adults and below the 90th percentile for age in children. In the patient with diabetes, angiotensin-converting enzyme (ACE) inhibitors are the first choice for treatment of hypertension.

*Comment*: Hypertension is a significant risk factor for many of the complications of diabetes, playing a role in the development of retinopathy, nephropathy, and cardiovascular disease. Because cardiovascular disease is the most significant contributor to the morbidity and mortality in patients with type 2 diabetes, aggressive regulation of blood pressure is advised. A recent clinical advisory from the National High Blood Pressure Education program (7) indicates that the coexistence of diabetes and hypertension warrants a lower blood pressure goal (135/80) than for the patient with hypertension who does not have diabetes (140/90). ACE inhibitors, and perhaps angiotensin-receptor blockers, offer many advantages in the treatment of hypertension in the patient with diabetes. There is evolving research examining the role of these agents in vascular reactivity, endothelial function, and fibrinolysis that may underlie the recent exciting observation from the MICRO-HOPE study of a protective role for ACE inhibitors against cardiovascular disease in persons with diabetes (8).

## SCREENING FOR NEPHROPATHY

A spot urine sample should be analyzed for albumin and creatinine and an albumin:creatinine ratio calculated on a yearly basis, beginning at diagnosis in those with type 2 diabetes and after 5 years of diabetes in those with type 1. A ratio of less than 30 mg albumin/g creatinine is considered normal. Microalbuminuria is 30–300 mg/g creatinine; more than 300 mg/g is considered macroalbuminuria. As there are many causes of transient proteinuria, including exercise, fever, and urinary-tract infections, it is suggested that this test be performed on three separate occasions (with two of the three positive) before the patient is considered to have clinically significant albuminuria.

Using this test, patients who require aggressive treatment can be identified, thereby minimizing the risk of progressive nephropathy. Factors important in the reduction of risk for diabetic nephropathy include the control of blood glucose and treatment of hypertension. As in hypertension, ACE inhibitors are the drugs of choice in the treatment of albuminuria. For patients who cannot tolerate ACE inhibitors, the September 20th, 2001, issue of the *New England Journal of Medicine* contained three papers showing the utility of angiotensin receptor blockers in diabetic nephropathy (9–11).

*Comment*: When to begin screening children with type 1 diabetes is a controversial topic. Although previously it was felt that duration of diabetes prior to puberty was not clinically significant, there is now increasing evidence that the duration of diabetes should be considered regardless of pubertal status, and it is recommended that all patients with type 1 diabetes be screened after 5 years of disease.

## SCREENING FOR RETINOPATHY

A yearly dilated fundoscopic examination is recommended, beginning at diagnosis in patients with type 2 diabetes and after 3–5 years in those with type 1 diabetes. It is recommended that this examination be done by an ophthalmologist or optometrist who is knowledgeable and experienced in the diagnosis of diabetic retinopathy.

*Comment*: When to begin screening children with type 1 diabetes is a controversial topic. Although previously it was felt that duration of diabetes prior to puberty was not clinically significant, there is now increasing evidence that the duration of diabetes should be considered regardless of pubertal status, and the screening of all patients with type 1 after 3–5 years of diabetes is recommended.

Yearly screening allows the detection of diabetic retinopathy at its earliest stages, permitting close follow-up and laser treatment, as appropriate. It also allows other types of diabetes-associated eye disease to be identified, such as cataracts, as well as common eye problems such as glaucoma. The availability of laser therapy for diabetic retinopathy has made a significant difference in preserving eyesight. Moreover, the detection of eye disease early in the course, when there is minimal to no functional disruption, offers the additional opportunity to motivate the patient to strive for optimal blood glucose and blood-pressure control to hopefully prevent more serious retinopathy.

## ASPIRIN USE

Patients with diabetes have a markedly greater risk of developing cardiovascular disease and its complications. It is therefore recommended that aspirin therapy be considered for most adult patients who have diabetes. Specifically, it is suggested that aspirin be used as secondary prevention if there is evidence of large-vessel disease (history of myocardial infarction, vascular bypass procedure, stroke, transient ischemic attack, peripheral vascular disease, claudication, or angina). In addition, aspirin should be considered in primary cardiovascular-risk reduction in patients at increased risk for macrovascular disease; so practically most experts recommend aspirin use in all adults with type 2 diabetes. Enteric coated aspirin in doses from 81 to 325 mg per day are suggested.

## FOOT CARE

Clinical assessment of the feet should be made on a regular basis to identify risk of or existing foot problems. A yearly, complete foot examination, including assessment of protective sensation (using a microfilament), foot anatomy and biomechanics, vascular status, and skin integrity is suggested. Patients at high risk for foot problems (established neuropathy, for example) should be examined at every office visit.

## SMOKING

Smoking should be actively discouraged, and all available methods for smoking cessation employed.

## INFLUENZA AND PNEUMOCOCCAL IMMUNIZATION

Yearly immunization against influenza is recommended in all patients with diabetes older than 6 months of age. Pneumococcal vaccine is also recommended because patients with diabetes are considered at high risk for serious disease. A one-time revaccination of patients above 64 years old is recommended 5 years after the initial vaccination.

## SUMMARY

Substantial evidence exists that adherence to standards of care improves clinical outcomes of patients with diabetes. However, much evidence also exists that care providers do poorly in consistently meeting these standards. The use of either a formal flowsheet in the medical record or a computerized database that contains a record of past diabetes care will maximize the likelihood that these standards will be followed by the practitioner. These tools are becoming more widely available and their use is strongly encouraged.

## REFERENCES

1. Clark NG. Standards of care in diabetes. In: Leahy JL, Clark NG, Cefalu W, eds. Medical Management of Diabetes Mellitus. New York: Marcel Dekker, pp. 41–49, 2000.
2. American Diabetes Association. Clinical practice recommendations 2001. Diabetes Care 24(suppl 1):S1–133, 2001.
3. American Association of Clinical Endocrinologists medical guidelines for the management of diabetes mellitus: the AACE system of intensive diabetes self-management—2000 update. Endo Prac 6:43–84, 2000.
4. National Cholesterol Education Program (NCEP). Highlights of the report of the expert panel on blood cholesterol levels in children and adolescents. Pediatrics 89: 495–501, 1992.
5. Executive summary of the third report of the National Cholesterol Education Program (NCEP) expert panel on detection, evaluation and treatment of high blood cholesterol in adults (adult treatment panel III). JAMA 285:2486–2497, 2001.
6. Haffner SM, Lehto S, Ronnemaa T, Pyorala K, Laakso M. Mortality from coronary heart disease in subjects with type 2 diabetes and in nondiabetic subjects with and without prior myocardial infarction. N Engl J Med 339:229–234, 1998.
7. The sixth report of the Joint National Committee on Prevention, Detection, Evaluation, and Treatment of High Blood Pressure. Arch Intern Med 157:2413–2446, 1997.
8. Heart Outcomes Prevention Evaluation Study Investigators. Effects of ramipril on cardiovascular and microvascular outcomes in people with diabetes mellitus: results of HOPE study and MICRO-HOPE substudy. Lancet 2000 355:253–259, 2000.
9. Lewis EJ, Hunsicker LG, Clarke WR, Berl T, Pohl MA, Lewis JB, Ritz E, Atkins RC, Rohde R, Raz I. Renoprotective effect of the angiotensin-receptor antagonist irbesartan in patients with nephropathy due to type 2 diabetes. N Engl J Med 345: 851–860, 2001.
10. Brenner BM, Cooper ME, de Zeeuw D, Keane WF, Mitch WE, Parving HH, Remuzzi G, Snapinn SM, Zhang Z, Shahinfar S. Effects of losartan on renal and cardiovascular outcomes in patients with type 2 diabetes and nephropathy. N Engl J Med 345:861–869, 2001.
11. Parving HH, Lehnert H, Brochner-Mortensen J, Gomis R, Andersen S, Arner P. The effect of irbesartan on the development of diabetic nephropathy in patients with type 2 diabetes. N Engl J Med 345:870–878, 2001.

# 3

## Insulin Syringes, Pens, and Glucose-Monitoring Equipment and Techniques

**Margaret Costello**
Vermont Regional Diabetes Center, Fletcher Allen Health Care,
University of Vermont College of Medicine, Burlington, Vermont

## DIABETES SELF-MANAGEMENT

Diabetes self-management education is performed by specially trained nurses, dieticians, pharmacists, and others to provide patients the skills, knowledge, and confidence to manage their own diabetes on a day-to-day basis through analysis of their lifestyle practices and blood glucose patterns to make informed decisions in their insulin doses or other therapy. Self-management education involves a continuum of services ranging from the teaching of survival skills to a comprehensive self-management program. Given the importance of self-management for the attainment of optimal glycemic control, it is recommended that specially trained licensed health-care professionals provide diabetes self-management education. Certified Diabetes Educators (CDEs) must accrue 1000 hours in direct diabetes education and pass a certifying exam from the National Certification Board for Diabetes Educators, with a recertifying exam every 5 years. Certification implies expertise in diabetes knowledge, skills, and the teaching of diabetes education based on national standards.

The steps in the educational process are:

1. Assessment of educational needs
2. Planning the teaching-learning process
3. Implementation
4. Documentation of the areas covered and the patient's progress
5. Evaluation

## Survival Skills

Instruction in survival skills should be given to all patients with diabetes who are unable to participate in a comprehensive self-management program. The following areas should be covered, using information that is consistent with national and regional standards of care:

- Disease basics
- Self-monitoring of blood glucose
- Exercise and activity
- Medication use
- Hypoglycemia
- Nutrition

## Comprehensive Self-Management Program

A comprehensive self-management program is contained in the curriculum designed by the American Diabetes Association. There are 15 core educational areas:

1. Diabetes overview
2. Stress and psychosocial adjustment
3. Family involvement and social support
4. Nutrition
5. Exercise and activity
6. Medications
7. Self-monitoring and use of results
8. Relationships among nutrition, exercise and activity, medication, and blood glucose levels
9. Prevention, detection, and treatment of acute complications
10. Prevention, detection, and treatment of chronic complications
11. Foot, skin, and dental care
12. Behavior-change strategies, goal setting, risk-factor reduction, and problem-solving skills
13. Benefits, risks, and management options for improving glucose control

14. Use of health-care systems and community support resources
15. Preconception care, pregnancy, and gestational diabetes

## INSULIN THERAPY

### Patient Education

Many individuals are reluctant to initiate insulin therapy. Openly discussing their concerns prior to technical training is of prime importance. In particular, a common fear is that the injections will be painful or complex. Discussing up front the convenience of modern injection systems, and injecting the patient with saline to show the painlessness of the needle may be all that is needed to gain his trust and acceptance. Common concerns and issues are discussed below.

- Needle phobias are common at any age. Ask about previous injection experiences patients may have had, or observed. Inform the patient that—unlike intramuscular (i.m.) injections, which are painful—subcutaneous (s.q.) insulin injections with today's syringes and pens are generally painless. Insulin doesn't sting (glargine occasionally causes minor local reactions because of its acidic buffer), but using of alcohol for skin cleansing can sting and is not necessary. Also, injection-assistance devices may help in extreme cases (discussed later).
- There may be concerns that insulin therapy is the treatment of last resort, and is permanent. Patients may view themselves as failures or struggle to accept that they cannot avoid insulin or diabetes self-care any longer.
- Patients may have memories of family members or friends who suffered complications or death that they associate with having started insulin. Their own use of insulin may trigger fears that they will have a similar fate. It is helpful to point out that insulin therapy is effective, relatively inexpensive, and generally well tolerated. Also, emphasize the patient's current lack of optimal glycemic control and the risk of microvascular complications that it creates, plus the ability to "fine-tune" insulin doses and regimens to exactly meet the patient's needs in order to maximize the benefits and minimize the difficulties.
- Many people fear that the inconvenience of carrying supplies and taking the time to prepare and administer insulin will be a major barrier. Reviewing with patients their lifestyle and schedule, and pointing out the relevant issues, will help them in choosing equipment and an insulin regimen that meets their needs.
- Most patients (whether they admit it or not) will have some anxiety about injecting themselves for the first time, which hinders them from thinking about much else. Preparing a saline injection and having them self-inject

as the first part of the teaching session can alleviate their anxiety, and allow them to concentrate on the information that must be learned when beginning insulin therapy.

Patients should never be expected to self-teach injection technique at home. Written literature and training tapes should be used only to complement, not replace, individualized live instruction. Referral to a trained diabetes educator is encouraged when first beginning insulin. If not possible, office staff should be formally trained in the proper techniques of injection, mixing, and self-blood-glucose monitoring; current equipment; detection, prevention, and treatment of hypoglycemia; sharps disposal; and insulin storage.

Patients already taking insulin who have an unexplained change in their blood glucose values or difficulty in attaining stable glycemia should be asked to demonstrate their syringe preparation and injection techniques, to describe their insulin storage practices, and to show their injection sites. This often uncovers problems, especially in self-taught or inadequately educated individuals and the elderly.

## Syringes

Gone are the days when patients boiled their glass syringes and needles, sharpened the needles with a whetstone, ran them through cotton to detect burrs, soaked everything in alcohol, and finally gave painful intramuscular injections. Now a variety of insulin-delivery systems exist that use disposable, wire-thin needles that have been laser-sharpened and silicon-coated so that injections are usually painless.

Today's disposable syringes come in multiple sizes (0.3 cc [doses up to 30 units], 0.5 cc [up to 50 units], and 1 cc [up to 100 units], needle thicknesses (28 to 30 gauge), and needle lengths (5/16'' and $^1/_2$''). Insulin in the United States is standardized to a concentration of 100 units per cc (U100), with syringes to match. However, some other parts of the world use other concentrations (mostly U40). Occasionally, foreign visitors call local pharmacies, physicians, or emergency departments because they have run out of insulin syringes. The concentration of their insulin needs to be determined. U40 syringes are available in the United States by special order, or U100 insulin may need to be given along with syringes. The 5/16'' needles are appropriate for children (unless obese) or, as a rule, individuals with a body mass index $< 27$ kg/m$^2$. Use in larger individuals can result in back-leakage and loss of insulin at injection sites, which can cause erratic or elevated blood glucose levels. Useful practices: blood glucose should be checked more frequently when changing syringes or needle lengths to make sure there is no deterioration in glycemic control; patients should be cautioned to check markings when changing syringes to avoid medication errors; be sure to order syringes that are large enough to hold increased or mixed doses.

*Reuse and Disposal*

Although syringe manufacturers recommend one-time usage of syringes, reuse is common and safe for most individuals if basic guidelines are followed. Immunocompromised patients or those with open wounds, poor hygiene, or acute concurrent illness should not reuse. It is generally recommended that syringes be used no more than three or four times (occasionally patients report longer usage without complaint or apparent problem), and that they be discarded if they come in contact with anything but skin. Recap the needles until the next use. Don't wipe the needle with alcohol; it results in a duller needle by removing the silicon coating faster. Patients who mix insulins dull their needles more quickly because of the puncturing of the rubber vial caps. Discuss needle reuse with your patients so you know exactly what they are doing.

Discarded sharps should be contained in a puncture-free container. Check with the local waste agency for specific instructions.

## Insulin Pens

Insulin pens are multidose devices in which a small disposable needle is twisted on and the dosage dialed in (Figure 1). Pens have been widely used in Europe

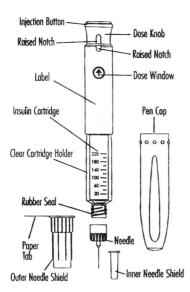

**FIGURE 1**  Schematic representation of the basic parts of an insulin pen (picture of a disposable pen taken from the product literature of Eli Lilly and Co.).

TABLE 1   Insulin Pen Manufacturers and Products

| Manufacturer | Product | Comments |
|---|---|---|
| Becton, Dickinson<br>800–237–4554 | B-D Pen | Uses any 1.5-cc cartridge—up to 30 units in 1-unit increments |
| | B-D Pen mini | Uses any 1.5-cc cartridge—up to 15 units in 1/2-unit increments |
| Disetronic<br>800–280–7801 | Disetronic Pen | Adaptor allows filling the reusable 3.15-cc cartridge with any manufacturer's insulin |
| Eli Lilly<br>800–545–5979 | Humalog<br>NPH<br>75% NPL/25% Humalog | Disposable pens filled with 3 cc delivered in 1-unit increments |
| | Cartridges | 1.5-cc cartridges of Humalog, Regular, NPH, 70/30 for nondisposable pens from other companies |
| Novo Nordisk<br>800–727–6500 | Innovo | Uses 3-cc cartridges; built-in memory with last dosage and elapsed time since last injection |
| | Novopen 3 | Uses 3-cc cartridges—up to 70 units in 1-unit increments |
| | Novopen 1.5 | Uses 1.5-cc cartridges—up to 40 units in 1-unit increments |
| | Novopen prefilled | Disposable pens of Regular, NPH, 70/30 filled with 1.5 cc delivered in 2-unit increments |
| | Cartridges | 1.5-cc and 3-cc Regular, NPH, 70/30 cartridges for nondisposable pens |
| Owen Mumford<br>800–421–6936 | Autopen | Uses any 1.5- and 3-cc cartridge; four models with different dosing range |

Pen products available in the U.S. at the time this table was produced. Refer to manufacturers for current products and specifications. Insulin aspart is not shown but should soon be available from Novo Nordisk. Also, glargine from Aventis is available only in vials but reportedly pen-based delivery is under development. Pen and cartridge volumes are based on U100 insulin (100 units per cc).

and other parts of the world for many years, and are rapidly gaining popularity in the United States. The available pens in the United States are shown in Table 1.

### Advantages

- Portable and self-contained, so no need to carry syringes and vials.
- Convenient. Takes less than 1 minute to prepare and easy to use, so ideal for starting insulin.
- Accurate dosing. Especially helpful for the elderly or patients with de-

creased dexterity or vision. Most pens have 1-unit increments, but 1/2-unit increments (BD Pen Mini) and 2-unit increments also exist (Novo prefills).

- Discreet, so injections can be given in public unnoticed.
- Multiuse, with less waste.
- Reduced chance of dosage errors related to air bubbles.
- Often cheaper for patients who take small doses of insulin because the smaller volume of pen cartridges or prefilled pens (150–300 units versus bottles that contain 1000 units) means less wastage due to expiration of the opened insulin before being used up.
- Smaller (31 gauge) and shorter (1/3″) needles are available than can be found in syringes.

### Disadvantages

- Insulin cannot be mixed in pens. However, many patients prefer to take multiple pen shots at one time rather than mixing in a syringe.
- Some pens have a shorter recommended lifespan (Table 2) once they are opened compared with vials of the same insulin, potentially resulting in increased wastage and cost.
- Some insulins are not available in pen form. However, this can be circum-

**TABLE 2** Manufacturer's Recommended Expiration Times for Insulin Pen Products

| Pen product | Days at room temperature | |
|---|---|---|
| | Opened | Unopened |
| Novolin Prefilled Pen 1.5 ml Regular | 28 | 28 |
| Novolin Prefilled Pen 1.5 ml NPH | 7 | 7 |
| Novolin Prefilled Pen 1.5 ml 70/30 | 7 | 7 |
| Novo 3 cartridge—Regular | 28 | 28 |
| Novo 3 cartridge—NPH | 14 | 14 |
| Novo 3 cartridge—70/30 | 10 | 10 |
| Novolog | 28 | 28 |
| Lilly Humulin cartridge 1.5 ml—Humalog | 28 | 28 |
| Lilly Humulin Prefilled Pen 3 ml—Humalog | 28 | 28 |
| Lilly Humulin Prefilled Pen 3 ml—NPH | 14 | 14 |
| Lilly Humulin Prefilled Pen 3 ml—75/25 | 10 | 10 |

Unused products that are refrigerated can be utilized to the expiration date on the pen/packaging. Once opened or removed from refrigeration, the times listed above apply. Room temperature is 59° to 86°F.

vented with the Disetronic pen, which can draw up any type of insulin into its reservoir.

- Some insurance companies won't reimburse pen costs.
- Patients on large insulin doses may exceed the maximal insulin delivery of the pen, or they may find them technically hard to use for large doses.
- On average, insulin cartridges and disposable pens are approximately 25% more expensive per unit than vials so they may be cost-prohibitive for patients on large doses.

### General Considerations for All Pens

- Use a fresh needle each time since there is no way to cover the needle once opened.
- At each usage, the pen must be primed by expelling 2 units to purge the needle of air. Then dial in the dosage to be injected.
- Always remove the needle between injections, as air can be drawn in and distort the chamber pressures.
- Never use a syringe to draw insulin out of a pen.
- Keep a record of the expiration date when a cartridge or disposable pen is opened, and follow the manufacturer's recommendations on when to discard it.
- Most pen needles are interchangeable, but the pen manufacturer may not honor the pen warranty unless its needles are used.
- Follow the manufacturer's directions on how to prepare the pen and administer the injection. Note especially how to determine when the full dose has been delivered. After injecting the insulin, be sure to leave the needle in for *at least 5 seconds*. Premature needle removal may result in leakage from the skin (a common complaint of patients when first starting pen use), resulting in a decreased dosage.
- The FDA has not approved pens for the visually impaired, and pen clicks should not be used to count the dose. However, pens are frequently very useful for low-vision patients after their ability to prepare the pen and inject accurately has been confirmed.

## Insulin Storage

Improperly stored insulin is a common cause of erratic or high blood sugars, and should be considered if there is a change in the patient's glycemic control, or if a patient does not seem to be responding to his insulin as usual, especially when traveling. Patients should be given the following instructions:

- Do not leave insulin in luggage or a car that might be exposed to extreme temperatures.

- Unopened vials, pens, and pen cartridges should be stored in the refrigerator at 36°F–46°F (2°C–8°C) until the expiration date.
- Once opened (when the stopper or seal has been punctured with a needle), insulin pens are kept at room temperature. Vials can be refrigerated or unrefrigerated, depending on what is more convenient for the patient. Once opened, vials are ''fresh'' for 28 days if stored at less than 86°F (15°C–30°C) and protected from bright sunlight. In contrast, pen products vary in the manufacturers' allowable time before discarding (Table 2).
- Insulin that has passed the expiration date, or has been exposed to other than recommended temperatures, will lose potency and should be discarded.
- Shaking or agitating insulin, such as when carrying it in a purse or loose in a car glove box, can reduce its potency. Hard shaking of long-acting insulin suspensions prior to drawing it up in a syringe can have the same effect. Cold insulin can be irritating to inject. Thus, patients should be told to *roll* the vial in their hands 10 times prior to drawing it up in the syringe (after letting it sit 30 minutes at room temperature if the vial is stored in the refrigerator).
- Drawing up several days' worth of syringes is a common practice, especially for individuals who require assistance from home health workers, visiting nurses, or family. Prefilled syringes should be kept refrigerated, stored vertically with the needles pointing up to prevent needle clogging by insulin crystals, and used within 21 days. Always label them carefully.

## Insulin Injection Technique

1. Collect supplies. Inspect the vial for any crystallization, clumping, or discoloration. If present, discard and open a new vial.
2. Wash hands.
3. Roll vial 10 times; excess agitation can damage the insulin and cause precipitation.
4. Wipe top of bottle with alcohol or cotton ball soaked in alcohol.
5. Push plunger up and then down to the number of units to be drawn up. Insert needle into vial and push plunger to empty the air into the vial.
6. Pull plunger down to the prescribed number of units. Draw 1–2 units extra to make up for insulin bubbles to be pushed out.
7. Inspect the syringe for any bubbles and tap with a finger or against a table to drive them to the top of the syringe, and then push out. Be sure the correct dose is still in the syringe; if it isn't, draw more. Many patients have an unfounded fear of injecting air by mistake but are afraid to discuss it. *Every patient should be reassured that in-*

*jecting air in the subcutaneous tissue does no harm other than de-creasing the intended dose.*

8.  Lightly pinch up the skin; holding the syringe like a pencil, insert the needle to the hub and push the plunger slowly. Wait 5 seconds and pull out the syringe.
9.  Dispose of sharps in the recommended way.
10. Do not massage the area. Note any back-leakage of insulin.

## Mixing Insulins

If possible, avoid teaching patients to mix when first initiating insulin therapy, as the extra steps can overwhelm and confuse them. Emphasize use of a consistent technique. Commercial premixed insulin (70/30, 75/25, 50/50) is useful as interim therapy, or for individuals who cannot master accurate mixing.

It was identified a decade ago that mixing long-acting insulin with Regular insulin slows the effect of the Regular insulin through microcrystallization; most problematic are Ultralente and Lente, with NPH causing less of this effect. The precipitation starts in a few minutes and takes up to 24 hours to be complete. (Commercially prepared mixes are not subject to this issue as the manufacturers' formulations create stable ratios of 70/30, 50/50, etc.) It was thus recommended that insulin injections be administered immediately after mixing. Also, commercial mixes or the use of multiple syringes, each containing only one kind of insulin, were suggested for those who were having syringes prepared ahead of time by family or home health workers. This "contamination" effect of long-acting insulin on Regular insulin is now less of an issue because it does not occur with the rapid-acting analogs, lyspro and aspart. However, caution should still be taken when mixing. NPH should never be mixed with Lente or Ultralente because of precipitation. Also, glargine cannot be mixed with any other insulin because of the low pH of the glargine buffer (pH 4) necessary to keep it soluble for injection. As new insulins come to market, it is important to consult with the manufacturer for correct mixing practices.

### Technique for Mixing Insulin

Guidelines for mixing insulins are similar to those for a single-drawn dose, with a few exceptions.

1.  Insert air into each vial before drawing any insulin. The amount inserted per vial should equal the insulin dose to be withdrawn. Insert air into the long-acting (cloudy) insulin vial first.
2.  After the remaining air is put into the short-acting (clear) insulin, draw up the prescribed dose and remove the needle. *The short-acting insulin should always be drawn up first* to prevent possible contamination of the vial with long-acting insulin, which could alter its kinetics of action.

3. Expel any remaining air, and inspect that the correct dose was taken.
4. Draw up the long-acting insulin, being careful not to overdraw.

## Injection Difficulties

*Bruising* at injection sites may be related to nicking superficial vessels, and is usually not due to poor injection technique. However, the problem may be worsened in patients taking anticoagulants, corticosteroids, or nonsteroidal anti-inflammatory drugs, and in the elderly.

*Painful injections* may be related to the use of alcohol at the site—if the site is dirty, patients should wash it with soap and water prior to injection but otherwise no skin preparation is recommended. Injection of cold insulin, or syringes that have been reused too many times so the needle is dulled, can also cause pain. So can a technically correct injection in patients who are nervous or hypersensitive to pain. Use of an ice cube on the site for a few minutes prior to injection often helps. When the problem is extreme, applying Emla cream 30 minutes before the injection can be beneficial. Also, switching to the thinnest available needle (31 gauge for insulin pens and 30 gauge for syringes) should be tried.

An important cause of painful injections is when they are i.m. Insulin is designed to be given s.q., which is generally painless. Kinetic properties of the different insulins are determined by how they exist in the subcutaneous space (crystals, hexamers, dimers, monomers). Only monomers and dimers can be absorbed into the blood; lyspro and aspart exist as monomers, accounting for their rapid action; Regular as dimers and hexamers, causing its multihour effect; and intermediate and long-acting insulins as crystals, so the effect is much longer. If patients inadvertently inject i.m.—that is, do not pinch the skin enough, causing them to go through the subcutaneous space—absorption into the blood is faster than usual, resulting in a quick effect and occasionally frank hypoglycemia. Intramuscular injections hurt. A useful way to identify i.m. injections is to differentiate pain on inserting the needle into the skin—any of the previous causes, including pain hypersensitivity—from pain when the plunger is pushed in—i.m. injection. To avoid this problem, injections are generally given at a 90° angle, but children or thin adults may need a 45° angle, especially in areas with little subcutaneous fat. The practice of pinching a small fold of skin should be reinforced.

*Allergic reactions* are rare and usually localized. Rubber and latex allergies related to latex in syringes or rubber stoppers on vials can be mistaken for an insulin allergy. Latex-free syringes are available (Terumo Corporation). Preservatives or other chemicals in the buffer, such as zinc or protamine, can cause allergic reactions, but this is rare. Since human insulin has come to the market, serious insulin allergies are quite rare.

*Lipoatrophy* is a sinking or pitting of the subcutaneous tissue around an injection site that is believed to be an allergic response to a specific insulin species or poor purity. It was relatively common a few years ago, especially in women and children and during the first year of therapy. Its occurrence has markedly decreased with today's use of highly purified human insulin.

*Lipohypertrophy* is a fatty buildup of subcutaneous tissue, usually related to overuse of an injection site, often because the frequent use causes it to become insensitive to pain. It remains relatively common, but is decreasing in frequency as patients are being urged to rotate their sites (Figure 2). Also important is the relative painlessness of today's syringes and pens. Thus, when lipohypertrophy is identified, causative factors besides the pain desensitizing effect must be considered. Patients may have a favorite site because of easy access, convenience, better visualization, or simply habit. Alternatively, difficult-to-see areas such as the buttocks may have lipohypertrophy without the patient's knowing it. It is important to educate patients that insulin absorption is erratic from hypertrophied

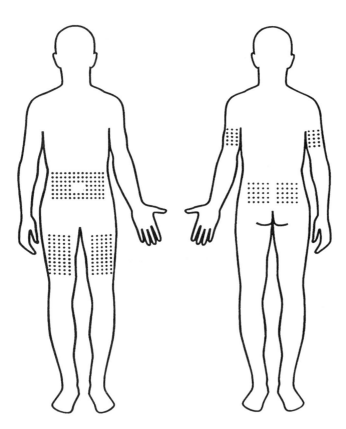

FIGURE 2   Stippled areas indicate recommended insulin injection sites.

sites, and to discuss alternative sites and proper site rotation. Lipohypertrophy usually resolves if the site is not used for several months. It is essential that providers inspect injection sites routinely. Also, patients will often state that they use their abdomen, but on inspection and more careful discussion, it is discovered that only a small area is used, which is hypertrophied. Individuals on multiple daily injections who use only one or two sites (especially arms and legs) are at the highest risk. Patients should be taught to rotate among individual sites.

## Insulin Absorption

Insulin absorption, and thus the timing of its action, is affected by many variables.

- The insulin formulation. The protamine in NPH and the excess zinc in Lente and Ultralente promote crystallization, which causes the cloudy appearance and slower absorption compared with Regular insulin or the rapid-acting analogs ("clear insulins").
- Raising skin temperature, such as by taking a shower or hot tub after an injection, increases absorption. Similarly, massaging the injection site increases local circulation and speeds absorption. Both are to be discouraged.
- Exercise increases blood flow, and thus absorption of locally injected insulin. It is recommended that patients be taught not to inject into a limb that recently has been exercised, or will be exercised within the next hour. Instead, the abdomen is the most neutral site in terms of this effect, and best used when physical activity is planned.
- Intramuscular injections increase the absorption rate, as already discussed.
- Subcutaneous injection sites vary in absorption rates (from fastest to slowest: abdomen, arms, legs, and buttocks). It's useful to match sites to a desired effect, e.g., use of the stomach before meals, and giving the evening shot in the buttocks or leg so it lasts through the night. However, it is important to realize that this effect does not occur with the rapid-acting analogs lyspro and aspart or the long-acting analog glargine; all are considered to have absorption rates that are unaffected by where they are injected.
- Sites of lipohypertrophy can cause unpredictable absorption. Also, patients should be instructed to avoid the umbilical area and any scars by at least two inches (stretch marks are not a concern).

## Injection Aids

A variety of devices are available to help those with technical or emotional difficulties with injections, including insulin pens, automatic needle injectors, needle-free jet injectors, and aids for the visually impaired (Table 3). Also, contact your local or state Division of the Blind to learn about local resources.

**TABLE 3** Insulin-Delivery Assistance Devices

| Type | Manufacturer | Product |
|---|---|---|
| Jet injectors—needleless injection systems | Activa 800–991–4464 | AdvantaJet, Advanta JetES, GentleJet |
| | Bioject 800–683–7221 #436 | Vitajet 3 |
| | Equidyne 877–474–6539 | Injex 30 |
| | Medi-Ject 800–328–3074 | Medi-Jector VISION |
| Automatic injectors— enable using needles more easily | Becton, Dickinson 800–237–4554 | Inject-Ease Automatic injector (conceals insulin syringe) |
| | Medicool 800–433–2469 | InstaJect injector (adjusts for depth of needle penetration) |
| | Owen Mumford 800–421–6936 | Autoject, Autoject 2 (injects needle at prescribed depth) |
| | Sherwood 314–621–7788 | Monoject Injectomatic (spring-loaded for monoject syringes) |
| Aids that enable syringe loading and insulin dose measurement in the visually impaired | Becton, Dickinson 800–237–4554 | Magni-Guide (2.5× scale magnifier and needle guide) |
| | Jordan Medical 800–541–1193 | Count-a-Dose (syringe filling and mixing devise) |
| | Meditec 303–758–6978 | Holdease (needle guide and syringe/vial holder) |
| | | Insulgage (allows tactile draw-up of preset dose) |
| | Palco 800–346–4488 | Inject-Eze 6000 (low-vision loading devise with 2× lens) |
| | | Insulcap (tactile-cue vial cap for ease in inserting a syringe) |
| | | Load Matic (syringe loader) |

Shown are insulin-delivery assistance devices by category. Refer to manufacturers for current products and specifications.

## SELF-BLOOD-GLUCOSE MONITORING

Self-blood-glucose monitoring (SBGM) is an essential part of any diabetes management program. It provides quick, reliable data for problem solving and decision making, and it is invaluable for detecting or confirming hypoglycemia and analyzing blood glucose patterns to adjust treatment. This relatively painless technique involves pricking the finger with a lancet device to obtain a drop of blood, which is placed on a reagent strip in a handheld meter to quantify the glycemia concentration. Two measurement technologies are commonly used: color-reflectance meters, which use strips impregnated with the enzyme glucose oxidase and a color indicator system for the chemical reaction, and meters that measure electrical current produced by the chemical reaction. Visual-read test strips are also available, but are not nearly as accurate as meter-read samples. Urine glucose testing is obsolete because it cannot detect hypoglycemia or even assess blood sugars in the recommended range since most individuals start spilling glucose into their urine when glycemia exceeds 180 mg/dl. However, urine testing is better than nothing for individuals who refuse blood glucose monitoring.

## Indications and Rationale

Essentially all individuals with diabetes should monitor their blood glucose level. SBGM is invaluable because of the instant and accurate data it provides, plus patient acceptance has been helped by the ease of use and accuracy of modern meters. Common objectives of its use are:

- Detection of hypoglycemia, especially in individuals with hypoglycemia unawareness.
- Improved decision making regarding adjustments of care in response to dietary and exercise changes.
- Enhanced effectiveness of patient–provider dialog regarding efficacy of the current therapy, and help in designing strategies to attain the glycemia targets.
- A level of patient self-sufficiency and problem solving that did not exist prior to their being able to determine a blood glucose level. This is true in emergent situations; when patients don't feel well, they can determine what role, if any, glycemia is playing. Also, patients can be safely managed at home during illness or acute hypo- or hyperglycemia that before SBMG would have led to seeking emergent medical attention. This concept is true for chronic management as well. Intensive diabetes management strategies and the current mantras of ''self-care'' and ''self-management'' could not exist without SBMG.

### Advantages

- Allows the patient to practice self-management, resulting in increased independence, self-confidence, and motivation.
- Provides reliable, objective, and quick test results for improved treatment decisions.
- Instant feedback on diet, exercise, and medication effects, anytime, anywhere.
- Detects or confirms asymptomatic hypoglycemia or hyperglycemia.

*Disadvantages*

- Discomfort of pricking the finger. Meters have recently come onto the market that use alternative sites (most commonly the forearm) that are advertised as being painless. However, these alternative sites are not as accurate as fingertip testing when blood glucose levels are rapidly changing, such as after meals or during the development of hypoglycemia.
- Cost is a major barrier for many people. Although insurance reimbursement for diabetes medications is growing, many plans still do not cover test strips, which cost $0.60 to $0.80 each.
- Requires a degree of mental acuity and manual dexterity that is sometimes lacking in the chronically ill or elderly.
- Incorrect technique or equipment malfunction can lead to erroneous test results and inappropriate decision making. However, over the last few years meters have become easier to use and more reliable, and require less blood for accurate testing. In the past, using too small a blood sample was a major cause of inaccurate results.
- Persistently high or labile blood sugars can lead to patient frustration. Paradoxically, the patient's motivation for better diabetes control can be hurt by ''bad blood sugars,'' leading to avoidance of testing.
- Inconvenience of carrying supplies and taking the time to test and record information. Most meters now have memories that allow later written documentation.

## Patient Education

Individualized instruction in product selection and use of the equipment is key, as is ensuring that patients know their glycemia targets and how to apply the data for better glycemic control. This can greatly increase patient motivation to test as well as improve the quality of the data, and decrease costly product waste. Exploring in a nonjudgmental manner the reasons for a patient's not testing as recommended often uncovers barriers that can be addressed through a change in equipment, helping them obtain affordable supplies, or re-emphasizing the necessity of testing for attaining the goals of therapy. Diabetes educators are trained to help patients identify and overcome barriers, and to teach blood glucose interpretation for problem solving. Instruction should include correct usage of the meter and its care, calibration, and use of control fluids; technique for finger pricking; proper disposal of sharps; the testing schedule; their blood glucose goals; record keeping; glucose-pattern interpretation, and how to use their SBGM data for diet, medication, or exercise insulin adjustments. Further, patients should know to bring their testing equipment and glucose diaries to each visit. They should be regularly asked to demonstrate their testing technique, and their meters should be checked for accuracy, especially when their log results are inconsistent with other indices of glycemia such as $HbA_{1c}$.

## Meter Selection

Meters have become smaller, faster, and easier to use, and require less blood. A large selection with various features are on the market, and it's best to be familiar with several models or refer to a diabetes educator. Meter kits also include lancet devices for finger pricking. It is important to determine that not only the meter but also the lancing device suits the patient. Getting input from the patient regarding meter selection is key, as their perception of what determines ease of use or a particularly desirable feature can greatly affect their motivation to test.

Meter features to consider include the required sample size, ease of use, "sipping strips" which use capillary action as opposed to direct application of a drop of blood on the strip, test time, meters that use sites other than the fingertip, accuracy and glucose range, meters that measure levels of whole-blood versus plasma glucose, memory capacity, available data-management software and its ease of use, temperature and altitude range, meter size and weight, large versus small screen and number size, ease of opening test-strip packages, individual foil-wrapped strips versus those stored in a vial, meter and strip costs, ease of coding the meter, and quality-control testing (Table 4).

Patient variables to consider include dexterity, cognitive abilities, visual acuity, frequency of testing, motivation, lifestyle, concerns about compactness, privacy, and how they wish to keep a record of their blood glucose results.

## Special Populations

The *elderly* are often undertreated in regard to blood glucose monitoring. Avoidance of hypoglycemia is of particular importance in this population. Moreover, labile blood glucose patterns and a tendency to hypoglycemia are a feature of many elderly patients as they become insulin-dependent. Thus, age should not be a limiting factor when considering fingerstick usage and frequency. Patient, personalized education is often required. Also, special attention should be paid to the patient's manual dexterity, vision, and potential memory deficits. Simplicity of use and need for only a small blood drop are particularly useful meter features for older patients.

*Children* often do best with equipment that hides the lancet, minimizes discomfort, and requires a small sample size. Meters with quick results are especially helpful to parents. Also, memory recall is a useful meter feature for children who report blood glucose results that are not consistent with their $HbA_{1c}$ value.

Major obstacles for the *visually impaired* (including fluctuating and low vision) are obtaining an adequate blood sample and correct placement on the test

**TABLE 4** Blood-Glucose-Monitoring Systems (refer to manufacturers for current products and specifications)

| Meter mfr. and name | Sample size (µl) | Glucose range (mg/dl) | Test time (seconds) | Strip name | Plasma/ whole blood | Memory (no. of tests) | Comments |
|---|---|---|---|---|---|---|---|
| Amira (877–264–7263) | | | | | | | |
| AtLast | 2 | 40–400 | 15 | AtLast | Plasma | Last 10 | Capillary action strip; alternative site options |
| Bayer Corporation (800–888–5957) | | | | | | | |
| Glucometer Dex | 3–4 | 10–600 | 30 | Sensor Disc | Plasma | 100 (date/time) | Capillary-action strip |
| Glucometer Elite | 2 | 20–600 | 30 | Elite | Plasma | 20 | Capillary-action strip |
| Glucometer Elite XL | 3 | 20–600 | 30 | Elite | Plasma | 120 (date/time) | Capillary-action strip |
| Home Diagnostics (800–342–7226) | | | | | | | |
| Prestige LX(HDI) | 5 | 25–600 | 10–50 | Prestige Smart System | Whole blood | 365 | Capillary-action strip; large, easy-to-read display |
| Hypoguard Corporation (800–888–5957) | | | | | | | |
| Assure Hypoguard | 10 | 30–550 | 35 | Assure | Whole blood | 180 | |
| Select GT Hypoguard | 9 | 30–600 | Within 50 | SelectGT | Plasma or whole blood | 100 | |
| Lifescan Corporation (800–227–8862) | | | | | | | |
| Fast Take | 15 | 20–600 | 15 | Fast Take | Plasma | 150 (date/time) | Capillary-action strip |
| One Touch Basic | 10+ | 0–600 | 45 | One Touch | Whole blood | 75 (date/time) | |
| One Touch Profile | 10+ | 0–600 | 45 | One Touch | Whole blood | 250 (date/time) | |
| Sure Step | 10–35 | 0–500 | Avg. 30 | Sure Step | Plasma | 150 (date/time) | Blood drop is smeared directly on strip |
| Ultra | 1 | 20–600 | 5 | Ultra | Plasma | 150 | Capillary-action strip; alternative site options |

| | | | | | | | |
|---|---|---|---|---|---|---|---|
| LXN Corporation (888–596–8378) | | | | | | | |
| Duet (LXN) | Glucose 10 Glucoprotein 25 | 20–600 | 8–30 | Duet Glucose | Whole blood | 200 glucose, 50 glucoprotein | Measures fructosamine (glucoprotein) as well |
| In Charge (LXN) | 6 | 20–600 | 5–20 | In Charge Glucose | Plasma | 200 glucose, 50 glucoprotein | Measures fructosamine (glucoprotein) as well |
| Medisense (Abbott) (800–527–3339) | | | | | | | |
| ExacTech RSG | 10–50 | 40–450 | 30 | ExacTech RSG | Whole Blood | 1 | |
| Precision Extra | 3.5 | 20–600 | 20 | Precision Extra | Plasma | 450 (date/time) 10 meter, 125 software | |
| Precision QID | 3.5 | 20–600 | 20 | Precision QID | Plasma | | |
| Sof-Tact IQ | 3 | | 15 | | Plasma | | |
| Roche Diagnostics (800–858–8072) | | | | | | | |
| Accu-Chek Advantage | 9 4 | 10–600 | 40 | Advantage Comfort Curve | Plasma | 100 (date/time) | Advantage top-load, Comfort Curve capillary-action strips; large, easy-to-read display |
| Accu-Chek Complete | 9 4 | 10–600 | 40 | Advantage Comfort Curve | Plasma or whole blood | 1000 | More complete data management |
| Therasense (888–522–5226) | | | | | | | |
| FreeStyle | 0.3 | 20–500 | 15 | TheraSense | Plasma | 250 (date/time) | Capillary-action strip; alternative site options |

Visual-read test strips

Bayer Corporation (800–348–8100)
Glucostix Reagent Strips
Roche Diagnostics (800–858–8072)
Chemstrip BG

strip. Talking meters are available. State associations for the visually impaired are excellent resources for training and product information.

## Recommended SBGM Test Frequency

Experience has shown that frequent monitoring augments patients' ability to meet their treatment goals and provides the needed feedback to pursue self-management. Still, the times and frequency of testing vary widely among individual patients, depending on their treatment goals, treatment regimen and its complexity, motivation, variability of dietary and exercise habits, physical and cognitive abilities, financial constraints, and concerns for hypoglycemia. It is generally recommended that patients test often enough to be familiar with their usual glycemia pattern, including testing under various dietary, work, and exercise conditions. The most common practice is testing before meals and at bedtime, and occasionally between 1 and 3 A.M. Also, 2-hour post-meal testing is being increasingly recommended to ascertain postprandial glucose control, especially in patients taking rapid-acting insulin analogs or oral agents such as Repaglinide and Nateglinide. All patients should have testing equipment and supplies on hand, and know how to use them, even if used only for emergent situations.

### Common Testing Patterns

- Stable-diet-controlled—test pre-breakfast and 2 hours post-breakfast or dinner two or three times per week.
- Oral agents alone or insulin/orals combination therapy—pre-breakfast four to seven times per week, pre-lunch two or three times per week, 2 hours post-breakfast or -dinner two or three times per week.
- Insulin therapy—the frequency is based somewhat on the insulin regimen and blood sugar stability:
    One daily injection—one to three tests daily (at least two recommended).
    Two daily injections—four tests daily (before meals and at bedtime). Stable patients on fixed doses can perform four times per day, three days a week, including some weekends.
    Intensive therapy (multiple injections or insulin pump)—four to seven times per day. Stabilized patients on fixed insulin doses may test four times daily three days per week, including a weekend day.
- Patients with asymptomatic nocturnal hypoglycemia should perform their bedtime fingerstick measurement $1^{1}/_{2}$ hours after their evening snack. They should also check between 1 A.M. and 3 A.M. on days following unusual exercise.
- Patients who test infrequently should increase the frequency when ill, traveling, changing daily routine, or having problems with hypo- or hyperglycemia, or after intense exercise.

## Technique for Self-Blood-Glucose Monitoring

1. It is recommended that hands be washed to remove any food or chemical residue. Infections are rare with fingersticks. Washing also increases the circulation, which can help if obtaining an adequate sample is a problem. Alcohol is not recommended because it toughens the skin.

2. Remove a test strip from the vial and recap immediately. Exposure to air and light can damage strips in as little as an hour.

3. Turn meter on, and prepare the lancet device and a strip according to the manufacturer's directions. Lancet devices should be used to decrease tissue trauma and discomfort. Newer models have adjustable depth penetration. Lancets and lancet devices should never be shared; there are reported cases of communicable diseases spread via lancet devices.

4. Shake hand at side below waist and milk the finger to be pricked if needed. Place the tip of the lancet on the side of the finger opposite the nail bed with firm pressure, and release the button. Because the sides of the fingers have fewer nerve endings than the tips, they are less sensitive. Meters that allow for alternative test sites, most commonly the forearm, have recently become available. However, some patients find it difficult to obtain an adequate sample at the alternative sites. It is advisable to have patients demonstrate their technique before prescribing any meter, especially when alternative sites are to be used.

5. Once the site has been lanced, gently squeezing the finger is generally adequate to obtain a drop. If not, running the finger under warm water and milking it prior to lancing the finger followed by lowering the hand almost to the floor while squeezing usually works.

6. Place the sample on the strip as directed. If the strip is not completely covered, the meter may report inaccurate results. Too small a blood drop is the most common cause of sampling error, although this happens less often with the newer meters, which require less blood, and also with the advent of capillary-action strips.

7. Record test results, including interpretation comments.

## Record Keeping

Record keeping is a critical part of diabetes self-care. Patients often rely on the meter memory to store information for their provider instead of writing down results. However, the meter memory is not a replacement for a written record. Ideally, the blood glucose values should be analyzed by the patient on an ongoing basis to determine the adequacy of glycemic control, and to make adjustments in insulin doses when necessary. This requires comparing several days' results to look for recurring problems that suggest a need to change the insulin doses (so-called *pattern management*), which underscores the need for a written record. An underutilized part of the record is the comment section in which pertinent information should be recorded. Comments about unusual diet, activity, stress, or medication changes can help to determine the cause of abnormal blood glucose values and the effectiveness of corrective actions. Also, it is important that the provider review the glucose log at each visit as this can increase patient motivation and aid in their learning how to solve problems and self-manage. Thus, regularly recording and analyzing their blood glucose values allows patients to become proactive rather than reactive in their diabetes management.

Noncompliance is an overused word. If an individual does not test or keep written records, exploring his or her reasons in a nonjudgmental way can provide insight. Common causes include inadequate education as to the importance of SBGM, testing burnout, frustration at test results, cost, discomfort, inconvenience of carrying equipment or taking the time to test, hiding the diagnosis from others, and denial. Monitoring can elicit unpleasant emotions from patients who view their results as unacceptable. These patients may need counseling to help them understand that their results are a feedback tool for problem solving, not a reflection of themselves for overly critical self-judgment.

## Meter Accuracy

Patients may question the accuracy of their meter after comparing the results of tests done simultaneously on two different glucose meters. Questions to ask include:

- Are the test strips within the expiration date, and have they been stored properly?
- Has fresh control fluid been used to check the system? Most vials of control fluid expire 3 months after being opened. Often patients have not been taught the purpose or technique of quality-control testing. It is useful to keep control fluids for commonly used meters in the office and to check meters with questionable accuracy.
- Is their meter coded correctly for the currently used strips? Most meters must be recoded each time a new vial of strips is opened.
- Did the patient obtain an adequate drop of blood and properly apply the sample? Inadequate samples are the most common cause of inaccurate results. It is advised that each patient's technique be checked regularly. For patients who have trouble getting an adequate sample, the newer meters that use capillary action to obtain the sample are usually preferable to the traditional hanging-drop method.
- Is the patient aware of anything that might have damaged the meter?
- Is the patient comparing whole-blood and plasma-read meters? Comparing

a meter's results with a lab measured plasma glucose is the only valid method for determining accuracy—a variance of less than 20% is considered acceptable meter performance. However, glucose meters use whole blood, and vein-drawn lab samples use the plasma portion. Newer meters mostly report plasma glucose measurements, but there are still many on the market that report whole-blood results, which are approximately 12% lower. Each mode of measurement is considered accurate. However, meters that report plasma results are generally preferable for patients in intensive treatment programs to allow easier matching of meter-read and lab-measured glycemia values. Also, a useful practice for patients who have more than one meter is to use the same brand or at least the same manufacturer for ease in comparing results.

## SICK-DAY MANAGEMENT

All diabetic patients should increase their monitoring of blood glucose—patients with type 1 diabetes should also start urine ketone measurements—during suspected or acute illness. Often glycemia values will increase before there are signs and symptoms of a developing illness. Patients need to be given specific instructions on how to monitor and adjust their therapy during periods of illness (''sick-day rules'').

- Blood glucose should be checked every 2 to 4 hours, or until the symptoms diminish.
- Urine ketones should be tested at least every 4 hours during acute illness.
- Increased insulin is often needed (10–20%). This must be stressed with patients who often want to reduce or eliminate their dosage because they are vomiting and not eating, and do not understand the body's need for *more* insulin when under stress, even if carbohydrate intake is decreased. Insulin omission is a common cause of diabetic ketoacidosis (DKA).
- Adequate hydration is critical. Patients should drink 8 ounces of calorie-free fluids (e.g., water, broth, or diet drinks) every hour while they are awake. Also useful are fluids that contain electrolytes, such as canned clear soups, bouillon, consommé, and sports drinks. A ''sipping diet'' consisting of 15 grams of carbohydrates, such as Gatorade every 1 to 2 hours, can be effective in patients with nausea and vomiting. Caffeine is a diuretic and should be avoided. Antiemetics or i.v. fluids may also be needed.
- Many over-the-counter cough and cold medications contain sugar and alcohol, and can increase blood glucose. Advise patients to use sugar-free preparations if available.
- Most situations can be managed by phone if the patient is monitoring and reporting his status. However, patients are often reluctant to contact their

provider until symptoms are severe. They should be instructed to contact their provider when:

They vomit more than once.
Diarrhea persists for more than 24 hours or occurs five times or more.
Blood glucose levels are higher than 300 mg/dl on two consecutive measurements which do not respond to insulin.
They observe moderate or large ketones.
They have unexplained chest pain and/or difficulty in breathing.
They should be seen for medical evaluation if:
They are unable to tolerate fluids or have persistent vomiting or diarrhea.
They report progressive weakness.
They are experiencing rapid and labored respirations or other significant difficulty in breathing.
There is a change in mental status.
Moderate or large urinary ketones do not improve after 12–24 hours of treatment.

## Urine Ketone Testing

Urine ketone testing is often overlooked, but it is an essential part of care for patients with type 1 diabetes. The individually foil-wrapped strips are convenient to carry. Type 2 diabetes patients are normally ketosis-resistant, but during periods of severe trauma, infection, or illness can become ketotic and even develop full-blown DKA. Thus, a useful practice is to have *all* diabetic patients monitor urine ketones during severe illness.

- Patients with type 1 diabetes should check urine ketones when their blood sugars are consistently over 240 mg/dl. This is especially critical for patients on insulin pumps since it may indicate malfunction of their pump delivery system.
- Pregnant women (including those with gestational diabetes) are advised to monitor urine ketones every morning.
- Positive urinary ketones do not always indicate sickness. Ketones are a byproduct of fat metabolism, and their presence with normal blood sugars can indicate fat mobilization in a patient who is actively trying to lose weight by restricting calories. However, patients with type 1 diabetes who are restricting their calories for weight management may also restrict their insulin, resulting in metabolic decompensation and DKA in the absence of marked hyperglycemia. This is especially common in teenage girls who desire rapid weight loss such as during prom season. Thus, patients should carefully monitor urinary ketones and glycemia during periods of caloric restriction.

## BIBLIOGRAPHY

American Association of Diabetes Educators. A Core Curriculum For Diabetes Education. 3rd ed. Chicago: AADE, 1998. Call 800-338-3633, press 1, and enter document no. 9001 to request a product order form.

American Diabetes Association. Clinical Practice Recommendations 2001. Diabetes Care 24(suppl 1), 2001.

American Diabetes Association. Medical Management of Type 1 Diabetes. 3rd ed. Alexandria, VA: ADA, 1998.

American Diabetes Association. Medical Management of Type 2 Diabetes. 4th ed. Alexandria, VA: ADA, 1998.

Edelman SV, Henry RR. Assessment of the treatment regimen. In: Diagnosis and Management of Type 2 Diabetes. 3rd ed. Caddo, OK: Professional Communications, pp 131–160, 1999.

LifeScan. Is My Blood Glucose Meter Accurate? Patient education brochure. Milpitas, CA: LifeScan, Inc., 1999.

Tobin CT. Diabetes self-management education and the diabetes team. In: Medical Management of Diabetes Mellitus. Leahy JL, Clark NG, Cefalu WT, eds. New York: Marcel Dekker, pp 51–56, 2000.

# 4

## Nutrition Assessment and Therapy

**Linda Tilton**

Vermont Regional Diabetes Center, Fletcher Allen Health Care,
University of Vermont College of Medicine, Burlington, Vermont

### INTRODUCTION

Nutrition therapy is a key component of the American Diabetes Association's (ADA) diabetes-care and self-management guidelines for patients with diabetes who are receiving insulin therapy. Nutrition assessment, along with the development and implementation of individualized nutrition goals and meal-planning guidelines, is as important to the successful management of diabetic patients treated with insulin as it is for patients who manage their diabetes with diet and exercise or oral medications. Although essential to optimal diabetes care, following nutrition recommendations and meal-planning strategies can often be the most challenging part of diabetes self-management for patients.

Diabetic patients treated with insulin find it difficult to understand and follow the nutrition component of their diabetes management plan for many reasons. Some examples of those reasons are:

- Diabetic patients and health-care practitioners often do not understand the current ADA nutrition recommendations.
- Health-care practitioners often do not emphasize nutrition therapy for diabetic patients treated with insulin.
- Diabetic patients often do not receive education on nutrition management of diabetes in the primary-care setting.

- Many diabetic patients find it difficult to follow a meal plan that they perceive limits their food choices.

As a result of these factors, many diabetic patients treated with insulin therapy do not optimize the nutrition component of diabetes management (1).

## HISTORICAL PERSPECTIVE

The ADA's nutrition recommendations for diabetes management have changed a great deal since the first recommendations were introduced in the 1920s. Some of the more recent changes directly contradict long-established standards of diabetes nutrition care.

In 1971, the ADA's nutrition recommendations for diabetes management called for a moderate carbohydrate intake of approximately 45% of total calories, 20% of calories from protein, and 35% from fat. Diabetic patients were encouraged to avoid sucrose and concentrated sweets; however, little emphasis was placed on the amount of protein and both total and saturated fat included in the diet. In 1986, the ADA's nutrition recommendations were revised to encourage a carbohydrate intake of approximately 60% of calories, along with reductions in protein and fat intake to 12–20% and less than 30% of total calories, respectively. The amount of protein and fat recommended in the meal plan was decreased to limit the risk of cardiac and renal complications of diabetes. Patients with diabetes were also encouraged to consume a diet high in fiber and to limit their intake of sucrose and foods that contained sugar (2).

In 1994, the ADA significantly revised its nutrition recommendations for diabetes management to reflect current research that indicated good blood glucose control can be achieved with varying percentages of calories from carbohydrate, protein, and fat in the meal plan. The ADA's nutrition recommendations currently emphasize a flexible approach to the nutrition prescription, with a meal plan that includes varying amounts of macronutrients based on a nutrition assessment and individualized treatment goals. Sucrose and foods containing sugar can now be consumed as part of the total carbohydrate content of the meal plan. Diabetic patients are also encouraged to moderate the amount of protein and limit both the total fat content and the amount of saturated fat in their diet (2).

These repeated revisions have resulted in confusion for health-care practitioners and patients, which often limits a diabetic patient's ability to optimize his or her diabetes control.

## ADA RECOMMENDATIONS

Although controversy continues to exist concerning the ideal percentage of protein, carbohydrate, and fat for a diabetic patient's nutrition prescription, nutrition

therapy is recognized as a key component of the successful management of insulin-treated diabetic patients. There is now general agreement that a generic diabetic diet that applies to all patients with diabetes simply does not exist. Physicians or health-care practitioners should no longer give their diabetic patients
standardized preprinted meal plans, with a one-size-fits-all calorie level and carbohydrate, protein, and fat percentages, without an assessment of their current
food intake, exercise habits, and diabetes treatment goals. Current ADA guidelines focus on the development of individual nutrition goals and meal plans (3).
The current ADA guidelines for macronutrients are listed below (2).

- Protein
    10–20% of total calories in patients without nephropathy
    In patients with overt nephropathy a limitation of protein intake to the
        Recommended Dietary Allowance (RDA) for adults of 0.8 g/kg/day
- Fat
    Approximately 30% of total calories, with the exact percentage based
        on lipid levels and weight-management goals
    Saturated fat less than 10% of total calories, less that 7% if LDL choles-
        terol is elevated
    Cholesterol less than 300 mg/day, less than 200 mg/day if LDL choles-
        terol is elevated
- Carbohydrate
    The percentage of total calories will vary based on treatment goals
    Makes up the remainder of calories after protein and fat percentages are
        met
    Sucrose and foods containing sugar may be included as part of the carbo-
        hydrate content of the meal plan

## THE ROLE OF THE REGISTERED DIETITIAN

The dietitian works in collaboration with the physician, nurse practitioner, physician's assistant, diabetes nurse educator, and patient as part of the diabetes management team. The role of the dietitian is to assess the patient's present nutritional
status, body weight, food intake, and exercise level, along with the patient's readi-
ness and ability to make behavior changes related to his or her present food
choices and exercise habits. An individualized assessment by a registered dietitian with training and expertise in diabetes self-management is the basis for the
development and implementation of individualized nutrition treatment goals and
meal plans.

After the initial assessment, the dietitian works closely with the patient and
the other members of the diabetes management team to establish and prioritize
goals, and then to develop strategies to achieve those goals. As an effective coun-

selor, the registered dietitian must include the patient in the process of developing nutrition goals and the individualized meal plan. It is important for the dietitian to provide close patient follow-up and to help motivate the behavior changes needed to optimize the patient's glycemic control (3).

## GOALS OF NUTRITION THERAPY

Nutrition goals for the insulin-treated diabetic patient are based on 1) the behavior changes that the individual with diabetes is willing and able to make and 2) the type of insulin program the patient is following. Goals are based on a patient's blood glucose, $HbA_{1c}$, serum lipid, blood pressure, and body weight goals. The type of insulin program is also an important consideration in the development of nutrition goals and the initiation of an individualized meal plan.

Achievement of nutrition goals is measured by assessing objective outcomes, such as self-monitored blood glucose levels or changes in $HbA_{1c}$ and serum lipid levels, and changes in body weight and exercise habits. If diabetes management goals are not achieved, the diabetes management team then re-evaluates the plan.

The overall goal of nutrition therapy in the insulin-treated diabetic patient (as in all patients with diabetes) is to assist the patient in making diet and exercise changes to improve metabolic control of his or her disease. The specific goals of nutrition therapy are as follows (2):

- To balance food intake and activity level with insulin and oral medications, if applicable, to achieve and maintain near normal blood glucose levels
- To achieve and maintain optimal serum lipid levels
- To achieve and maintain a reasonable body weight in adults; provide adequate calories for normal growth and development in children and adolescents; and meet the increased nutritional needs of pregnancy, lactation, and illness
- To prevent and treat the acute complications of diabetes such as hypoglycemia and the long-term complications such as cardiac and renal disease
- To improve overall health through optimal nutrition

## NUTRITION STRATEGIES FOR INSULIN THERAPY

Strategies for nutrition management as part of insulin therapy will vary based on whether the patient has type 1 or type 2 diabetes and whether he or she is following a conventional or intensive insulin program (2).

In either case, an individualized meal plan based on the patient's food preferences and usual pattern of daily meals and snacks should be developed with a registered dietitian, and agreed to by the patient prior to initiating insulin therapy. It is important for the patient to consistently follow the meal plan as the insulin program is initiated and insulin doses are adjusted. Consistent timing of meals and snacks as well as the quantity of foods consumed (especially carbohydrates) will help to optimize glycemic control. As the patient learns the onset, peak, and duration of his or her insulins, adjustments can be made in the meal plan, insulin program, or both to achieve target blood glucose levels (2).

## NUTRITION STRATEGIES FOR TYPE 1 DIABETES

The goals of nutrition therapy for the type 1 diabetic patient are listed in Table 1. The usual food intake and exercise habits should be determined prior to the initiation of either conventional or intensive insulin therapy, because it is important to integrate insulin therapy into the patient's accustomed routine. It is recommended that all patients starting insulin therapy meet with a registered dietitian to develop an individualized meal plan that incorporates their food preferences, usual pattern of meals and snacks, and exercise habits. An initial meal plan should

**TABLE 1**  Goals for Nutrition Strategies

| Type 1 diabetes | Type 2 diabetes |
| --- | --- |
| The ideal meal plan integrates insulin therapy into usual eating and exercise habits | Primary nutrition goals are to achieve and maintain normal blood glucose and lipid levels, and to control blood pressure |
| Patients on conventional insulin therapy need to eat at consistent times to coordinate with the action time of insulin | Spread food intake, especially of carbohydrates, throughout the day |
| Adequate calories should be provided to maintain a reasonable body weight in adults and meet the nutritional needs for growth, development, pregnancy, lactation, and illness | Moderate calorie restriction and weight reduction; weight goals based on a *reasonable body weight*, not ideal body weight; increased physical activity and exercise level |
| Patients learn to adjust insulin doses by evaluating blood glucose patterns | Monitor blood glucose levels to determine whether goals are achieved |
| Patients on intensive insulin regimens have more flexibility in timing of meals and snacks and the amount of food eaten | Nutrition and exercise remain primary therapy, even when oral medication and/or insulin are added |

be developed and communicated to the provider initiating the insulin therapy so that the insulin program can be tailored to the patient's usual patterns of eating and exercise. Patients with type 1 diabetes on a conventional insulin program, such as twice-daily injections of short- and intermediate-acting insulin, should exercise and eat their meals and snacks at the same time each day so that the insulin action can be coordinated with their food intake and activity levels. Following a consistent meal plan and exercise program will help optimize glycemic control and decrease the risk of hypoglycemic events in the patient following a conventional insulin program (4).

Type 1 diabetic patients following conventional insulin-therapy programs need to monitor their blood glucose levels, as instructed by their physician or health-care practitioner, to identify blood glucose patterns. Blood glucose patterns are then used to adjust insulin doses and modify the insulin program or meal plan to achieve target blood glucose levels and glycemic control. Although many newly diagnosed type 1 diabetic patients are well managed on a conventional insulin program, many patients change to an intensive insulin program to achieve blood glucose goals and increase the flexibility of their food choices and lifestyle. Intensive insulin therapy allows the patient more flexibility in the timing of meals and exercise as well as in the composition of meals, and the ability to minimize or eliminate snacks. Intensive insulin programs include multiple daily injections with basal insulin and rapid- or short-acting pre-meal insulin or the use of an insulin pump with rapid- or short-acting insulin given as a pre-meal bolus. The amount of pre-meal rapid- or short-acting insulin can be adjusted based on the amount of food eaten (specifically, the carbohydrate content of the meal), the addition of snacks, and changes in exercise or activity levels. The patient can choose if and when to eat a meal or snack and use an algorithm or a carbohydrate-to-insulin ratio to calculate his or her pre-meal dose of rapid- or short-acting insulin (4). While a meal plan is often used as a guide to food choices, the patient who selects intensive therapy is able to enjoy flexibility of food choices and variability in the timing of meals, snacks, and exercise that would not be possible on a conventional insulin program.

## NUTRITION STRATEGIES FOR TYPE 2 DIABETES

Nutrition therapy is a key component of the management of type 2 diabetes. Because type 2 diabetes is a complex and diverse disease, it is important that nutrition therapy be individualized for each patient and based on specific goals to improve metabolic control. The goals of nutrition therapy for the type 2 diabetic patient are listed in Table 1. Reduction in calorie intake, moderate weight loss, and maintenance of a reasonable body weight are all effective nutrition strategies to improve metabolic control in the overweight type 2 diabetic patient.

A moderate weight loss of 5–10 kg (approximately 10–20 lb), regardless of initial weight, has been shown to improve glycemic control and to reduce serum lipid levels and blood pressure (2). For this reason, weight control continues to be an important strategy in nutrition management of type 2 diabetes.

Patients often experience difficulty in achieving weight loss and maintaining a reasonable body weight through traditional nutrition strategies, such as calorie-restricted diets. Therefore, the focus of nutrition therapy for type 2 diabetes is on achieving target blood glucose levels and improving metabolic control. Type 2 diabetic patients should be encouraged to monitor blood glucose levels because nutrition therapy and lifestyle changes often have a positive effect on blood glucose levels before weight loss goals are achieved. The focus of nutrition assessment and therapy for type 2 diabetes is to identify a reasonable body weight for the patient, and to encourage diet and lifestyle changes to achieve and maintain weight loss goals, blood glucose targets, and blood-pressure levels, and to improve metabolic control. Nutrition strategies encourage a moderate reduction in daily calorie intake, usually a reduction of 250–500 calories per day from the patient's usual daily intake, as assessed by a registered dietitian. In addition to nutrition therapy, a regular program of exercise is also encouraged to promote weight loss, achieve target blood glucose levels, and optimize metabolic control of type 2 diabetes. Increased physical activity can help to decrease insulin resistance, lower blood glucose levels, and improve overall health in addition to facilitating weight loss.

Because of the complex and diverse nature of type 2 diabetes, it is important to individualize the macronutrient composition of the meal plan based on each patient's goals, to improve metabolic control and limit long-term complications of the disease. In patients with hyperlipidemia, a reduction in both total and saturated-fat intake is usually recommended to help achieve serum lipid goals and decrease the risk of cardiac disease. A useful nutrition strategy to both optimize blood glucose control and improve serum lipid levels is to reduce the carbohydrate content of the diet to 40–45% of calories and to space meals and snacks throughout the day. Because carbohydrate-containing foods have the largest effect on blood glucose levels, blood glucose control can often be improved by spacing the carbohydrate intake at regular intervals. These meal-planning strategies can limit the rise in blood glucose levels after meals and snacks and optimize the benefits of endogenous insulin production and hypoglycemic medications in blood glucose control. The results of blood glucose monitoring are often used to adjust the amount of carbohydrates consumed and the timing of meals and snacks to achieve target blood glucose levels (5).

Because many type 2 diabetic patients are unable to achieve optimal metabolic and glycemic control through diet and exercise modifications and oral medications, insulin therapy is often started. However, it is important for both the patient and the health-care practitioner to recognize the continued benefits of diet, exercise, and lifestyle modifications—too often, patients and health-care practitioners place less emphasis on meal planning and exercise after a type 2 diabetic patient is started on insulin therapy. The key to achieving blood glucose targets with the addition of insulin therapy is for the patient to follow a meal plan with a consistent carbohydrate intake and to eat and exercise at consistent times each day. Consistent food intake and exercise habits will help match blood glucose levels with the action of hypoglycemic medications and insulin to achieve target blood glucose levels and limit hypoglycemic reactions (5).

## MEAL-PLANNING STRATEGIES

A meal plan is an individualized guide to daily food choices that incorporates an individual's food preferences, blood glucose targets, and nutrition goals of diabetes management. A meal plan is designed to achieve blood glucose goals by matching food intake—specifically, carbohydrate foods—to the action of oral medications and endogenous or exogenous insulin. An individualized meal plan also incorporates other specific nutrition goals, such as a reduction in calorie level or total and saturated-fat intake to promote weight loss or control serum lipid levels.

There is no one specific approach to meal planning that will meet the needs and nutrition goals of all diabetic patients. As part of the initial nutrition assessment, the registered dietitian determines the optimal meal-planning approach based on the needs and goals of the patient. The plan should be easily understood by the patient and serve as a useful guide to his or her daily food choices. Meal-planning methods are an important tool to help optimize glycemic and metabolic control for type 1 or type 2 diabetic patients on insulin therapy. Frequently used meal-planning methods are listed in Table 2.

Patients often begin diabetic meal planning with a simplified approach to their daily food choices based on a modification of the USDA Food Guide Pyramid (see Figure 1). *First Steps in Diabetic Meal Planning* is a pamphlet (developed jointly in 1995 by the American Dietetic Association and the American Diabetes Association) that bases the choice of food groups and portion control on the Food Guide Pyramid (6). Many diabetic patients quickly learn to use this

TABLE 2   Meal-Planning Methods

Food Guide Pyramid
Exchange-List-based meal plans
Consistent-carbohydrate meal plans
Carbohydrate counting

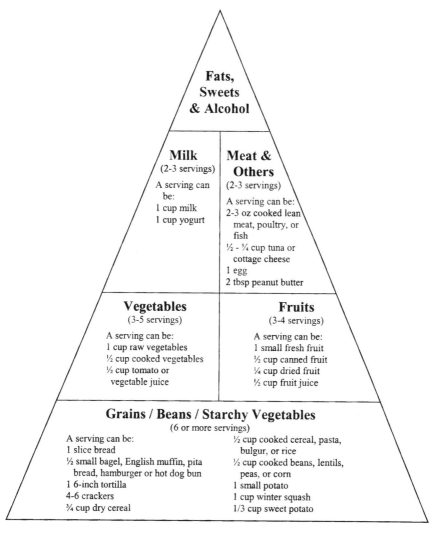

**Fats,
Sweets
& Alcohol**

**Milk**
(2-3 servings)

A serving can be:
1 cup milk
1 cup yogurt

**Meat &
Others**
(2-3 servings)

A serving can be:
2-3 oz cooked lean
  meat, poultry, or
  fish
½ - ¾ cup tuna or
  cottage cheese
1 egg
2 tbsp peanut butter

**Vegetables**
(3-5 servings)

A serving can be:
1 cup raw vegetables
½ cup cooked vegetables
½ cup tomato or
  vegetable juice

**Fruits**
(3-4 servings)

A serving can be:
1 small fresh fruit
½ cup canned fruit
¼ cup dried fruit
½ cup fruit juice

**Grains / Beans / Starchy Vegetables**
(6 or more servings)

A serving can be:
1 slice bread
½ small bagel, English muffin, pita
  bread, hamburger or hot dog bun
1 6-inch tortilla
4-6 crackers
¾ cup dry cereal

½ cup cooked cereal, pasta,
  bulgur, or rice
½ cup cooked beans, lentils,
  peas, or corn
1 small potato
1 cup winter squash
1/3 cup sweet potato

**FIGURE 1**  USDA Food Guide Pyramid.

pamphlet as a guide to their daily food choices. An individualized diabetic meal plan can be developed by the registered dietitian to identify healthy food choices and specify portions of each food group at meals and snacks. Meals and snacks can be planned with a consistent carbohydrate content spaced throughout the day to match food intake with the peak action of insulin therapy. The Food Guide Pyramid can also be used to achieve other nutrition goals such as weight loss and controlling serum lipid levels by identifying portion size and emphasizing low-fat food choices and limited intake of added fats.

As patients move to more intensive diabetes management, they usually progress to a more intensive program of insulin therapy that includes more frequent injections and a combination of different types of insulin to achieve target blood glucose levels. A more individualized and detailed system of meal planning is often required. The American Diabetes Association Exchange Lists for Meal Planning (see Table 3) form the basis for carbohydrate counting and are frequently used when a patient desires a meal-planning approach that provides more detailed information on the macronutrient content of each food group and a more precise system for measuring food portions. The Exchange Lists for Meal Planning were revised in 1995 to combine the starch, fruit, and milk groups, along with the new other-carbohydrate group containing sweets and snack foods, into the Carbohydrate Group. The Meat and Meat Substitute Group was divided into categories of very lean, lean, medium, and high-fat, and the Fat Group was broken down into monounsaturated, polyunsaturated, and saturated lists to encourage a decreased intake of both total and saturated fat (7).

The Exchange Lists for Meal Planning encourage flexibility in food choices and provide a more precise system of portion control to match the carbohydrate content of meals and snacks with the insulin therapy. These are used to more precisely define the carbohydrate content of each meal and snack for more effective use of the patient's intensified insulin program. The calorie level along with the protein and both total and saturated-fat content of the meal plan can be more precisely defined using the exchange system.

''Carbohydrate counting'' is a meal-planning system in which the primary emphasis is placed on the total carbohydrate content of foods rather than on other macronutrients. The total carbohydrate content of meals and snacks, regardless of the carbohydrate source, is assumed to have a greater effect on postprandial blood glucose levels than protein and fat do. Meal plans are developed with a

TABLE 3   Nutrient Content of Exchange Groups

| Exchange group | Carbohydrate (g) | Protein (g) | Fat (g) |
|---|---|---|---|
| Starch | 15 | 3 | Trace |
| Fruit | 15 | 0 | 0 |
| Milk (skim) | 12 | 8 | 0 |
| Other carbohydrates | 15 | Varies | Varies |
| Vegetables | 5 | 2 | 0 |
| Meat (lean) | 0 | 7 | 3 |
| Fat | 0 | 0 | 5 |

Source: Ref. 8.

consistent carbohydrate content at each meal and snack to achieve target blood glucose levels and to form a basis for adjustments in insulin therapy. The total carbohydrate content of the meal or snack determines the amount of rapid- or short-acting insulin required for blood glucose control, while the intermediate- or long-acting insulin covers the glycemic effect of protein and fat intake. Adjustments in insulin therapy are made based on carbohydrate intake at meals and snacks, along with the results of blood glucose monitoring to achieve target blood glucose levels.

The carbohydrate content of each food is precisely measured by either counting carbohydrate grams or using a modification of the American Diabetes Association exchange system based on carbohydrate groups or exchanges (8). Patients choose to count either carbohydrate grams or carbohydrate groups in which one carbohydrate group is equal to 15 grams of carbohydrate. Meal planning is simplified because food selection is focused primarily on carbohydrates, and postprandial blood glucose levels are more consistent as a result of the more precise method to determine carbohydrate intake. Carbohydrate counting can be used to ensure a consistent carbohydrate intake for a diabetic patient on conventional insulin therapy or to make adjustments in pre-meal rapid- or short-acting insulin doses based on the amount of carbohydrate consumed by patients on intensive insulin programs.

## HYPOGLYCEMIA ASSOCIATED WITH INSULIN THERAPY

A hypoglycemic reaction can vary in severity and may occur in anyone with diabetes. Insulin therapy significantly increases the risk, incidence, and severity of hypoglycemic reactions.

Hypoglycemia can be the result of too much insulin, too little food (i.e., skipped or delayed meals and snacks), alcohol intake, or exercise. It can often be prevented by monitoring blood glucose levels, taking insulin and oral medications as prescribed, following a meal plan, limiting alcohol intake, and planning extra snacks if needed to cover the hypoglycemic effects of exercise. The symptoms of hypoglycemia include hunger, headache, irritability, confusion, lethargy, and, in severe cases, seizure or loss of consciousness. Patients treated with insulin or oral hypoglycemic medications should know how to recognize and promptly treat hypoglycemic reactions.

Hypoglycemia should be treated immediately if the blood glucose level is less than 70 mg/dl, even if the patient is not experiencing symptoms. The patient's first step in treating hypoglycemia is to check his or her blood glucose level if possible. Foods and beverages that contain quick-acting carbohydrates are recommended to treat hypoglycemic reactions because foods that are high in fat take longer to elevate blood glucose levels. Patients should always keep a source of quick-acting carbohydrate on hand to treat hypoglycemic reactions. If

TABLE 4  Foods Containing 15 Grams of
Carbohydrate for Treating Hypoglycemia

| Food source | Amount |
| --- | --- |
| Glucose tablets | Three or four |
| Glucose gel | 1 tube |
| Hard candy | 4–6 pieces |
| Fruit juice | 4 oz |
| Sports drinks | 8 oz |
| Honey or corn syrup | 1 tbsp |
| Raisins | 2 tbsp |
| Skim milk | 8 oz |
| Regular (non-diet) soda | 4 oz |

the blood glucose level is between 50 and 70 mg/dl, the patient will need to consume a food or beverage containing 15 grams of quick-acting carbohydrate. Examples of such foods and beverages and the appropriate amount to consume are listed in Table 4. This treatment should increase the blood glucose level by 30–45 mg/dl over 15 minutes.

If the initial blood glucose level is less than 50 mg/dl, 30 grams of quick-acting carbohydrate should be consumed. The blood glucose level should be re-checked after 15 minutes and an additional 15 grams of quick-acting carbohydrate consumed if the blood glucose level is still below 70 mg/dl. If a meal is not planned within 1–2 hours of treating a hypoglycemic reaction, a snack containing 15–30 grams of carbohydrate should be consumed to prevent another hypoglycemic reaction. For many years, consuming a protein-containing snack was recommended to prevent recurrent hypoglycemia. However, current guidelines indicate that this is not necessary (4).

## SUMMARY

Nutrition therapy is a key component to the successful management of diabetes treated with insulin therapy. Whether a patient has type 1 or type 2 diabetes, nutrition assessment along with the development of individualized nutrition treatment goals, and meal plans to achieve those goals, is crucial to the successful initiation of insulin therapy. There is no longer one single generic diabetic diet or one approach to meal planning that will meet the needs of all diabetic patients. The overall goal of nutrition therapy is to improve metabolic control. To this end it is recommended that nutrition therapy be individualized for all diabetic patients and based on specific goals to improve metabolic control.

## REFERENCES

1. Bantle JP. A physician's perspective on medical nutrition therapy for diabetes. In: Franz MJ, Bantle JP, eds. American Diabetes Association Guide to Medical Nutrition Therapy for Diabetes. Alexandria, VA: ADA, 1999, pp 18–25, 1999.
2. Nutrition recommendations and principles for people with diabetes mellitus. Diabetes Care 23(suppl 1):S43–46, 2000.
3. Franz MJ. A dietitian's perspective on medical nutrition therapy for diabetes. In: Franz MJ, Bantle JP, eds. American Diabetes Association Guide to Medical Nutrition Therapy for Diabetes. Alexandria, VA: ADA, pp 3–17, 1999.
4. Kulkarni K, Franz MJ. Nutrition therapy for type 1 diabetes. In: Franz MJ, Bantle JP, eds. American Diabetes Association Guide to Medical Nutrition Therapy for Diabetes. Alexandria, VA: ADA, pp 26–45, 1999.
5. Beebe C. Nutrition therapy for type 2 diabetes. In: Franz MJ, Bantle JP, eds. American Diabetes Association Guide to Medical Nutrition Therapy for Diabetes. Alexandria, VA: ADA, pp 46–68, 1999.
6. American Diabetes Association. The American Dietetic Association: First Steps in Diabetes Meal Planning. Alexandria, VA: ADA, 1995.
7. American Diabetes Association. Exchange Lists for Meal Planning. Alexandria, VA: ADA, revised 1995.
8. American Diabetes Association. Carbohydrate Counting Level 1: Getting Started. Alexandria, VA: ADA, 1995.

# 5

## Physiology of Glucose Homeostasis and Insulin Secretion

**Robert A. Ritzel and Peter C. Butler**
University of Southern California, Los Angeles, California

### INTRODUCTION

In health, blood glucose concentration is closely regulated. Since low blood sugar is life-threatening, it is not surprising that there are numerous mechanisms to prevent hypoglycemia (1). There are fewer systems in place to prevent hyperglycemia, explaining the relatively high frequency of the clinical syndrome of diabetes mellitus. In this chapter we first review the metabolic pathways that regulate glucose metabolism. We then review the regulation of insulin secretion and, finally, examine how these processes are coordinated to maintain blood glucose concentration in the fasting and fed states.

### METABOLIC PATHWAYS

Blood glucose is constantly being removed into tissues and simultaneously replenished, in a process called glucose turnover. Glucose can enter the blood by absorption from the gut following a meal, or be released from the liver into the blood. Glucose released from the liver is either mobilized from glycogen stores (glycogenolysis) or newly synthesized (gluconeogenesis). Together, glycogenolysis and gluconeogenesis constitute hepatic glucose release.

TABLE 1   Hormonal Control of Glucose Homeostasis

| Effect | Insulin | Glucagon | Epinephrine | Growth hormone | Cortisol |
|---|---|---|---|---|---|
| Glucose uptake | ↑ | ↓ | ↓ | ↓ | ↓ |
| Glucose production | | | | | |
|   Glycogenolysis | ↓ | ↑ | ↑ | ↑ | ↑ |
|   Gluconeogenesis | ↓ | ↑ | ↑ | ↑ | ↑ |

## Hepatic Glucose Release

In the overnight fasted state, the liver has ~50 g of glucose stored as glycogen (2). Glycogen breakdown to glucose-6-phosphate in the liver is stimulated by glucagon, epinephrine, growth hormone, and cortisol (Table 1) (1). The concentration of these hormones increases with duration of fasting. After ~40 hours of fasting, the liver glycogen stores are largely depleted and gluconeogenesis becomes the predominant source of hepatic glucose release. Gluconeogenesis is the synthesis of glucose-6-phosphate from three carbon precursors, such as glycerol, lactate, and amino acids. Both gluconeogenesis and glycogenolysis to generate glucose-6-phosphate occur in almost all tissues. However, glucose-6-phosphate cannot be released from the cell into the circulation until the phosphate is removed. The enzyme required to facilitate this (glucose-6-phosphatase) is abundant in liver but not present in fat or muscle. Therefore, in the fasting state almost all glucose released into the blood arises from the liver (so-called hepatic glucose release). In health, after an overnight fast the liver releases glucose at ~2 mg/kg/min, which approximates the rate of glucose uptake (3). In patients with diabetes, fasting hyperglycemia is due to increased hepatic glucose release. The fasting blood glucose concentration is correlated with the rate of hepatic glucose release, and so the higher the rate of hepatic glucose release the higher the blood glucose concentration (4).

It follows that to decrease the fasting blood glucose concentration to normal in patients with diabetes it is necessary to decrease the rate of hepatic glucose release to ~2 mg/kg/min.

## Glucose Uptake by Insulin-Sensitive Tissues

Glucose is removed from the blood into the extracellular space by passive diffusion and then into the intracellular space via membrane glucose transporter proteins. Because the glucose concentration in most cells is barely detectable, the glucose concentration gradient from outside to inside a cell (~90 mg/dl) strongly favors inward diffusion. However, since glucose is soluble in water but not fat, glucose cannot cross the lipid bilayer cell membrane. To allow this, a water "pore" spanning the membrane is required. This barrier to diffusion presents an opportunity to regulate glucose uptake.

Glucose transport into cells is permitted by glucose transporter proteins, which span the membrane and provide the aqueous pore through which glucose can pass (5). Distinct forms of these proteins allow for differential regulation of glucose uptake in different tissues. For example, in muscle and fat tissue the glucose-4-transporter protein subtype is predominant. Following exposure to insulin, the glucose-4-transporter proteins rapidly move to the cell surface, allowing glucose transport into the cell. This action by insulin to stimulate glucose uptake in tissues with insulin-sensitive glucose-4-transporter proteins defines muscle and fat as so-called insulin-sensitive tissues.

However, even in insulin-sensitive tissues, insulin levels are not the only factor that regulates glucose uptake. Exercise also facilitates glucose transporter availability at the muscle cell membrane, increasing the rate of glucose uptake (6). Also, the glucose concentration *per se* regulates the rate of glucose uptake (7). At any given insulin level, glucose uptake increases with increasing glucose concentrations (so-called mass action of glucose). The action of glucose to promote glucose uptake results in *increased* rates of glucose uptake in diabetic patients, with hyperglycemia versus nondiabetic controls, provided that at least some insulin is present (8). This increased rate of glucose uptake matches the increased rate of hepatic glucose release that has caused the hyperglycemia, with the net effect that the blood glucose concentration remains stable but high.

### Glucose Uptake by Insulin-Independent Tissues

Some glucose transporter isoforms do not require insulin in order to be translocated to the cell membrane. For example, the glucose-2-transporter protein—the predominant form in the liver and the endocrine pancreas—remains in the cell membrane independent of insulin action. As a result, glucose is taken up passively down its concentration gradient into cells by these constantly available glucose transporter proteins. This allows the liver to take up glucose when the blood glucose concentration is high after a meal, and so replenish liver glycogen stores. Likewise, it allows the pancreatic endocrine cells to "sense" the blood glucose concentration and release insulin (β cells) and glucagon (α calls) accordingly.

## INSULIN SECRETION

### Proinsulin Biosynthesis, β-Cell Mass, and Insulin Secretion

Insulin is synthesized in pancreatic β cells, where it is processed from its precursor, proinsulin, into c-peptide (connecting peptide) and insulin (9). Processed insulin is stored in insulin vesicles. There are ~2000 β cells in an islet and ~1 million islets in the pancreas of an adult human. The β cell is shaped like a truncated cone, with the base of the cell exposed first to the blood flowing into the islet capillary bed. The membrane at the base of the cell has the glucose-2-transporter proteins that permit glucose access to the cell. Metabolism and oxidation of this glucose to carbon dioxide and water generate ATP. The increased ATP prompts exocytosis of stored insulin vesicles that discharge insulin from the apex of the β cell into the capillary and then into the portal vein. Although the prevailing glucose concentration is the best-recognized stimulant for insulin secretion, fatty acids are also important regulators of insulin secretion.

Evidence is increasing that the β-cell mass is regulated in adult life with new islet formation from exocrine ducts as well as β-cell replication within islets (10). Chronic insulin resistance leads to an adaptive increase in β-cell mass. Animals and humans with a partial decrease in β-cell mass as a consequence of a partial pancreatectomy have impaired insulin secretion, with an increased proinsulin-to-insulin ratio suggestive of inadequate processing of insulin. Leahy and colleagues (11) have shown somewhat paradoxically, that partial inhibition of insulin secretion can overcome diabetes under conditions of decreased β-cell mass. This intriguing observation implies that the pattern of insulin release may be more important than the absolute amount.

## Pattern of Insulin Secretion

Insulin secretion has a diurnal rhythm, with an increased rate of secretion during the day and decreased secretion at night (12). Also, insulin is secreted in both an ultradian (13) and a high-frequency pulsatile pattern (14). The ultradian pulses occur with a frequency of one pulse each 40 minutes, a rate that is decreased in patients with type 2 diabetes. The high-frequency pulses occur at one pulse per 6 minutes. Almost all insulin is secreted in these high-frequency discrete insulin secretory pulses. The amplitude of the resulting insulin concentration oscillations in the portal vein (1000–4000 pmol/L) is very large, but hepatic insulin clearance results in a marked attenuation of these oscillations by the time they reach the systemic circulation (amplitude ~10 pmol/L) (15). The pacemaker responsible for generating this high-frequency pulsatile rhythm is unknown, but each islet independently secretes insulin in a comparable pulsatile manner so the property must be present within islets. Also, the mechanism that allows the 1 million islets to be coordinated to secrete pulses in a synchronous manner is not known although the intrapancreatic neural network is believed to be important. Transplanted islets in the liver secrete insulin in a coordinate fashion once the islets have been reinnervated (16).

The significance of these high-frequency insulin oscillations for insulin action is not fully understood, although there is some evidence that they are important. Clearly, reproducing the insulin-concentration profile present in the portal vein in humans—either in the fasting state or, particularly, after a meal—would be impossible with insulin exogenously injected into the subcutaneous tissue or even the systemic circulation. Consistent with the observations of Leahy and colleagues that β-cell rest can overcome diabetes in animal models with a partial pancreatectomy, overnight β-cell rest can at least temporarily restore pulsatile insulin secretion in patients with type 2 diabetes (17). It is therefore rational to increase insulin sensitivity in patients with a partial decrease in β-cell mass (such as those with type 2 diabetes). This strategy is likely to at least partially restore the pattern of insulin secretion toward normal, and the available evidence suggests that the pattern of insulin secretion is important for effective insulin action.

## REGULATION OF GLUCOSE METABOLISM IN THE FASTED AND FED STATE

### Fasting

In health, the blood glucose concentration remains remarkably stable even after prolonged fasting (Figure 1). After an overnight fast, basal insulin concentrations are relatively low, and insufficient to stimulate glucose uptake by muscle and fat. Under these conditions glucose uptake is primarily by insulin-independent tissues such as brain, red blood cells, and the kidney. With fasting, insulin-dependent tissues rely primarily on free fatty acids for energy. These free fatty acids are derived from breakdown of fat stores (triglyceride). Blood glucose remains constant because the liver releases glucose derived initially from glycogenolysis—and, with time, increasingly from gluconeogenesis—at a rate that matches that of glucose uptake.

The basal rate of insulin is sufficient to constrain the rate of hepatic glucose release to match that of glucose uptake. In the absence of this basal insulin, the rate of hepatic glucose release would be much greater and the blood glucose concentration would increase. The basal rate of insulin is also sufficient to constrain levels of lipolysis to provide sufficient FFA for oxidation by muscle and fat. In the complete absence of insulin, lipolysis would occur at much higher rates and excessive FFA would be converted to ketones in the liver, resulting in diabetic ketoacidosis (18).

### Replacement of Basal Insulin

Basal insulin is provided by either a continuous subcutaneous infusion from an insulin pump or intermittent injection (daily or twice daily) of insulin formulated to be released slowly from this site (19). Replacement insulin therapy in the basal state (between meals and overnight) has the object of constraining hepatic glucose release to match glucose uptake by non-insulin-independent tissues (Figure 2).

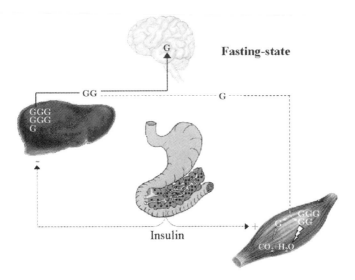

**FIGURE 1** In the fasting state, glucose enters the circulation from the liver (from stored glycogen or newly formed glucose) and is taken up predominately by non-insulin-sensitive tissues (such as the brain). Relatively little glucose is taken up by insulin-sensitive tissues such as muscle. The blood glucose is maintained by the actions of insulin to restrain hepatic glucose release to match the rate of glucose uptake. This is the *basal* insulin component required in insulin-replacement therapy.

The amount of insulin required to this end varies from person to person (depending on hepatic insulin sensitivity). It will also vary according to both the time of day and the duration of the fast. For example, at night insulin requirements fall but in the morning they rise. This is presumably a consequence of the circadian rhythm of growth hormone and cortisol, hormones that increase the requirements of insulin by increasing the rate of gluconeogenesis (cortisol and growth hormone) and glycogenolysis (growth hormone). The advantage of an insulin pump over injection of a sustained-release form of insulin for provision of basal insulin supply is that it can be programmed to vary according to these circadian changes.

Long-acting insulin preparations available for intermittent subcutaneous injection include NPH insulin, which requires twice-daily injections; Ultralente insulin, which results in rather variable day-to-day insulin-concentration profiles; and recently an insulin analog, insulin glargine, modified to provide a slow release from the site of injection (20). Some patients prefer not to wear a pump and prefer intermittent insulin injections. Also, an advantage of the intermit-

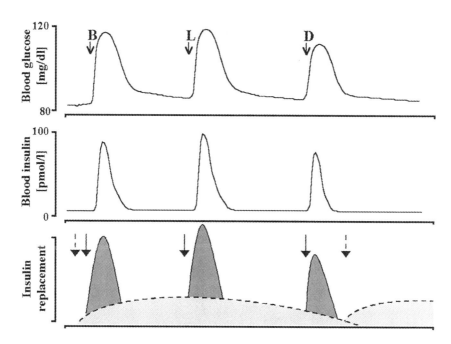

**FIGURE 2**   Insulin replacement. In health (top panel), blood glucose remains stable between meals and only increases transiently after a meal (B-breakfast; L-lunch; and D-dinner or evening meal). This is because the circulating insulin concentration (middle panel) restrains glucose output between meals to match glucose uptake (*basal insulin*) and increases abruptly with meals to further inhibit hepatic glucose release and stimulate glucose uptake by insulin-sensitive tissues (Figure 1). Insulin replacement (bottom panel) is designed to reproduce this pattern of insulin secretion. Basal insulin replacement (light shaded area) is given by either twice-daily NPH insulin injections (broken arrows in lower panel) or once-daily Ultralente or insulin glargine or by a continuous infusion by a pump. The meal-related insulin boluses of insulin might be given either as intermittent injections of rapidly acting insulin (e.g., lispro or aspart insulin) just prior to meals (solid arrows) or as boluses from a continuous pump.

tent injection of longer-acting insulin preparations is that the patient is less vulnerable to the sudden loss of insulin availability that occurs with undetected pump failure.

However, as day-to-day variation in levels of stress, exercise, illness, etc., induce variable levels of growth hormone, cortisol, and epinephrine, optimal basal insulin requirements inevitably vary from day to day as well. Ultimately, provision of an optimal basal insulin supply will require a system that responds to the prevailing blood glucose (a closed-loop feedback system).

## Meal Ingestion

Following a meal, glucose is absorbed over a period of ~180 minutes, most quickly in the first hour (Figure 3). In health, the resulting glycemic excursion is limited, whereas in diabetes both the peak and the duration of the glycemic response are markedly increased.

In health, following meal ingestion insulin secretion is rapidly increased through the mechanism of both hyperglycemia and the incretin hormones such as GIP and GLP-1 (21). In contrast, the glucagon concentration tends to be suppressed initially as a consequence of the hyperglycemia but increases later due to the rising concentration of circulating amino acids. Both of these hormonal

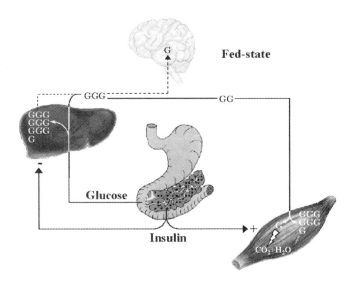

FIGURE 3 Fed state—following meal ingestion, glucose enters the circulation from both the meal and the liver. In health, in response to the resulting increment in blood glucose, there is a prompt increase in insulin secretion (Figure 2). As a consequence, hepatic glucose release is suppressed and glucose uptake by insulin-sensitive tissues such as skeletal muscle is rapidly increased. As a result of these combined actions, the increment in blood glucose concentration is restrained and the glucose concentration rapidly restored to fasting levels. Bolus insulin treatment at meals (Figure 2) seeks to reproduce these actions.

responses to meal ingestion are abnormal in people with diabetes (22). The post-prandial increment in insulin secretion is blunted in type 2 diabetes and absent in type 1 diabetes. The basal glucagon levels tend to be higher in patents with diabetes, and the glucagon concentrations are not appropriately suppressed after meal ingestion.

In health, the postprandial glycemic response is constrained by extraction of ~40% of the meal glucose by the liver, suppression of hepatic glucose release, and stimulation of glucose uptake by insulin-sensitive tissues (muscle and fat). Theoretically any of these could contribute to the postprandial hyperglycemia in diabetes. Hepatic extraction of meal glucose is not impaired in diabetes (23). Glucose is taken up by the liver, provided that at least some insulin is present, and patients with poorly controlled diabetes tend to have increased rather than decreased liver glycogen stores.

The primary mechanism subserving postprandial hyperglycemia is failure to adequately suppress hepatic glucose release. Given the impaired insulin secretion after meal ingestion, and failure to suppress glucagon secretion, the failure to suppress hepatic gluconeogenesis and glycogenolysis is not surprising.

Provided that at least basal insulin levels are present, glucose uptake by insulin-sensitive tissues is *greater* in patients with diabetes than in nondiabetics after meal ingestion, and so impaired glucose uptake is not responsible for post-prandial hyperglycemia. The increased rate of glucose uptake is due to the mass action effect of glucose to promote glucose uptake in insulin-sensitive tissues (skeletal muscle, fat) in the presence of some insulin.

## Meal-Related Insulin Replacement

In contrast to basal insulin, the primary goal for insulin-replacement therapy after meal ingestion is to provide insulin with a rapid increase that will as closely as possible reproduce that seen in vivo from the intact pancreas (Figure 2). With Regular (soluble) insulin this is problematic because the peak insulin concentration after subcutaneous insulin injection is not achieved until ~2 hours after injection. Insulin analogs are now available (lispro and aspart) that are formulated not to form hexamers and so are released rapidly from the injection site, reaching a peak ~ 30–60 minutes after injection. These analogs are most frequently used in insulin pumps. Therefore, the most effective means of providing insulin for meals is either intermittent injection of a subcutaneous injection of a rapidly absorbed insulin analog or a bolus of insulin from an insulin pump.

Several groups are currently investigating inhaled insulin as an alternative to meal-related subcutaneous insulin. Absorption is not as fast as with analog insulin injected subcutaneously, and concerns about possible pulmonary complications will have to be ruled out.

## SUMMARY AND CONCLUSIONS

In healthy individuals, blood glucose concentration is tightly regulated. Insulin is secreted in a basal rate between meals that is sufficient to constrain the rate of hepatic glucose release to match the rate of glucose uptake. After meal ingestion, the insulin secretion rate is promptly increased and leads to further suppression of hepatic glucose release, increased glucose uptake by insulin-sensitive tissues, and restoration of blood glucose levels to fasting levels. In patients with diabetes, the mechanism of hyperglycemia in the fasting and fed states is excess hepatic glucose release. This is due to inadequate insulin delivery to the liver along with hepatic insulin resistance. Treatment strategies to restore the blood glucose concentration to normal require provision of an adequate amount of insulin to appropriately inhibit hepatic glucose release in the basal fasting state and after meal ingestion.

## ACKNOWLEDGMENTS

The laboratory of Dr. Peter Butler is funded by NIDDK grant 1R01–59579–01, National Institutes of Health.

## REFERENCES

1.  Butler PC, Rizza RA. Regulation of carbohydrate metabolism and response to hypoglycemia. Endocrinol Metabolism Clin North Am 18:1–25, 1989.
2.  Nilsson L, Hultman E. Liver glycogen in man: the effects of total starvation on a carbohydrate-poor diet followed by carbohydrate refeeding. Scand J Clin Lab Invest 32:325–330, 1973.
3.  DeBodo RC, Steele R, Altszuler N, On the hormonal regulation of carbohydrate metabolism: studies with [14]C glucose. Recent Prog Horm Res 19:449–488, 1963.
4.  Butler PC, Rizza RA. Contribution to postprandial hyperglycemia and effect on initial splanchnic glucose clearance of hepatic glucose cycling in glucose-intolerant or NIDDM patients. Diabetes 40:73–81, 1991.
5.  Joost HG, Weber TM. The regulation of glucose transport in insulin-sensitive cells. Diabetologia 32:831–838, 1989.
6.  Goodyear LJ, Kahn BB. Exercise, glucose, transport, and insulin sensitivity. Annu Rev Med 49:235–261, 1998.
7.  Verdonk CA, Rizza RA, Gerich JE. Effects of plasma glucose concentration on glucose utilization and glucose clearance in normal man. Diabetes 30:535–537, 1981.
8.  Firth RG, Bell PM, Marsh HM, Hansen I, Rizza RA. Postprandial hyperglycemia in patients with noninsulin-dependent diabetes mellitus: role of hepatic and extrahepatic tissues. J Clin Invest 77:1525–1532, 1986.
9.  Steiner DF, James DE. Cellular and molecular biology of beta cell. Diabetologia 35(suppl 2):S41–48, 1992.

10. Nielson JH, Galsgaard ED, Moldrup A, Friedrichsen BN, Billestrup N, Hansen JA, Lee YC, Carlsson C. Regulation of beta-cell mass by hormones and growth factors. Diabetes 50(suppl 1):S25–29, 2001.
11. Leahy JL, Bumbalo LM, Chen C. Diazoxide causes recovery of β-cell glucose responsiveness in 90% pancreatectomized diabetic rats. Diabetes 43:173–179, 1994.
12. Boden G, Ruiz J, Urbain JL, Chen X. Evidence for a circadian rhythm of insulin secretion. Am J Physiol 271 (Endcrinol Metab 34):E246–E252, 1996.
13. Shapiro ET, Tillil H, Polonsky KS, Fang VS, Rubenstein AH, Cauter EV. Oscillations in insulin secretion during constant glucose infusion in normal man: relationship to changes in plasma glucose. J Clin Endocrinol Metab 67(2):307–314, 1988.
14. Lang DA, Matthews DR, Burnett M, Ward GM, Turner RC. Pulsatile, synchronous basal insulin and glucagons secretion in man. Diabetes 31:22–26, 1982.
15. Song SH, McIntyre SM, Shah H, Veldhuis, JD, Hayes, PC, Butler, PC. Direct measurement of pulsatile insulin secretion from the portal vein in human subjects. J Clin Endocrinol Metab 85:4491–4499, 2000.
16. Pørksen N, Munn S, Ferguson D, O'Brien T, Veldhuis J, Butler PC. Coordinate pulsatile insulin secretion by chronic intraportally transplanted islets in the isolated perfused rat liver. J Clin Invest 94:219–227, 1994.
17. Laedtke T, Kjems L, Pørksen N, Schmitz, O, Veldhuis JD, Kao PC, Butler, PC. Overnight inhibition of insulin secretion restores pulsatility and the proinsulin/insulin ratio in Type 2 diabetes. Am J Physiol Endocrinol Metab 279:E520–E528, 2000.
18. Laffel L. Ketone bodies: a review of physiology, pathophysiology and application of monitoring to diabetes. Diabetes/Metab Res Rev 15(6):412–426, 1999.
19. Silverstein JH, Rosenbloom AL. New developments in type 1 (insulin-dependent) diabetes. Clin Pediatr 39(5):257–266, 2000.
20. Buse J. Insulin glargine (HOE901): first responsibilities: understanding the data and ensuring safety. Diabetes Care 23:576–578, 2000.
21. Doyle ME, Egan JM. Glucagon-like peptide-1. Recent Prog Horm Res 56:377–399, 2001.
22. Perley MJ, Kipnis DM. Plasma insulin responses to oral and intravenous glucose: studies in normal and diabetic subjects. J Clin Invest 46:1054–1962, 1967.
23. Firth R, Bell P, Marsh M, Rizza RA. Effects of tolazamide and exogenous insulin on pattern of postprandial carbohydrate metabolism in patients with non-insulin-dependent diabetes mellitus: results of randomized crossover trial. Diabetes 36:1130–1138, 1987.

# 6

## Insulin Pharmacokinetics

**Steven D. Wittlin, Hans J. Woehrle, and
John E. Gerich**
University of Rochester School of Medicine and Dentistry,
Rochester, New York

### OVERVIEW

A variety of insulin preparations are now available that differ in times of onset, peak effect, and duration of action, enabling the clinician to more appropriately satisfy their patients' requirements in a safe and effective manner (1,2). Insulin, which first became available for patients with diabetes mellitus in 1922 (3,4), was originally extracted from porcine and bovine pancreases and differed in structure from human insulin by one and three amino acids, respectively. The early preparations were dilute (1 unit/ml), of crude purity, and short-acting. Patients had to inject themselves four to six times a day with relatively large volumes, which made the injections painful. Local cutaneous reactions at injection sites (inflammation, lipoatrophy, and lipohypertrophy) were common due to contaminants. Moreover, because the preparations were antigenic, most patients developed insulin antibodies, which delayed the onset and prolonged the duration of insulin action. Development of antibodies sometimes caused severe immune insulin resistance that necessitated desensitization and the use of corticosteroids or specifically modified insulins (e.g., sulfated insulins).

As technology advanced, the preparations were standardized and became available in concentrations of 40 and 80 units/ml. Insulin in the United States is now uniformly 100 units/ml (U100). By the 1950s, longer-acting preparations were developed by adding chemicals to the buffer, which caused microcrystallization of the insulin, slowing absorption from the subcutaneous space into the blood (so-called "cloudy insulins"). Zinc was added to the Lente preparations (Lente and Ultralente), and protamine and a small amount of zinc to NPH (neutral protamine Hagedorn) (5). Combining these long-acting preparations with a fast-acting insulin such as Regular or Semilente permitted fewer injections and improved dosage individualization. Also, formulations of already-mixed short- and intermediate-acting insulins ("premixes") eventually came to market.

In the 1970s, advances in tissue chromatography led to preparations of higher purity, which markedly decreased antibody generation and immune insulin resistance, as well as local and systemic reactions. By the late 1980s, manufacture of human insulin using recombinant DNA technology became possible, so in most Westernized countries usage of animal insulin has mostly ceased. Human insulin has a slightly more rapid onset and shorter duration of action than the animal insulins, although the effect is of modest clinical significance. The one exception is Ultralente. Beef Ultralente, which is no longer available in the United States, was a peakless insulin that lasted over 24 hours, whereas human Ultralente has a peak and duration of action that resembles those of animal NPH (peak 8–10 hours, duration 15–20 hours).

With the development of the radioimmunoassay for insulin in 1960, it became apparent that the normal secretion of insulin was mainly regulated by, and paralleled, changes in blood glucose levels. With meal ingestion, plasma insulin levels increase three- to fivefold to peak within 30–60 minutes, and return to premeal levels within 2–3 hours. Initially, twice-daily (before breakfast and supper) injections of mixtures of a fast-acting and intermediate-acting insulin were used in patients with type 1 diabetes, who have no endogenous insulin, in an attempt to simulate the physiological delivery of insulin. Later, this regimen was improved by using pre-meal injections of Regular or Semilente insulin with once- or twice-daily long-acting preparations such as Ultralente. An alternative to this "basal-bolus" approach came into use in the 1980s with insulin pumps—continuous subcutaneous insulin infusion (CSII)—that deliver a bolus of Regular insulin prior to meals superimposed on a basal rate and that can be preprogrammed to deliver an amount that varies according to the time of day. Regardless of whether the short-acting insulin was given by syringe, pen, or pump, the resultant plasma insulin levels and biological effect did not perfectly simulate the normal pattern, because the slow absorption of Regular or Semilente insulin required that it be taken 30–45 minutes prior to meals for optimal prevention of post-meal hyperglycemia (6). The required delay was inconvenient, and in practice few patients actually waited that long. Moreover, the resultant plasma insulin levels did not generally peak until 60–120 minutes postprandially and remained elevated for up to 6 hours (7). Therefore, attempts to limit postprandial increases in plasma glucose by increasing insulin doses often resulted in hypoglycemia prior to the next meal. This was a serious limitation—it is now well recognized that hypoglycemia is the rate-limiting factor for achieving optimal glycemic control in patients with type 1 diabetes and in many patients with type 2 diabetes who take insulin.

Another problem was the variability in the day-to-day insulin profiles of the available insulins (8,9). The short-acting insulins (Regular and Semilente) have coefficients of variation in peak levels of 20–30%, whereas the longer-acting preparations (NPH, Lente, and Ultralente) have variations that are twice as great. Other factors affect the absorption characteristics (Table 1). The one of greatest clinical significance is variable absorption from different injection sites: insulin onset is quickest and its duration of action shortest from the abdomen, followed by the arms and then the buttocks and thighs (10).

The past decade has seen the development of insulins with amino acid substitutions that alter the absorption characteristics: "insulin analogs," or "designer insulins" (11–15). There are now two preparations—lispro and aspart—that are absorbed faster and have a shorter duration of action than Regular human insulin, and another with a longer duration of action (>24 hours) than Ultralente that is essentially peakless—glargine (Table 2). These analogs have overcome many of the limitations of native human insulin: they have excellent day-to-day consistency in absorption characteristics, their absorption rates are minimally affected by the anatomical injection site, and the fast on–off effect of the rapid-acting preparations allows injecting at the time of eating and minimizes postprandial hypoglycemia. Thus, in many patients, the analogs have provided the first opportunity to design insulin programs that mimic normal patterns of physiological insulin delivery.

TABLE 1   Some Variables
Influencing Insulin Absorption

1. Site of injection
2. Local heat
3. Insulin dose
4. Depth of injection
5. Exercise
6. Insulin species
7. Insulin mixtures

TABLE 2   Action Profiles of Various Insulin Preparations

| Type of insulin | Onset | Peak | Duration |
|---|---|---|---|
| Human Regular | 15–30 min | 120 min | 6–8 hr |
| Lispro insulin | 15 min | 60 min | 3–4 hr |
| Aspart insulin | 15 min | 60 min | 3–4 hr |
| Human NPH | 2 h | 5–7 hr | 13–16 hr |
| Human Lente | | | |
| Human Ultralente | 1 hr | 10 hr | 20 hr |
| Insulin glargine | 1.5 hr | Peakless | 24 hr at least |

## SHORT-ACTING INSULINS

Regular human insulin exists mostly as complexes of six insulin molecules (hexamers) because of spontaneous self-association, and a smaller proportion of singles (monomer) and doubles (dimers). When given intravenously, Regular human insulin rapidly dissociates into monomers. However, after subcutaneous injection, dissociation is much slower. Because insulin needs to be monomeric for absorption from the subcutaneous space into the blood, this slow dissociation delays the appearance of insulin into the blood, and thus its onset of action (16). As shown in Table 2, the onset of action of subcutaneously injected Regular human insulin is approximately 15–30 minutes, its peak action occurs at about 120 minutes, and the duration of action at doses used clinically is generally between 6 and 8 hours. These values relate to abdominal subcutaneous injection, which is the preferred site of injection. Absorption from the abdomen is more rapid than that following subcutaneous injection in the arm, which in turn is more rapid than that following subcutaneous injection in the thigh (10).

As a result of studying the structural basis for the self-association of human insulin, analogs with amino acid substitutions were developed that eliminate self-aggregation. Two of these, lispro and aspart, are commercially available (12,15).

Insulin lispro (Humalog) is the result of altering the 28th and 29th B-chain amino acids from proline, lysine to lysine, proline, which eliminates the ability to self-aggregate so only monomers exist after injection in the subcutaneous space. Absorption is thus much faster than with Regular insulin (17). Lispro binds to the insulin receptor with approximately the same affinity as native human insulin, but has a slightly higher affinity for the IGF-1 receptor. The clinical significance of the latter remains to be determined. Euglycemic clamp studies in normally glucose-tolerant subjects reveal that when given subcutaneously, lispro results in two- to threefold higher peak serum insulin levels sooner (42 versus 101 minutes) than Regular, and its duration of action is shorter at 3–4 hours (17). Importantly, there is no significant difference in total hypoglycemic potency between these two insulins. Other clinically useful differences from Regular insulin are fewer anatomical effects on absorption (18), and the time to peak activity is not dose-dependent as it is with Regular (2).

Large clinical trials that compared insulin lispro with Regular insulin have shown lower postprandial glucose rises in type 1 and type 2 patients with lispro, although overall glycemic control as measured by $HbA_{1C}$ is not substantially different. One explanation may be that lispro is less likely to cause mild hypoglycemia than Regular insulin when used in doses that yield comparable postprandial control in type 1 patients (19–22), which results in a reduced need for between-meal snacks. Also, meta-analysis in type 1 patients suggests that lispro reduced severe hypoglycemia (23). No difference in serum lipid concentrations has been demonstrated. In both type 1 and type 2 patients, insulin antibody concentrations with lispro use was no different than with Regular insulin (24). Initial studies in patients treated with CSII suggest a benefit of insulin lispro over Regular insulin in reduction of both $HbA_{1C}$ and postprandial glycemia (25,26). In most patients, doses of lispro and Regular insulin are comparable, although minor adjustments may be required in individual patients. Insulin lispro should be given up to 15 minutes before a meal (27).

In summary, advantages of insulin lispro are its ease of use with no need to wait before eating and better prandial control in type 1 patients with less hypoglycemia than Regular insulin. Disadvantages relate to the rapidity of onset and short duration. Type 1 patients may "run out" of insulin if sufficient basal insulin or mixture with Regular insulin is not used. Finally, its safety in pregnancy has not been established.

Insulin aspart (Novolog) is similar in concept to lispro, and was created by substituting aspartic acid for proline at position 28 on the B chain (15,28). Self-association is decreased similarly to insulin lispro, resulting in a monomeric/dimeric insulin analog. Because aspartic acid is negatively charged, the lack of association may be charge-mediated rather than steric. Potency of aspart is similar to that of human insulin, with approximately 90% binding affinity to the insulin receptor (29). Also, binding to the IGF-1 receptor is similar to human insulin.

Insulin aspart is absorbed twice as fast as Regular insulin (30). Site effects in terms of absorption and glucose-lowering action are negligible (31). The peak insulin levels attained are approximately twice as high for aspart versus Regular insulin at 52 minutes and 109 minutes, respectively. The duration of action is 3–4 hours. A study comparing aspart and lispro showed no major clinical differences (32).

A brief clinical trial of insulin aspart versus Regular insulin showed the expected reduction in postprandial glycemia (33). However, after 1 month no difference in fructosamine (a measure of overall glycemia like $HbA_{1C}$, but for the last 7–10 days) was noted. A longer, 6-month trial showed a small 0.15% reduction in $HbA_{1C}$ with insulin aspart versus Regular, the former being given at mealtime and the latter 30 minutes before meals (34). Also, there were fewer episodes of severe hypoglycemia.

Overall, the pharmacodynamics of lispro and aspart in terms of rapidity of action and short duration are similar, and, not surprisingly, their advantages, disadvantages, and how they are used are comparable. Both appear to reduce postprandial glycemia and lessen the risk for hypoglycemia. Both should be administered 0 to 15 minutes before a meal, and no dosing adjustment is generally made when switching from Regular insulin to aspart or lispro. Studies support the use of either in insulin pumps (25,26,35). In contrast, there is no advantage of the monomeric analogs during intravenous infusion, which should probably be reserved, at present, for Regular insulin.

## INTERMEDIATE-ACTING INSULINS

The initial purpose for the development of long-acting insulin preparations was to minimize the number of daily injections needed for glycemic control. Ideally, the action of such an insulin preparation should reflect naturally occurring changes in insulin requirements throughout the day. This would be particularly important during the overnight period, when longer-acting insulins are required to suppress endogenous glucose production. Additionally, the kinetics and dynamics should be highly reproducible so that day-to-day variation in absorption/activity is as low as possible.

Two intermediate-acting insulins have been widely used: the zinc-precipitated Lente insulin and the protamine-precipitated NPH insulin (5). Although pork insulin preparations are still available, since the introduction of human insulin to the U.S. market the use of animal insulin has markedly decreased. Overall, human insulin has a somewhat earlier peak of onset and shorter duration of action compared with pork insulin. However, the clinical implications of this finding are probably small; clinical studies have shown essentially equivalent glycemic control with pork and human insulin. Only human insulins are discussed in the remainder of this section.

## LENTE INSULIN

Lente insulin was invented in 1952 by Hallas-Moller (36), who observed that the addition of zinc in the presence of acetate buffer at neutral pH caused insulin to crystallize, markedly prolonging its action after subcutaneous injection. Two forms of insulin appear: an amorphous precipitate called Semilente, which has a duration of action similar to that of Regular insulin, and stable crystals of insulin called Ultralente. Commercial preparations of Lente insulin are standardized to a mixture of 30% Semilente and 70% Ultralente. Early formulations of this mixture combined beef and pork insulin, because the conditions caused the porcine insulin to become amorphous and the beef to crystallize (5). Human Lente is now available. Its kinetics of action are similar to those of NPH, although it peaks a little more slowly than the NPH, and a biphasic pattern in the systemic insulin appearance of Lente insulin has been described, probably due to the different kinetics of the amorphous and crystalline compounds. Duration of action is 13–16 hours, and the maximal blood-glucose-lowering effect is seen around 6 hours after injection. It is noteworthy that the zinc insulins are not miscible with non-zinc insulins such as Regular or NPH, because the high zinc content can lead to unpredictable microcrystallization and prolongation of the effect of the non-zinc insulin.

## NEUTRAL PROTAMINE HAGEDORN INSULIN

The most commonly used intermediate-acting insulin is neutral protamine Hagedorn (NPH) insulin (isophane). It was developed in the Novo-Hagedorn laboratories in Denmark in 1946 by Krayenbuhl and Rosenberg (37), based on the original observation of Hagedorn that insulin's effect was prolonged when combined with proteins such as protamine (38), and that of Scott and Fisher showing that small amounts of zinc lengthened the action of protamine insulin (39). NPH contains equal amounts of protamine and insulin with a small amount of zinc at neutral pH. Protamine is a basic, highly negatively charged protein derived from fish sperm. It is essentially nonimmunogenic. The commercial preparations of NPH are a suspension of oblong tetragonal crystals with essentially no unprecipitated (Regular) insulin (5). Because of the symmetric, even structure of the insulin-protamine crystals, and because protamine and insulin are used in equimolar amounts, the term *isophane* (Greek *iso*, ''even'' and *phane*, ''appearance'') is often used for this insulin preparation. For both forms of crystallized insulin (NPH and the Lente), the insulin crystals may sediment soon after agitating the bottle. To ensure accurate dosing, then, care must be taken to gently, but thoroughly, mix the vial prior to drawing it up in the syringe. Sedimentation of insulin crystals may in part explain the described day-to-day variability of insulin action for the longer-acting insulins. Also, commercially available NPH preparations contain very small amounts of nonbound protamine—too little to bind significant amounts of Regular insulin when mixed with the NPH—so NPH–Regular mixtures are much more stable than Lente– or Ultralente–Regular mixtures. This has allowed development of commercial fixed mixtures of NPH and Regular insulin. In the United States, 70/30 and 50/50 (%NPH/%Regular) are available, while in other parts of the world many more proportions are obtainable. The onset of action and duration of the preparation depend on the relative amounts of NPH and Regular insulin in the mixture. In general, the more NPH, the later the onset and the longer the duration of action. A similar mixture using 75% neutral protamine lispro (NPL) and 25% lispro has recently been marketed.

The absorption of both NPH and human Lente insulin follows a monoexponential course, as does Regular insulin. For the most part, there seem to be no clinically important differences in absorption between these two insulin preparations, although NPH insulin has been reported to have a somewhat faster onset and shorter duration (40). Both insulins after subcutaneous injection have a slow on–off pattern that is interspersed by a considerable peak, plus there is a large day-to-day variability of up to 50% for both NPH and Lente (9). It therefore seems that neither Lente nor NPH fulfills the criteria for an ideal basal insulin.

In summary, NPH and Lente have been mainstays of insulin regimens for a half-century. They provide basal insulin coverage, but at a price: absorption is variable, they have a distinct peak, and human preparations generally last for considerably less than 24 hours, necessitating multiple injections.

## LONG-ACTING INSULINS

The long-acting insulin used in the United States is Ultralente. As indicated above, it is an insulin–zinc crystalline preparation that was developed to be a basal, long-acting insulin because in animal form its duration of action when injected subcutaneously exceeds 24 hours and is relatively peakless. Because human Ultralente is more soluble, its duration of action is significantly shorter (Table 2). In a recent study (9), human Ultralente was shown to have an onset of action of $1.0 \pm 0.2$ hour and a duration of action of $19 \pm 5.8$ hours. Peak action was at 10–12 hours. Moreover, the intersubject variability was twice that seen with a subcutaneous insulin pump. Other sources show that intrasubject variability is very high with Ultralente. Disappointingly, when twice-daily Ultralente was compared to twice-daily Lente insulin in 66 patients in a double crossover study, the major clinical difference was more severe hypoglycemia with Ultralente treatment, mostly between 5 A.M. and breakfast (41).

Because of the above-indicated drawbacks of NPH, Lente, and Ultralente as basal insulins, long-acting insulin analogs have been developed to try to better mimic physiological basal insulin secretion. The only commercially available long-acting analog at the time of this writing is insulin glargine (14). It is produced by modifying insulin at position 21 of the A chain by substituting glycine for asparagine, and also at the amino-terminus of the B chain by adding two arginines. This shifts the isoelectric point, causing glargine to be virtually insoluble at a physiological pH. It is kept soluble within the bottle by using a buffer with a pH of 4. When injected into the neutral pH of the subcutaneous space, glargine precipitates, markedly delaying absorption. The result is a nearly peakless insulin analog, with onset of action in 2–4 hours and a duration of action more than 24 hours. In the previously mentioned study of Lepore at al. (9), glargine's onset of action was $1.5 \pm 0.3$ hours and duration $20.5 \pm 3.7$ hours. Plus, its effect was essentially peakless, and there was no fall-off in action at 24 hours. Intersubject variability was ~60% that of NPH.

Three clinical trials with insulin glargine for type 1 diabetes have been published. A phase 3 multicenter trial that compared glargine and bolus lispro with NPH and bolus lispro showed lower fasting blood glucose levels and more patients reaching target fasting glucose in the glargine group. Further, the glargine group showed less variability in fasting blood glucose and less weight gain (42). A 28-week study by Ratner et al. (43) compared glargine and NPH for basal insulin coverage. It showed a greater reduction in fasting plasma glucose, and there were fewer episodes of symptomatic or nocturnal hypoglycemia in the glargine group. A 4-week trial by Rosenstock et al. (44) showed better control of fasting blood glucose with glargine than with NPH.

In type 2 diabetes, a 1-year study compared bedtime NPH and bedtime glargine in 426 patients failing oral agents, and showed similar improvements in $HbA_{1C}$ but less nocturnal hypoglycemia and lower post-dinner glucose levels in the glargine group (45). Rosenstock et al. (46) performed a 28-week open-label trial in patients with type 2 diabetes who were already taking NPH so they continued the NPH or were switched to glargine. Once-daily bedtime glargine was found to be as effective as once- or twice-daily NPH in terms of glycemic control, with a lower risk of nocturnal hypoglycemia and less weight gain.

Compared to NPH insulin, glargine causes more pain at the injection site (as many as 6.1% of patients versus 0.3% for NPH), which may reflect its mild acidity. Glargine is clear, whereas other long-acting insulins such as NPH and the Lentes are milky, requiring care in the labeling and in patients' handling of the glargine vials. It cannot be mixed with other insulins because of the need to keep the pH at 4 to preserve solubility for injection. It has 60% of the lipogenic potency of human insulin but 783% the mitogenic potency (29). The mitogenic potency has, thus far, not been a clinical problem but long-term follow-up is needed. A problem—not unique to glargine—is that its profile does not perfectly mimic the dawn phenomenon seen in some patients with type 1 diabetes. Regardless, insulin glargine appears to provide a more predictable, longer-duration, peakless profile compared with the other available basal insulins (9,47).

## SUMMARY AND CONCLUSION

The major short-acting insulin and analogs are Regular, aspart, and lispro. Aspart and lispro have a faster onset and shorter duration of activity that more closely mimic the "normal" insulin response to a meal, which is viewed as their major advantage. However, somewhat paradoxically, their major drawback is also the short duration, which may result in periods of "underinsulinization" in some patients with type 1 diabetes. This may be obviated by the longer-acting analog insulin glargine (42–44,47). The latter has a longer duration and is more predictable than the other intermediate- and longer-acting insulins: NPH, Lente, and Ultralente. Newer analogs are in development to address problems of stability, variability of absorption, and selectivity. An example is Insulin detemir (Lys $B^{29}[N^{\varepsilon}$-tetradecanoyl] des B30) human insulin. In the presence of zinc and phenol it is mainly hexameric, and it also has a fatty-acid side chain. This results in aggregation of hexamers, resulting in a slowly and more predictably absorbed insulin-like molecule (48). It is less potent than NPH, but less mitogenic than insulin glargine (29). Hopefully, newer analogs will provide even better tools for mimicking the physiological insulin profile.

## REFERENCES

1. Burge MR, Schade DS. Insulins. Endocrinol Metab Clin North Am 26:575–598, 1997.
2. Davidson JK, Anderson JHJ Jr, Chance RE. Insulin therapy. In: Davidson JK, ed. Clinical Diabetes Mellitus: A Problem-Oriented Approach. 3rd ed. New York: Thieme, pp 329–403, 2000.
3. Bliss M. The Discovery of Insulin. Toronto: McClelland and Stewart, 1982.
4. Best CH. The first clinical use of insulin. Diabetes 5:65–67, 1956.
5. Deckert T. Intermediate-acting insulin preparations: NPH and lente. Diabetes Care 3:623–626, 1980.
6. Dimitriadis GD, Gerich JE. Importance of timing of preprandial subcutaneous insulin administration in the management of diabetes mellitus. Diabetes Care 6:374–377, 1983.
7. Heinemann L, Richter B. Clinical pharmacology of human insulin. Diabetes Care 16(suppl 1):90–100, 1993.
8. Galloway JA, Spradlin CT, Nelson RL, Wentworth SM, Davidson JA, Swarner JL. Factors influencing the absorption, serum insulin concentration, and blood glucose responses after injections of regular insulin and various insulin mixtures. Diabetes Care 4:366–376, 1981.
9. Lepore M, Pampanelli S, Fanelli C, Porcellati F, Bartocci L, Di Vincenzo A, Cordoni C, Costa E, Brunetti P, Bolli GB. Pharmacokinetics and pharmacodynamics of subcutaneous injection of long-acting human insulin analog glargine, NPH insulin, and ultralente human insulin and continuous subcutaneous infusion of insulin lispro. Diabetes 49:2142–2148, 2000.
10. Berger M, Cuppers HJ, Hegner H, Jorgens V, Berchtold P. Absorption kinetics and biologic effects of subcutaneously injected insulin preparations. Diabetes Care 5:77–91, 1982.
11. Barnett AH, Owens DR. Insulin analogues. Lancet 349:47–51, 1997.
12. Holleman F, Hoekstra JB. Insulin lispro. N Engl J Med 337:176–183, 1997.
13. Bolli GB, Di Marchi RD, Park GD, Pramming S, Koivisto VA. Insulin analogues

and their potential in the management of diabetes mellitus. Diabetologia 42:1151–1167, 1999.

14. Bolli GB, Owens DR. Insulin glargine. Lancet 356:443–445, 2000.
15. Setter SM, Corbett CF, Campbell RK, White JR. Insulin aspart: a new rapid-acting insulin analog. Ann Pharmacother 34:1423–1431, 2000.
16. Brange J, Owens DR, Kang S, Volund A. Monomeric insulins and their experimental and clinical implications. Diabetes Care 13:923–954, 1990.
17. Howey DC, Bowsher RR, Brunelle RL, Woodworth JR. [Lys(B28), Pro(B29)]-human insulin: a rapidly absorbed analogue of human insulin. Diabetes 43:396–402, 1994.
18. Ter Braak EW, Woodworth JR, Bianchi R, Cerimele B, Erkelens DW, Thijssen JH, Kurtz D. Injection site effects on the pharmacokinetics and glucodynamics of insulin lispro and regular insulin. Diabetes Care 19:1437–1440, 1996.
19. Anderson JH Jr, Brunelle RL, Koivisto VA, Pfutzner A, Trautmann ME, Vignati L, DiMarchi R. Multicenter Insulin Lispro Study Group. Reduction of postprandial hyperglycemia and frequency of hypoglycemia in IDDM patients on insulin-analog treatment. Diabetes 46:265–270, 1997.
20. Anderson JH Jr, Brunelle RL, Keohane P, Koivisto VA, Trautmann ME, Vignati L, DiMarchi R. Multicenter Insulin Lispro Study Group. Mealtime treatment with insulin analog improves postprandial hyperglycemia and hypoglycemia in patients with non-insulin-dependent diabetes mellitus. Arch Intern Med 157:1249–1255, 1997.
21. Heller SR, Amiel SA, Mansell P. U.K. Lispro Study Group. Effect of the fast-acting insulin analog lispro on the risk of nocturnal hypoglycemia during intensified insulin therapy. Diabetes Care 22:1607–1611, 1999.
22. Gale EA. The UK Trial Group. A randomized, controlled trial comparing insulin lispro with human soluble insulin in patients with type I diabetes on intensified insulin therapy. Diabet Med 17:209–214, 2000.
23. Brunelle BL, Llewelyn J, Anderson JH Jr, Gale EA, Koivisto VA. Meta-analysis of the effect of insulin lispro on severe hypoglycemia in patients with type I diabetes. Diabetes Care 21:1726–1731, 1998.
24. Fineberg NS, Fineberg SE, Anderson JH, Birkett MA, Gibson RG, Hufferd S. Immunologic effects of insulin lispro [Lys (B28), Pro (B29) human insulin] in IDDM and NIDDM patients previously treated with insulin. Diabetes 45:1750–1754, 1996.
25. Renner R, Pfutzner A, Trautmann M, Harzer O, Sauter K, Landgraf R. German Humalog-CSII Study Group. Use of insulin lispro in continuous subcutaneous insulin treatment: results of a multicenter trial. Diabetes Care 22:784–788, 1999.
26. Hanaire-Broutin H, Melki V, Bessieres-Lacombe S, Taiber JP. The Study Group for the Development of Pump Therapy in Diabetes. Comparison of continuous subcutaneous insulin infusion and multiple daily injection regimens using insulin lispro in type I diabetic patients on intensified treatment: a randomized study. Diabetes Care 23:1232–1235, 2000.
27. Rassam AG, Zeise TM, Burge MR, Schade DS. Optimal administration of lispro insulin in hyperglycemic type I diabetes. Diabetes Care 22:133–136, 1999.
28. Simpson KL, Spencer CM. Insulin aspart. Drugs 57(5):759–765, 1999.
29. Kurtzhals P, Schaffer L, Sorensen A, Kristensen C, Jonassen I, Schmid C, Trub T.

Correlations of receptor binding and metabolic and mitogenic potencies of insulin
analogs designed for clinical use. Diabetes 49:999–1005, 2000.

30. Heinemann L, Heise T, Jorgensen LN, Starke AA. Action profile of the rapid acting
    insulin analogue: human insulin B28Asp. Diabet Med 10:535–539, 1993.

31. Mudaliar SR, Lindberg FA, Joyce M, Beerdsen P, Strange P, Lin A, Henry RR.
    Insulin aspart (B28 asp-insulin): a fast acting analog of human insulin: absorption
    kinetics and action profile compared with regular human insulin in healthy nondia-
    betic subjects. Diabetes Care 22:1501–1506, 1999.

32. Hedmann CA, Lindstorm T, Arnqvist HJ. Direct comparison of insulin lispro and
    aspart shows small differences in plasma insulin profiles after subcutaneous injection
    in type I diabetes. Diabetic Care 24:1120–1121, 2001.

33. Home PD, Lindholm A, Hylleberg B, Round P. UK Insulin Aspart Study Group.
    Improved glycemic control with insulin aspart: a multicenter randomized double-
    blind crossover trial in type I diabetic patients. Diabetes Care 21:1904–1909, 1998.

34. Raskin P, Guthrie RA, Leiter L, Riis A, Jovanovic L. Use of insulin aspart, a fast-
    acting insulin analog, as the mealtime insulin in the management of patient with
    type I diabetes. Diabetes Care 23:583–588, 2000.

35. Bode BW, Strange P. Efficacy, safety and pump compatibility of insulin aspart used
    in continuous subcutaneous insulin infusion therapy in patients with type 1 diabetes.
    Diabetes Care 24:69–72, 2001.

36. Hallas-Moller K, Petersen K, Schlichtkrull J. Crystalline and amorphous insulin-
    zinc compounds with prolonged action. Science 116:394–398, 1952.

37. Krayenbuhl C, Rosenberg T. Crystalline protamine insulin. Rep Steno Mem Hosp
    1:60–73, 1946.

38. Hagedorn HC. Modification of insulin. Phys Bull 12:26–33, 1947.

39. Scott DA, Fisher AL. Studies on insulin with protamine. J Pharmacol Exp Ther 58:
    78–92, 1936.

40. Heine RJ, Bilo HJ, Fonk T, van der Veen EA, van der Meer J. Absorption kinetics
    and action profiles of mixtures of short and intermediate-acting insulins. Diabeto-
    logia 27:558–562, 1984.

41. Tunbridge F, Newens A, Home P, Davis S, Murphy M, Burrin JM, Alberti KG,
    Jensen I. A comparison of human ultralente- and lente-based twice-daily injection
    regimens. Diabet Med 6:496–501, 1989.

42. Raskin P, Klaff L, Bergenstal R, Halle J, Donley D, Mecca T. A 16-week comparison
    of the novel insulin analog insulin glargine (HOE 901) and NPH human insulin used
    with insulin lispro in patients with type 1 diabetes. Diabetic Care 23:1666–1671,
    2000.

43. Ratner R, Hirsh I, Neifing J, Garg S, Mecca T, Wilson C. Less hypoglycemia with
    insulin glargine in intensive insulin therapy for type 1 diabetes. Diabetes Care 23:
    639–643, 2000.

44. Rosenstock J, Park G, Zimmerman J. U.S. Insulin Glargine (HOE 901) Type I Diabe-
    tes Investigator Group. Basal insulin glargine (HOE 901) versus NPH insulin in
    patients with type 1 diabetes on multiple daily insulin regimens. Diabetes Care 23:
    1137–1142, 2000.

45. Yki-Jarvinen H, Dressler A, Ziemen M. Less nocturnal hypoglycemia and better
    post-dinner glucose control with bedtime insulin glargine compared with bedtime

NPH insulin during insulin combination therapy in type 2 diabetes. Diabetes Care 23:1130–1136, 2000.

46. Rosenstock J, Schwartz SL, Clark CM Jr, Park GD, Donley DW, Edwards MB. Basal insulin therapy in type 2 diabetes: 28-week comparison of insulin glargine (HOE 901) and NPH insulin. Diabetes Care 24:631–636, 2001.

47. Heinemann L, Linkeschova R, Rave K, Hompesch B, Sedlak M, Heise T. Time-action profile of the long-acting insulin analog insulin glargine (HOE 901) in comparison with those of NPH insulin and placebo. Diabetes Care 23:644–649, 2000.

48. Hermansen K, Madsbad S, Perrild H, Kristeusen A, Axelsen M. Comparison of the soluble basal insulin analog insulin detemir with NPH insulin. Diabetes Care 24:296–301, 2001.

# 7

## Intensive Insulin Therapy in Type 1 Diabetes Mellitus

**Jack L. Leahy**

University of Vermont College of Medicine, Burlington, Vermont

### INTRODUCTION

There are few bigger challenges for medical practitioners than taking care of patients with type 1 diabetes mellitus. The difficulties are numerous. Glucose homeostasis is normally controlled by a complex physiology of precise variations in insulin secretion that exactly counter the wide swings in nutrient intake, physical activity, and stress of modern society. Attempts over the years to approximate this system using subcutaneous insulin have suffered from insulin preparations that lack the pharmacokinetics of the normal system. In addition, the average physician received little training in insulin usage during his or her internship and residency, and there have been few CME programs in this area. Also, there is a clear understanding by most physicians that if they aggressively push insulin doses to tolerance, the result too often is hypoglycemia that can vary anywhere from annoying to life-threatening. Finally, patients are not always advocates for their care; sometimes the attitude is "The fewer shots, the better" or "I feel great, so why must I do so many finger sticks?" The net consequence is that premixed insulins are the most prescribed insulin preparations in the United States, and national surveys continue to show distressingly high $HbA_{1c}$ values.

To paraphrase Bob Dylan, ''The times, they are changing.'' A number of events occurred in the 1990s that provided us the tools, know-how, and incentive to do better. Best known is the demonstration in both type 1 and type 2 diabetes of the benefits of intensive glycemic control for the prevention of microvascular complications (1–3), a fact that is understood and expected by many patients. Parenthetically, the long-term risk of suboptimal glycemic control, which was also made obvious by these studies, underlies the diabetes treatment guidelines and performance measures that have become widespread. New insulin preparations are now available that better approximate normal insulin secretion (4–7; reviewed in Chapter 6)—intensive treatment programs (often termed ''basal-bolus'') that combine these insulins into physiologically correct 24-hour insulin exposure are increasingly being used. Also, insulin-delivery systems (pens, syringes with ''skinny'' and short needles, pumps) and blood glucose monitoring equipment have become easier to use, more reliable, and less painful.

This chapter is intended to demystify insulin therapy in type 1 diabetes (and diabetes in general) by providing a conceptual framework for what to do and how to do it. This is not to say it is easy. Obtaining the target $HbA_{1c}$ (generally less than 7%) without significant hypoglycemia in a patient with type 1 diabetes often requires a team of experts—physician, registered dietician (RD), and certified diabetes educator (CDE)—to analyze diet and lifestyle practices and look for clues to day-to-day variations in glycemia. Whether the primary physician or a diabetes specialist is the main caregiver will depend on many factors. This chapter does not dictate who it should be. What it does espouse is that insulin programs be used that are based on the unique diet, exercise, and work habits of each patient, i.e., that we get away from the one-size-fits-all approach to insulin treatment. Patients may go through a difficult time for a while trying to cope with all the things asked of them with an intensive treatment program. However, over the long term, they will have a better understanding of their diabetes and how to manage it, and a greater chance for a life unencumbered by hypoglycemia and end-organ complications.

## NORMAL INSULIN SECRETION

A key principle for physiological insulin delivery is to mimic the normal pattern of β cell function as closely as possible. Figure 1 shows insulin secretion in a healthy individual, measured every 10 minutes over a normal 24-hour period that included three standard meals—the top panel shows the actual data; the bottom panel is a stylized version used in this chapter as insulin programs are discussed. The multiple arrows in Figure 1A are large spikes of insulin secretion that occur every 1–3 hours and are called ''ultradian oscillations''; the study from which the figure was taken investigated these oscillations (8). Instead, view the figure for the 24-hour pattern of insulin secretion.

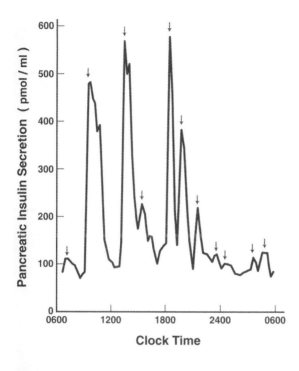

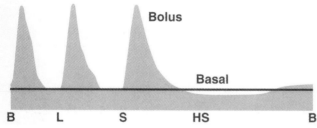

FIGURE 1   Insulin secretion measured in a healthy individual every 10 minutes over a normal 24-hour period that included three standard meals. The top panel is the actual data taken from Ref 8. The multiple small arrows identify large spikes of insulin secretion that occur every 1–3 hours, called ultradian oscillations; the study from which the figure was taken investigated these oscillations. The bottom panel is a stylized version of the same data for use in Figures 2 and 3, which pertain to insulin treatment.

The following features of Figure 1 should be noted:

- There are three large peaks of insulin release that rise rapidly and then wane over 2–3 hours, corresponding to the meals. Also evident is a relatively constant secretion of insulin over the 24-hour period that is not food-related. The latter is critically important during the night and between meals to regulate glucose output from the liver; without it, hepatic glucose release increases markedly, resulting in high fasting and pre-meal blood glucose levels. These two components as applied to insulin treatment are termed "basal" (non-food-related) and "bolus" (meal-induced) insulin secretion.
- Quantitative insulin release for the meals is similar. This seems counterintuitive since caloric intake for supper is generally many-fold that for breakfast. The explanation is the "dawn phenomenon"—a lowering of tissue insulin sensitivity in the early morning hours because of the nighttime diurnal rise in cortisol and growth hormone. Thus, we require more insulin secretion/injected per breakfast calorie than for supper. This underlies the confusion of many new insulin users about why the breakfast dose of rapid insulin typically equals or exceeds that for supper. It also explains why persons who use carbohydrate counting to determine meal insulin doses often use a lower ratio of grams of carbohydrate/insulin unit for breakfast than supper.
- Insulin secretion returns to the basal rate between meals. In other words, people are *not* designed to have much circulating insulin between meals. This has important implications for the common usage of breakfast-time NPH in the United States, which produces a nonphysiological sustained insulin effect from midmorning to late afternoon, necessitating between-meal snacks to prevent hypoglycemia.

A useful analogy is that people function like an automobile in terms of insulin secretion/needs—idle between meals, with a rapid burst when the pedal is pushed by an influx of foodstuffs. In the average person, about half of the insulin released in a day is meal-related, the other half is basal. This fact is often used in the design of insulin programs: 50% of the insulin is given as basal coverage and the other 50% at meals. However, these proportions can be varied according to the habits of the individual. Males in their late teens and early 20s often consume huge numbers of calories in many snacks and meals such that food-related insulin needs far exceed basal insulin needs. Similarly, in highly physically active, insulin-sensitive individuals, the amount of basal insulin can be modest compared to that at meals. *Thus, both meal-related and basal insulin needs must be met for an insulin program to work, and caregivers need to know their patients' dietary habits (meal sizes, times, snacks, variations) and exercise patterns (when, what, how often) as well as other relevant factors (work shifts, alcohol) when designing an insulin regimen.*

## BASAL-BOLUS INTENSIVE INSULIN THERAPY

### What Is Basal-Bolus Insulin Treatment?

Basal-bolus coverage combines the available insulin preparations (Table 1) into programs that take into account the unique dietary, exercise and other habits of your patient to mimic as closely as possible physiological insulin delivery—i.e., provide insulin in approximately the correct amount when needed, and *not* provide it when unnecessary—in order to attain near-normal daytime and nighttime glycemia. By necessity, multiple shots and frequent self-blood-glucose monitoring (SBGM) are required. Diabetes education is also a core element along with dietary instruction in how to regularize nutritional intake or, alternatively, how to use analysis techniques such as "carbohydrate counting" to determine insulin dosages for meals (see Chapter 4).

### Who Is Eligible?

*Every* person with type 1 diabetes should be a candidate for intensive insulin therapy unless there is a contraindication. Exclusions can be medical (history of severe hypoglycemia, too old or too young, illnesses in which hypoglycemia could be life-threatening such as severe coronary, cerebrovascular, or hepatic disease) or nonmedical (unwillingness or inability to follow the program, drug or alcohol abuse, etc.). However, it must be emphasized these factors do not *de facto* exclude a candidate. There are many elderly patients who do spectacularly well on multishot insulin programs, and many persons with debilitating hypogly-

**TABLE 1**  Pharmacokinetics of Subcutaneous Insulin

| Insulin | Onset | Peak action | Duration |
|---|---|---|---|
| Short-acting | | | |
| Lispro/aspart | 5–15 min | 1–2 hr | 3–4 hr |
| Regular | 30–60 min | 2–4 hr | 6–8 hr |
| Intermediate-acting | | | |
| NPH | 1–3 hr | 5–7 hr | 13–16 hr |
| Lente | 1–3 hr | 4–8 hr | 13–20 hr |
| Long-acting | | | |
| Ultralente | 2–4 hr | 8–14 hr | <20 hr |
| Glargine | 1–2 hr | Peakless | >24 hr |

cemia on a standard insulin regimen who see a major improvement when switched to a physiologically correct program. Thus, most patients with type 1 diabetes should be receiving intensive insulin therapy.

### What Are the Goals and Risks?

The blood glucose goals of the American Diabetes Association (9,10) are shown in Table 2. The listed HbA$_{1c}$ of less than 7% is accepted around the world based on the findings of the Diabetes Control and Complications Trial (DCCT) performed in type 1 diabetes (see Table 3), which showed an acceptable balance of protection against microvascular complications versus risk of severe hypoglycemia with this HbA$_{1c}$ level (1). Equally important is to prevent rigidity of lifestyle by providing flexibility for exercise, sports, diet, work, travel, or whatever the patient wants for a happy life.

The caregiver also needs to know the risks and problems with intensive insulin therapy so they can be openly discussed with the patient. Best known is the potential for hypoglycemia. The DCCT reported a threefold increase in severe hypoglycemia, which was defined as requiring aid from someone else, and a threefold increase in hospitalization for hypoglycemia, in patients with HbA$_{1c}$ of 7.2% versus 8.9% (1). Several subgroups were at particularly high risk: adolescents, males, those without residual c-peptide, and those with a prior history of severe hypoglycemia (11). The most important clinical predictor for high-risk patients is the presence of hypoglycemia unawareness—patients report that their reactions have changed so they no longer feel the sweats, shakes, or pounding heart (i.e., loss of the catecholaminergic symptoms) but instead experience

**TABLE 2** Goals for Glycemic Control Recommended by the American Diabetes Association

|  | Normal | Goal | Additional action suggested |
|---|---|---|---|
| Whole-blood values (mg/dl)[a] |  |  |  |
| Average preprandial | <100 | 80–120 | <80, >140 |
| Average bedtime glucose | <110 | 100–140 | <100, >160 |
| Plasma values (mg/dl)[b] |  |  |  |
| Average preprandial | <110 | 90–130 | <90, >150 |
| Average bedtime glucose | <120 | 110–150 | <110, >180 |
| HbA$_{1c}$(%)[c] | <6 | <7 | >8 |

[a] Measurement of capillary blood glucose.
[b] Values calibrated to plasma glucose.
[c] HbA$_{1c}$ is referenced to a nondiabetic range of 4.0–6.0%.
*Source*: Ref. 9.

**TABLE 3** The Diabetes Control and Complications Trial

| | |
|---|---|
| **Design** | |
| Intensive regimen | Minimum of three shots/day or a pump (35% used a pump) |
| | Four blood glucose measurements/day +1/week at 3 A.M. |
| | Blood sugar guidelines |
| | 70–120 mg/dl (3.9–6.7 mM) before meals |
| | <180 mg/dl (10 mM) 1–2 hr after a meal |
| | >65 mg/dl (3.6 mM ) at 3 A.M. |
| | Attained HbA$_{1c}$ of 7.2% (normal <6.05%) |
| Conventional | One or two insulin injections/day, no or only occasional self-blood-glucose monitoring |
| | Attained HbA$_{1c}$ of 8.9% |
| **Results** | |
| Retinopathy | Primary intervention: 50% incidence with conventional, 15% incidence with intensive therapy |
| | Secondary intervention: 54% less progression with intensive therapy and 54% less need for laser therapy with intensive therapy |
| Nephropathy | Primary intervention: rare events, not significant |
| | Secondary intervention to microalbuminuria: 40% conventional, 25% intensive, and to overt proteinuria: 10% conventional, 5% intensive |
| | Overall, 35% less microalbuminuria, 54% less proteinuria |
| Neuropathy | Primary intervention: 10% conventional, 3% intensive |
| | Secondary intervention: 16% conventional, 7% intensive |
| | Overall, 61% reduced |
| Macrovascular | No statistical difference between conventional and intensive treatment groups because too few events in either group—44% fewer events in intensive group |
| **Problems** | |
| Weight gain | Intensive group gained an average of 10 lb (4.5 kg) versus 5 lb in conventional group |
| Hypoglycemia | Threefold increased incidence of severe hypoglycemia |

The DCCT (1985–1993) assessed the relationship in type 1 diabetes between blood glucose control and development/progression of microvascular complications. There were two groups: primary intervention (up to 5 years of diabetes with no known retinopathy) and secondary intervention (up to 15 years of diabetes with mild retinopathy). *Source*: Ref. 1.

subtle changes in mentation, ability to concentrate, or personality (discussed in Chapter 13). Its presence is not necessarily a contraindication for intensive insulin therapy, but these patients must be watched carefully for blood sugars of 30 or 40 mg/dl in their logbooks that may not be perceived by the patient as particularly problematic. Also, as extensively discussed in Chapter 13, recurrent hypoglycemia has been identified as an important cause of the impaired insulin counterregulation that leads to hypoglycemia unawareness. Indeed, it was observed some years ago that intensive insulin therapy *elicited* this effect in otherwise healthy patients with type 1 diabetes (12,13). However, as the importance of hypoglycemia's impairing insulin counterregulation became known, prevention of hypoglycemia became a prime goal when practicing intensive insulin therapy. Further, it is now understood that intensive insulin therapy is based on physiological insulin delivery that mutes both the hyper- and hypo- swings in glycemia. Indeed, a basal-bolus regimen is now often *recommended* for patients who are experiencing major hypoglycemia. Patients need a balanced discussion of this issue. For some, fear of hypoglycemia can be a major issue that stops them from fully following the prescribed diet and insulin program. They need to know that this may, paradoxically, worsen swings in glycemia and problems with hypoglycemia. Also, preventive measures need to be in place. Patients should be taught that alcohol and exercise can promote hypoglycemia, a bedtime snack is strongly recommended, and a glucagon emergency kit should be kept in the house and perhaps at work. To summarize, in many patients, an intensive insulin regimen has no major detrimental effect and may even alleviate problems with hypoglycemia.

The DCCT noted an average 10-pound weight gain in the intensively treated group versus 5 pounds in the group with conventional treatment (1). Patients with type 1 diabetes are usually of relatively normal weight and share the same body consciousness as young people in general—weight gain (or fear thereof) at times is the main factor that limits a patients willingness to undergo intensive therapy. The weight gain is multifactorial, including lessening of glycosuria, increasing calorie intake to treat or prevent hypoglycemia, and reversing the catabolic effect of poorly controlled diabetes. As glycemia is optimized, it is important to work with a dietitian to develop a meal plan for weight maintenance. Also, a major focus of "tweaking" the regimen once it has been started is to minimize hypoglycemia. In addition, it should be pointed out to the patient that basal-bolus regimens generally minimize or eliminate between-meal snacks, which helps with weight control.

Intensive glycemic control occasionally worsens pre-existing retinopathy (14), but the effect is generally short-lived and without functional significance although proliferative retinopathy and blindness have rarely been reported. It is suggested that patients with known retinopathy be evaluated by an ophthamologist prior to starting an intensive insulin program, and frequently thereafter.

## HOW TO START BASAL-BOLUS THERAPY

### Step 1: Minimize Variables

The previous section emphasized the importance of exercise and dietary habits for the timing and amount of needed insulin. Modern life for many people entails substantial day-to-day variations in eating and exercise. When beginning an insulin program, regularize these factors as much as possible, at least for the short term until the insulin program and approximate doses have been established.

- Have a detailed discussion with the patient about his normal day and how it is affected by habits, hobbies, sports, work, weekends, travel, etc. Identify the variables. Emphasize uniformity at work—avoid varying shifts, work trips, wide swings in physical work, and other changes during the transition onto insulin. Have the patient postpone vacations, stressful family events, and other nonessential happenings.
- Patients should see a registered dietitian for evaluation of their eating habits, and to be educated in the importance of consistency in their meals. The concept of carbohydrate counting can also be introduced (discussed in Chapter 4).
- Patients should receive basic diabetes education, preferably from a CDE, covering SBGM, proper injection technique, how to mix insulins if relevant, and how to recognize, avoid, and treat hypoglycemia.
- Identify factors that might influence insulin absorption—and thus kinetics of the insulin effect—such as massage, heat, and exercise. Also important is where one injects; insulin onset is quickest and its duration of action shortest from the abdomen, followed by the arms, then the buttocks and thighs. Practically, I generally recommend using the abdomen during the day and the thighs or buttocks for the bedtime injection.
- It is generally prudent to eliminate strenuous exercise for a while; when this is not possible, emphasize regularity of exercise in terms of intensity, timing, and doing it daily. Educating the patient about the effects of exercise on insulin dosing and absorption, risks of hypoglycemia and its avoidance, the best time to exercise, etc., will help avoid later confusion over the effect of variable exercise on the patient's glycemic response to the new insulin program.

### Step 2: Involve the Patient

The patient should have a role in establishing the treatment goals. Carefully discuss what you are doing and why. Identify what the patient wants to accomplish. You want a partnership with your patient that agrees on the desired goals and how they will be tracked, celebrates the same successes, and shares the same standards of when "good is not good enough."

## Step 3: Establish the 24-Hour Insulin Dosage

Next is calculation of the approximate 24-hour insulin need. It is done on a unit-per-kilogram basis by multiplying the body weight in kilograms by a factor that takes into account the patient's tissue insulin sensitivity. Suggested conversion factors are shown in Table 4. Thus, a 28-year-old 70-kg man who bikes or plays tennis on a daily basis would be started on 21 units of insulin per day (0.3 units/kg), while a man of the same age and height with a sedentary lifestyle would receive 35 units (0.5 units/kg). Other factors, such as eating habits, are considered but in more of a qualitative way—if that inactive patient is a "big eater" (maybe not gaining weight because of the out-of-control diabetes), then a slightly higher conversion factor (0.6 units/kg) might be tried, resulting in 42 units. In contrast, pre-existing impaired renal function would result in less insulin because of the reduced insulin clearance. The same approach would be taken if there is another illness that poses a danger with hypoglycemia such as severe cardiac, cerebral, or hepatic disease. Young people (arbitrarily, less than 30 years old) with new-onset type 1 diabetes are usually given less insulin as they typically experience a rather substantial reduction in insulin needs after starting insulin therapy ("honeymoon period"); a starting insulin dosage of 0.3 units/kg is suggested. Clearly, this is an inexact science, but it is a necessary starting point for calculating the initial insulin doses. After starting, doses are adjusted based on the SBGM results. It is obviously preferable to err on the low side with the starting doses, and use the SBGM results to adjust the insulin dosages upward.

## Step 4: Choose the Insulin Program and Calculate the Starting Insulin Doses

Several insulin programs are based on a basal-bolus approach. Three are shown in Figure 2, and are discussed in detail below: Ultralente and pre-meal lispro or aspart; glargine and pre-meal lispro or aspart; and pre-meal Regular and NPH at bedtime. Daytime NPH, which remains very popular in the United States, is also discussed; however, most experts view this program as not allowing intensive insulin coverage in the average patient with type 1 diabetes. Pluses and minuses of each programs are discussed, and specifics on how to calculate the starting insulin doses are provided. The patient should be presented with the different programs and choose the one that is of most interest and fits best with his or her lifestyle.

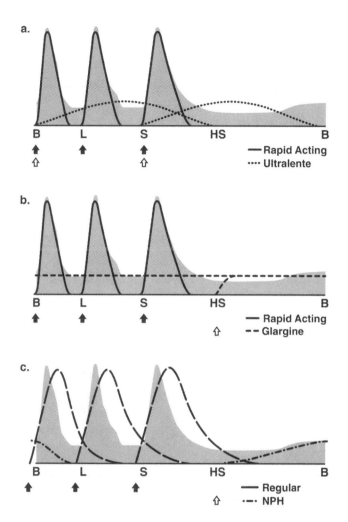

FIGURE 2   Basal-bolus insulin regimens showing the number of injections and time of administration relative to meals (B = breakfast; L = lunch; S = supper) and bedtime (HS). (Top) twice-daily Ultralente insulin and mealtime rapid-acting analog. (Center) bedtime glargine and mealtime rapid-acting analog. (Bottom) pre-meal Regular insulin and bedtime NPH insulin. The shaded area depicts the normal 24-hour pattern of insulin secretion from Figure 1. Insulin levels from each program are shown as broken or solid lines based on the pharmacokinetics of the different insulin preparations. Convergence of the perimeter of the shaded area and the insulin lines indicates correct insulin activity. Nonconvergence is too little, or too much, insulin effect.

## INSULIN PROGRAMS

### Ultralente and Pre-Meal Lispro or Aspart

#### Advantages

- Provides flexibility for varying dietary habits
- Short duration of action of lispro and aspart results in fewer between-meal "hypos"
- Insulin coverage for snacks or extra meals is easily provided by additional injections of the rapid-acting insulin
- No waiting time between the lispro or aspart injection and the meal

#### Disadvantages:

- Ultralente is the most variable of the available insulin preparations in terms of day-to-day consistency in insulin kinetics, and thus glycemic control
- Nocturnal hypoglycemia in some patients
- Difficult to compensate for variance in physical activity

#### Program

The use of Ultralente insulin for basal coverage and a rapid-acting insulin at meals has been the mainstay approach for intensive insulin therapy in the United States for many years. Figure 2A shows how it is generally done: Ultralente with lispro or aspart when beginning breakfast, lispro or aspart at lunch, and Ultralente with lispro or aspart at supper. Before the rapid-acting insulin analogs became available, Regular insulin was used for the mealtime coverage, and it was generally recommended that the Ultralente and Regular insulins be given as separate injections (five shots per day) to avoid the effect of Ultralente's slowing the kinetics of action of the Regular (15). This is now a moot issue because lispro and aspart are resistant to this effect (three shots each day). Also, the analogs provide other important benefits such as no waiting time between the injection and eating the meal, and a shorter duration of action for more focused mealtime insulin delivery and less risk of between-meal hypoglycemia than Regular insulin.

It confuses some practitioners that Ultralente is given twice daily, because they were taught it has a 24–36-hour duration of action. That was when the insulin in Ultralente was of beef origin. Human-based Ultralente has been available for several years, and its duration of action is considerably shorter. Further, many physicians believe that Ultralente is a peakless insulin when in fact there is a sizable peak effect, as shown in Figure 2A, that causes some patients to experience nocturnal hypoglycemia. Because of this, many experts advise a four-shot variation on this regimen: Ultralente and lispro or aspart at breakfast, Humalog or aspart at lunch, Humalog or aspart at supper, and NPH at bedtime.

*Overview*

This program is one of the best for patients who want flexibility for dietary habits in both when they eat and what they eat. By taking rapid-acting insulin for each meal, they can take exactly the right amount of insulin at exactly the right time. Also, snacks or extra meals are easily covered with additional injections of rapid-acting insulin. Furthermore, the use of separate basal and bolus insulin coverage means patients have near-total freedom over the timing of when they eat. Thus, this regimen is particularly useful for anyone with erratic eating habits.

The main disadvantages are twofold. Ultralente is the most inconsistent of the available insulin preparations in terms of its absorption (16), causing considerable day-to-day variability in insulin action and thus glycemia in some patients. This can be particularly problematic for patients who are highly physically active, and is generally not the best choice for them. The second issue regards the substantial peak effect of this insulin. Trying to optimize fasting blood glucose values by upward adjustments of the P.M. Ultralente dose causes nighttime hypoglycemia (with or without symptoms) in approximately 25% of patients. Changing to the four-shot variation listed above often eliminates this problem.

Is it necessary to use rapid-acting insulin analogs for the mealtime coverage over Regular insulin? Generally the answer is yes, as it has been repeatedly shown that there is less postprandial and middle-of-the-night hypoglycemia with the analogs (17–19). When should the analogs be injected? While there has been some disagreement, most studies suggest injecting anywhere from 15 minutes before the meal to when the patient starts to eat (20).

A complex issue is when to perform SBGM—pre-meal or post-meal? Because of the targeted effect of lispro and aspart for postprandial glycemic control, pre-meal glucose monitoring does not provide optimal information for determining the mealtime insulin dosages. Thus, when beginning the program, it is useful on some days to measure blood glucose values before a meal (goal 80–120 mg/dl) and other days 2 hours after meals (goal <140 mg/dl). However, once the program has been established, the use of algorithms for adjustments in the mealtime insulin dosage based on the glycemia at that time means that most testing is done pre-meal.

How do you do it?

1. Calculate the 24-hour insulin need as described in Table 4.
2. Give 50% of the 24-hour dosage as Ultralente split equally between breakfast and supper.
3. Give the remaining 50% of the 24-hour dosage at meals with, on average, 30–40% at breakfast, 30% at lunch, and 30–40% at dinner depending on the patient's eating habits.
4. Adjust these starting dosages if the patient has unusual eating, exercise, or work habits.

**TABLE 4**  Sensitivity Factors for Calculating 24-Hour Insulin Needs
(approximate figures to be used in calculating the starting 24-hour
insulin needs)

| | |
|---|---|
| Phenotype | |
|   Normal weight | |
|     Extremely physically active | 0.3 units/kg |
|     Moderately physically active | 0.4 units/kg |
|     Minimally active | 0.5 units/kg |
|   Obese | |
|     Extremely physically active | 0.5 units/kg |
|     Moderate physically active | 0.6 units/kg |
|     Minimally active | 0.8 units/kg |
| Renal failure | Subtract 0.2 units/kg |
| Coexisting illness raising risk of hypoglycemia | Subtract 0.2 units/kg |
| Eating habits ("big eater") | Add 0.1 unit/kg |
| New-onset type 1 diabetes <30 years old | 0.3 units/kg |

5.  Perform daily fasting, pre-meal or 2-hour postmeal, and bedtime SBGM along with weekly middle-of-the-night SBGM.

6.  Example: 70-kg male who is moderately physically active. Total daily insulin dose is 70 kg × 0.4 units/kg = 28 units. Total Ultralente: 28 × 50% = 14 units. A.M. and P.M. Ultralente: 14 × 50% = 7 units each. Total lispro or aspart: 28 × 50% = 14 units. Pre-breakfast lispro or aspart: 14 × 40% = 6 units. Pre-lunch and pre-supper lispro or aspart: 14 × 30% = 4–5 units. **Final**: 7 units Ultralente and 6 units lispro or aspart pre-breakfast, 4 units lispro or aspart pre-lunch, 6 units Ultralente and 4–5 units lispro or aspart pre-dinner. Adjust insulin doses as needed based on the SBGM values to attain the glycemia goals in Table 2.

## Glargine and Pre-Meal Lispro or Aspart

### Advantages

- Basal-bolus regimen with the same advantages as the Ultralente program
- Less middle-of-the-night hypoglycemic risk than Ultralente—24-hour near-constant effect of glargine makes for an ideal basal insulin
- Avoids mixing, because single insulins are given at each injecion—can thus use an insulin pen for all injections for maximal convenience and accuracy in dosing

*Disadvantages*

• Difficult to compensate for variances in physical activity

*Program*

This is a variation on the Ultralente program that substitutes glargine as the basal insulin. This insulin has only recently come to market, and experience with it is limited. However, what has been observed to date has raised considerable hope that it will be an ideal basal insulin because of its near-constant (''peakless'') effect over 24 hours (16,21), which should help lower or eliminate the nocturnal hypoglycemia that is sometimes seen with Ultralente (22–25).

Figure 2B shows the program: lispro or aspart insulin at each meal, and glargine at bedtime. It is a four-shot program because glargine *cannot be mixed with other insulins*; the manufacturer recommends that it be given at bedtime when other insulins generally are not given, to avoid inadvertent mixing. The restriction against mixing reflects its insolubility at a physiological pH, which accounts for the prolonged duration of action when injected into the subcutaneous space. The pH of the glargine bottle/cartridge is 4, which keeps it soluble for injection and explains why it cannot be mixed with other insulins. For most patients, four shots instead of three shots per day is only a minor annoyance because of the relative painlessness of modern injection systems. Moreover, many patients find insulin pens preferable to syringes (at the writing of this chapter, glargine is available only in vials but the manufacturer expects to have a pen system shortly).

*Overview*

This program has all the advantages of the previously described Ultralente regimen, and eliminates many of the disadvantages. It is excellent for patients who want maximal flexibility for dietary habits. Further, the studies to date have shown a high consistency of day-to-day insulin effect for glargine, and a nearly flat insulin profile over 24 hours (16,21), which makes for a near-perfect basal insulin. These characteristics avoid the main disadvantages of Ultralente—its day-to-day variability in insulin action, and the substantial peak that causes middle-of-the-night hypoglycemia in some patients. However, it should again be stated that glargine is very new to the market, and the reported benefits need to be confirmed in real-world clinical settings. On the other hand, the difficulty of using a long-lasting basal insulin in patients whose physical activity varies widely is as true with glargine as it is for Ultralente.

How do you do it?

1. Calculate the 24-hour insulin need as described in Table 4.
2. Give 50% of the 24-hour dosage as glargine at bedtime.
3. Give the remaining 50% of the 24-hour dosage at meals with, on aver-

age, 30–40% at breakfast, 30% at lunch, and 30–40% at dinner depending on the patient's eating habits.

4. Adjust these starting dosages if the patient has unusual eating, exercise, or work habits.
5. Perform daily fasting, pre-meal or 2-hour postmeal, and bedtime SBGM along with weekly middle-of-the-night SBGM.
6. Example: 70-kg male who is moderately physically active. Total daily insulin dose is 70 kg $\times$ 0.4 units/kg = 28 units. Total glargine: 28 $\times$ 50% = 14 units. Total lispro or aspart: 28 $\times$ 50% = 14 units. Pre-breakfast lispro or aspart: 14 $\times$ 40% = 6 units. Pre-lunch and pre-supper lispro or aspart: 14 $\times$ 30% = 4–5 units. **Final**: 6 units lispro or aspart pre-breakfast, 4 units lispro or aspart pre-lunch, 4–5 units lispro or aspart pre-dinner, and 14 units glargine at bedtime. Adjust insulin doses as needed based on the SBGM values to attain the glycemia goals in Table 2.

## Pre-Meal Regular and Bedtime NPH

### Advantages

- Provides more flexibility for varying exercise habits than Ultralente or glargine
- Less risk of nocturnal hypoglycemia than Ultralente
- An insulin pen can be used for all injections, for maximal convenience and accuracy in dosing

### Disadvantages

- Minimal flexibility for dietary variations
- Must wait 30 minutes between the Regular insulin injection and the meal
- Longer effect of Regular insulin versus lispro and aspart means greater risk of between-meal ''hypos''

### Program

This is a common intensive insulin program outside the United States (as already discussed, the United States uses Ultralente and rapid-acting insulin at meals; the difference reflects the insulin manufacturers that serve various geographical areas and the products they sell as opposed to any great advantage of one regimen over another). Figure 2C shows how it is done: Regular insulin 30 minutes before each meal and NPH at bedtime (by 11 P.M. even if staying up past that time). The 30-minute waiting period between taking the Regular insulin and eating is important in order to match the peak insulin effect and the postprandial rise in glycemia.

*Overview*

This program is based on a different principle than the previously discussed glargine and Ultralente regimens, as a single insulin is used for basal and bolus coverage during the day. This allows less dietary flexibility than with Ultralente or glargine, especially for variations in mealtimes. For example, eating lunch at 12:00 noon and dinner at 9:00 P.M. versus the usual 6:00 P.M. will be accompanied by substantial pre-dinner hyperglycemia because of waning of the Regular insulin effect. Some patients prevent this by taking an extra, small dose of Regular in the middle of the afternoon. The ability to compensate for variation in meal size is also limited with this regimen, as changing the Regular insulin dosage for a smaller or larger than normal meal affects basal insulin delivery at the same time. Thus, this is not the best regimen for patients who want substantial flexibility in their diet.

In contrast, it provides more flexibility for exercise and sports than either Ultralente or glargine, as the Regular insulin coverage is 5–6 hours compared with the much longer duration of glargine and Ultralente.

How do you do it?

1. Calculate the 24-hour insulin need as described in Table 4.
2. Give 30% of the 24-hour dosage for the breakfast injection, 25% at lunch, 25% at dinner, and 20% at bedtime. (The latter percentage is for insulin-sensitive patients, the usual case in type 1 diabetes. For a patient with type 2 diabetes, nighttime coverage usually requires a much higher percentage of the daily insulin because of the typical presence of insulin resistance.)
3. Adjust these starting dosages if the patient has unusual eating, exercise, or work habits.
4. Perform daily fasting, pre-meal or 2-hour postmeal, and bedtime SBGM along with weekly middle-of-the-night SBGM.
5. Example: 70-kg male who is moderately physically active. Total daily insulin dose is 70 kg × 0.4 units/kg = 28 units. First injection: 28 × 30% = 8 units. Second and third injections: 28 × 25% = 7 units. Fourth injection: 28 × 20% = 6 units. **Final**: 8 units Regular pre-breakfast, 7 units Regular pre-lunch, 7 units Regular pre-dinner, 6 units NPH at bedtime. Adjust insulin doses as needed based on the SBGM values to attain the glycemia goals in Table 2.

## Daytime NPH

*Advantages*

- No insulin at lunch
- Physicians most familiar with this program

- Can use insulin premixes for convenience and accuracy of insulin proportions

### Disadvantages

- No flexibility for dietary or exercise variations
- Morning NPH predisposes to late-morning and early-afternoon hypoglycemia requiring between-meal snacks
- Pre-supper NPH predisposes to middle-of-the-night hypoglycemia and/or inadequate control of fasting blood glucose level

### Program

Figure 3 shows how daytime NPH regimens are generally used—the two-shot program in Figure 3A is NPH with Regular or a rapid-acting analog before breakfast and supper (this is given as premixes in some patients), and the three-shot program in Figure 3B is NPH and Regular or a rapid-acting analog before breakfast, Regular or the rapid-acting analog at dinner, and NPH at bedtime (by 11 P.M. even if staying up past that time).

### Overview

No discussion of insulin therapy would be complete without including daytime NPH, the most popular insulin regimen in the United States. However, experts argue against its use in type 1 diabetes, because inherent limitations make it difficult, if not impossible, to obtain the glycemia goals in Table 2 without unacceptable hypoglycemia. Indeed, the DCCT study, which was begun in 1985 and planned a few years earlier, allowed *only* an Ultralente regimen or insulin pump in the intensively treated group and instead assigned NPH to conventional therapy (1). Thus, NPH-based regimens are generally appropriate only for patients who are *not* candidates for intensive glycemic control.

The major limitation of this regimen is having to use NPH in the morning to provide lunchtime insulin coverage through its "slow on, slow off" action. This leads to hyperinsulinemia from the midmorning to the late afternoon, which makes patients prone to hypoglycemia. Even with midmorning and midafternoon snacks, many patients still experience late-morning "shakes" or "jitters." To avoid this, they generally take insufficient NPH to cover the post-lunch glycemia, which protects against hypoglycemia but also results in hyperglycemia that continues through much of the afternoon. Further, wanting to alter the timing or type of lunch poses an insurmountable problem with this regimen. Exercise is also problematic because of the prolonged hyperinsulinemic effect of NPH, which promotes peri- or post-exercise hypoglycemia. Thus, patients are locked into a regimented lifestyle, with virtually no flexibility for variations in diet or exercise if they are to avoid hypoglycemia. Some patients expand the flexibility of this

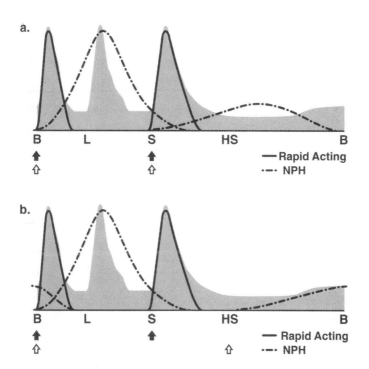

Figure 3    Conventional NPH insulin regimens showing the number of injections and time of administration relative to meals (B = breakfast; L = lunch; S = supper) and bedtime (HS). (Top) twice-daily NPH insulin and rapid-acting analog. (Bottom) the three-shot regimen, which splits the evening insulin into rapid-acting analog at supper and NPH at bedtime. The shaded area depicts the normal 24-hour pattern of insulin secretion from Figure 1. Insulin levels from each program are shown as broken or solid lines based on the pharmacokinetics of the different insulin preparations. Convergence of the perimeter of the shaded area and the insulin lines indicates correct insulin activity. Nonconvergence is too little, or too much, insulin effect.

regimen by using a dose of short-acting insulin at lunch to make it more of a basal-bolus program. However, Ultralente and glargine are better basal insulins, and it would seem preferable to use one of those regimens. Another approach is to use multiple small NPH dosages throughout the day, which produces an effective basal insulin (26)—however, this is complex for the average patient, and probably not needed now that glargine is available.

Use of NPH in the evening can also be problematic. Originally this regimen consisted of two shots, with the NPH given with the Regular insulin at supper

(Figure 3A). In most people, NPH is not a 12-hour insulin so fasting hyperglyce-mia occurs, and increasing the suppertime NPH dose to try to optimize the fasting blood glucose level often leads to middle-of-the-night hypoglycemia. An excep-tion is when the metabolism of insulin is slowed so the NPH activity persists until the next morning. This is seen in elderly patients because of their reduced glomerular filtration rate, which explains why twice-a-day premixed insulins are successful in some of those patients. Impaired renal function also slows insulin metabolism. Otherwise, it is recommended that the nighttime insulin be given in two injections: the short-acting insulin at supper and the NPH at bedtime (Figure 3B). Some practitioners are confused about the risk of nocturnal hypoglycemia with this three-shot program. If the NPH is taken at 10:00 P.M., and it has a 6–8-hour peak, they reason that the peak will be at 4–6 A.M. and cause prewaking hypoglycemia. Remember that insulin requirements begin to rise at 3:00 A.M. because of the dawn phenomenon; NPH peaking before we awake is in fact ad-vantageous for control of the fasting blood glucose level.

How do you do it?

1. Calculate the 24-hour insulin need as described in Table 4.
2. Give two-thirds of the 24-hour dosage in the morning, with two-thirds as NPH, the other one-third as Regular or a rapid-acting analog.
3. Give the remaining one-third of the 24-hour dosage in the P.M., with one-half as NPH and the other half as Regular or the rapid-acting ana-log. It is given as a single injection at supper in the two-shot program; in the three-shot program it is divided, with the Regular or rapid-acting analog given at supper and the NPH at bedtime (before 11 P.M. even if staying up later).
4. Adjust these starting dosages if the patient has unusual eating, exercise, or work habits,
5. Perform daily fasting, pre-meal or 2-hour postmeal, and bedtime SBGM along with weekly middle-of-the-night SBGM.
6. Example: 70-kg male who is moderately physically active. Total daily insulin dose is 70 kg $\times$ 0.4 units/kg = 28 units. Total A.M. insulin: 28 $\times$ 67% = 18 units. A.M. NPH: 18 $\times$ 67% = 12 units. A.M. Regular or rapid-acting analog: 18 $\times$ 33% = 6 units. Total P.M. insulin: 28 $\times$ 33% = 9 units. P.M. NPH: 9 $\times$ 50% = 5 units. P.M. Regular or rapid-acting analog: 9 $\times$ 50% = 5 units. **Final (two shots)**: 12 units NPH and 6 units Regular or rapid-acting analog at breakfast, and 5 units NPH and 5 units Regular or a rapid-acting analog at dinner. **Final (three shots)**: 12 units NPH and 6 units Regular or rapid-acting analog at breakfast, 5 units Regular or rapid-acting analog at dinner, 5 units NPH at bedtime. Adjust insulin doses as needed based on the SBGM values to attain the predefined glycemia goals.

## DOSAGE ADJUSTMENTS

Modern life entails sizable variations in daily diet, activity, and work demands. For most patients, using the same insulin doses day in and day out is not compatible with stable glycemic control. Further, an important goal of modern insulin therapy is to eliminate barriers to jobs, hobbies, sports, travel, or whatever the patient wants for a happy life. Thus, once the insulin regimen is in place, dose adjustments are typically built in to promote stable glycemia while allowing patients to live the kind of life they want.

### Pattern Management

Changes in a patient's activity, medical condition, or nutrition, or sometimes unknown factors, can result in the need to modify the basic insulin dosages and/ or program. This is recognized through *pattern management*, which uses the patient's blood glucose records to identify "problem" glycemia times and then adjust the dose of insulin that is active at that time. This is second nature to most patients and physicians. However, two aspects need highlighting. First, dosage changes should be made based on several days of SBGM; an inescapable characteristic of type 1 diabetes is variable blood sugars, and making a fundamental change in the insulin program because of a few days of surprising values is ill advised. Alternatively, if an event has occurred that explains the change in glycemia and is ongoing—the patient started a new sport or exercise program, went on a diet, etc.—it makes little sense to wait before making adjustments. Second, a key principle in blood sugar management is that the patient's blood glucose value *now* affects what it will be several hours from now. Stated another way, patients know that how they start the day in terms of glycemia affects their glucose values for the rest of the day. Thus, if the patient's log shows high or low blood glucose values throughout the day, change *only* the overnight insulin to optimize the fasting blood glucose level. Observe what happens to the blood glucose values later in the day, then, if necessary, change the insulin coverage one shot at a time (coverage for lunch, then supper, then bedtime) until day-long glycemia is optimized.

### Algorithms or Sliding Scales?

A common element of intensive insulin programs is "insulin algorithms": short-term adjustments in doses for variable activity, diet, etc. Unlike pattern management, the dose changes are made only once, to cover the event. Each patient's algorithms are unique, and are based on the patient's and caregiver's identification of diet, exercise, and other habits that cause the blood glucose values to deviate from the usual range, then designing and validating diet and/or insulin fixes. Algorithms are operative when patients tell you, "I play basketball two night a week after dinner with my friends. Dinner those nights is always pasta, and I reduce my lispro by 2 units. After the game I drink half a glass of Gatorade. Also, I always do a glucose test before the Gatorade and it's generally 130 to 150. Rarely it's less than that, and then I drink a full glass of Gatorade.'' The purpose of these short-term adjustments is to maintain stable glycemia. Thus, by necessity, the changes must be precise and based on testing—it needs to be proven that a 2-unit lowering of the pre-meal insulin dose following a 60-minute game of tennis works better than a 1- or 3-unit adjustment. In fact, as patients start frequent use of SBGM, identifying problem activities and ''fixes'' becomes second nature for many of them. Often the role of the physician is to make sure the changes are validated with blood glucose testing to prove they work.

Another common algorithm is to build in compensatory variations in the mealtime insulin dose for out-of-range blood glucose levels. An example is shown in Table 5. The dose changes are typically based on the rule of 1800, which states that the glycemia-lowering effect of a 1-unit change in lispro/aspart can be calculated as 1800 divided by the patient's 24-hour insulin dosage (1500

**TABLE 5** Sample Algorithm for Pre-Meal Adjustment Based on Self-Blood-Glucose Measurement

| Pre-meal blood glucose (mg/dl) | Lispro/aspart adjustment (units) |
|---|---|
| <60 | −2 |
| 61–80 | −1 |
| 81–140 | 0 |
| 141–200 | +1 |
| 201–260 | +2 |
| 261–320 | +3 |
| >321 | +4 |

An algorithm is a supplement or subtraction from the usual mealtime insulin dosage that compensates for the premeal glycemia level. The dosing range is calculated by the rule of 1800 for lispro or aspart insulins and 1500 for Regular insulin: divide the total 24-hour insulin dose by 1500 or 1800 to get the glucose-lowering effect of 1 unit of that insulin. This algorithm was for an individual taking 30 units of insulin daily—thus, adjustments of 60-mg/dl increments in glycemia per 1 unit lispro/aspart.

is used for Regular insulin). For example, if your patient takes 30 units of insulin each day, each unit of lispro/aspart will lower glycemia an average of 60 mg/dl. The scale in Table 5 is constructed with 1-unit adjustments of lispro/aspart for every 60-mg/dl increase or decrease from the ideal glycemia range. Key to this practice is appreciating that these are adjuncts to the patient's usual doses. Thus, my own practice introduces this insulin adjustment only *after* we have completed what has already been discussed: validation of the program and basic doses, pattern management for fine tuning, and introduction of algorithms for lifestyle variations.

In contrast to the above approach, "sliding scales" are not recommended although they are frequently used in primary-care settings. These are scales that patients use to determine their mealtime insulin dosage based *only* on their blood glucose level; their usual mealtime insulin need, what they are going to eat, recent activity, and other relevant factors are not considered. Further, sliding scales are rarely individualized or validated for a particular patient, so overdosing or under-dosing is common. Thus, in most patients the net result is that sliding scales promote erratic blood glucose control and/or an inability to get the target $HbA_{1c}$ without unpredictable hypoglycemia (27,28). For all these reasons, sliding scales are viewed by diabetes specialists as being generally detrimental to the patient and not recommended.

## SELF-BLOOD-GLUCOSE-MONITORING

SBGM is a necessary evil that makes having diabetes particularly difficult. Despite considerable improvement in meters over the past few years, the pain, inconvenience, expense, and sometimes emotional upset caused by a "bad blood sugar" make doing SBGM one of the most hated parts of the treatment program. Physicians need to discuss this issue openly with their patients. My own practice recommends four daily tests (pre-meal alternating with post-meal, and pre-bed) when insulin programs are initiated or changed, or when variable daily glycemia prevents obtaining the target $HbA_{1c}$. Also, the presence of hypoglycemia unawareness mandates frequent testing. I impress on patients that the tests are done for them—*they* need to know how different aspects of their lifestyle affect their blood glucose level. I also recommend the patient set aside a time to review and analyze that day's tests, often with the spouse so that there is a family approach to taking care of the patient's diabetes. Don't make the mistake of leaving analysis of the SBGM entirely up to patients and not reviewing their logs when they come to see you. You want to know that blood testing is being done, and that patients are correctly identifying problem patterns. Also, patients often complain, "I do my blood tests, but my doctor never looks at them." It's hard to convince a patient to make a change in his or her treatment program if the doctor is viewed as uninterested.

Once the target HbA$_{1c}$ is attained without problematic hypoglycemia, the frequency of SBGM is reduced for patients who find it onerous, although this ends up being relatively few. The common usage of mealtime algorithms based on glycemia requires testing at each meal. Also, persons with fluctuating blood sugars, a reduced perception of hypoglycemia, or lifestyles with sizable variations in diet or activity should continue to test frequently. In reality, this rarely is a contentious issue because most patients use their readings almost like a warning light in a car to know that their diabetes is under control.

## SUMMARY

I have tried to provide a conceptual framework for approaching insulin therapy in type 1 diabetes. This is not to say it is easy. One of the key messages is individualization—identify your patient's lifestyle and habits, and design an insulin program that incorporates these elements. Basal-bolus insulin regimens are not burdens for patients; they free them to live the kind of life they want. The concept of individualization should not be interpreted as lacking any principle as to how to design an insulin program, that we make it up as we go—just the opposite. This chapter provides a clear system that entails getting to know your patients, and their getting to know themselves better through intensive diabetes and dietary education. An insulin program is chosen that provides flexibility for the identified lifestyle factors, and starting dosages are calculated based on physiological and mathematical principles. SBGM is used to tweak the doses, and also to help the patient identify what factors vary their glycemia and require algorithm counteradjustments. Success is patients' attaining their target HbA$_{1c}$, relatively free of hypoglycemia and pursuing the kind of life they want.

## REFERENCES

1. The Diabetes Control and Complications Trial Research Group. The effect of intensive treatment of diabetes on the development and progression of long-term complications in insulin-dependent diabetes mellitus. N Engl J Med 329:977–986, 1993.
2. UK Prospective Diabetes Study (UKPDS) Group. Intensive blood-glucose control with sulphonylureas or insulin compared with conventional treatment and risk of complications in patients with type 2 diabetes. Lancet 352:837–853, 1998.
3. UK Prospective Diabetes Study (UKPDS) Group. Effect of intensive blood-glucose control with metformin on complications in overweight patients with type 2 diabetes. Lancet 352:854–865, 1998.
4. Barnett AH, Owens DR. Insulin analogues. Lancet 349:47–51, 1997.
5. Holleman F, Hoekstra JB. Insulin lispro. N Engl J Med 337:176–183, 1997.
6. Bolli GB, Di Marchi RD, Park GD, Pramming S, Koivisto VA. Insulin analogues and their potential in the management of diabetes mellitus. Diabetologia 42:1151–1167, 1999.

7. Bolli GB, Owens DR. Insulin glargine. Lancet 356:443–445, 2000.

8. Polonsky KS, Given BD, Van Cauter E. Twenty-four-hour profiles and pulsatile patterns of insulin secretion in normal and obese subjects. J Clin Invest 81:442–448, 1988.

9. American Diabetes Association. Standards of medical care for patients with diabetes mellitus. Diabetes Care 24(suppl 1):S33–S43, 2001.

10. American Diabetes Association. Postprandial blood glucose. Diabetes Care 24:775–778, 2001.

11. The Diabetes Control and Complications Trial Research Group. Hypoglycemia in the Diabetes Control and Complications Trial. Diabetes 46:271–286, 1997.

12. Simonson DC, Tamborlane WV, DeFronzo RA, Sherwin RS. Intensive insulin therapy reduces counterregulatory hormone responses to hypoglycemia in patients with type I diabetes. Ann Intern Med 103:184–190, 1985.

13. Amiel SA, Tamborlane WV, Simonson DC, Sherwin RS. Defective glucose counterregulation after strict glycemic control of insulin-dependent diabetes mellitus. N Engl J Med 316:1376–1383, 1987.

14. Reichard P, Nilsson BY, Rosenqvist U. The effect of long-term intensified insulin treatment on the development of microvascular complications of diabetes mellitus. N Engl J Med 329:304–309, 1993.

15. Colagiuri S, Villalobos S. Assessing effect of mixing insulins by glucose-clamp technique in subjects with diabetes mellitus. Diabetes Care 9:579–586, 1986.

16. Lepore M, Pampanelli S, Fanelli C, Porcellati F, Bartocci L, Di Vincenzo A, Cordoni C, Costa E, Brunetti P, Bolli GB. Pharmacokinetics and pharmacodynamics of subcutaneous injection of long-acting human insulin analog glargine, NPH insulin, and ultralente human insulin and continuous subcutaneous infusion of insulin lispro. Diabetes 49:2142–2148, 2000.

17. Brunelle BL, Llewelyn J, Anderson JH Jr, Gale EA, Koivisto VA. Meta-analysis of the effect of insulin lispro on severe hypoglycemia in patients with type 1 diabetes. Diabetes Care 21:1726–1731, 1998.

18. Heller SR, Amiel SA, Mansell P. Effect of the fast-acting insulin analog lispro on the risk of nocturnal hypoglycemia during intensified insulin therapy. U.K. Lispro Study Group. Diabetes Care 22:1607–1611, 1999.

19. Gale EA. The UK Trial Group. A randomized, controlled trial comparing insulin lispro with human soluble insulin in patients with Type 1 diabetes on intensified insulin therapy. Diabet Med 17:209–214, 2000.

20. Rassam AG, Zeise TM, Burge MR, Schade DS. Optimal administration of lispro insulin in hyperglycemic type 1 diabetes. Diabetes Care 22:133–136, 1999.

21. Heinemann L, Linkeschova R, Rave K, Hompesch B, Sedlak M, Heise T. Time-action profile of the long-acting insulin analog insulin glargine (HOE901) in comparison with those of NPH insulin and placebo. Diabetes Care 23:644–649, 2000.

22. Raskin P, Klaff L, Bergenstal R, Halle JP, Donley D, Mecca T. A 16-week comparison of the novel insulin analog insulin glargine (HOE 901) and NPH human insulin used with insulin lispro in patients with type 1 diabetes. Diabetes Care 23:1666–1671, 2000.

23. Rosenstock J, Park G, Zimmerman J. Basal insulin glargine (HOE 901) versus NPH

insulin in patients with type 1 diabetes on multiple daily insulin regimens. Diabetes Care 23:1137–1142, 2000.

24. Pieber TR, Eugene-Jolchine I, Derobert E. The European Study Group of HOE 901 in Type 1 Diabetes. Efficacy and safety of HOE 901 versus NPH insulin in patients with type 1 diabetes. Diabetes Care 23:157–162, 2000.

25. Ratner RE, Hirsch IB, Neifing JL, Garg SK, Mecca TE, Wilson CA. U.S. Study Group of Insulin Glargine in Type 1 Diabetes. Less hypoglycemia with insulin glargine in intensive insulin therapy for type 1 diabetes. Diabetes Care 23:639–643, 2000.

26. Lalli C, Ciofetta M, Del Sindaco P, Torlone E, Pampanelli S, Compagnucci P, Cartechini MG, Bartocci L, Brunetti P, Bolli GB. Long-term intensive treatment of type 1 diabetes with the short-acting insulin analog lispro in variable combination with NPH insulin at mealtime. Diabetes Care 22:468–477, 1999.

27. Gearhart JG, Ducan JL, Replogle JH, Forbes RC, Walley EJ. Efficacy of sliding-scale insulin therapy: a comparison with prospective regimens. Fam Pract Res J 14: 313–322, 1994.

28. Sawin CT. Action without benefit: the sliding scale of insulin use. Arch Intern Med 157:489, 1997.

# 8

# Insulin Therapy in Type 2 Diabetes Mellitus

**Andrew J. Ahmann**
**and Matthew C. Riddle**
Oregon Health and Science University, Portland, Oregon

## INTRODUCTION

The prevalence of type 2 diabetes mellitus is increasing at an alarming rate in the United States and around the world (1). It is a very costly disease, both monetarily and in terms of reduced quality of life (2). These costs are the consequence of the multiple debilitating chronic complications of hyperglycemia. The clinician's therapeutic goal is to avoid and mitigate these complications.

Just as the Diabetes Control and Complications Trial (DCCT) did for type 1 diabetes, the United Kingdom Prospective Diabetes Study (UKPDS) clearly demonstrated the significant benefit of improved glucose control in reducing the microvascular complications of type 2 diabetes (3). There was also a reduction in the rate of myocardial infarction (MI) among those treated with sulfonylureas or insulin, but it narrowly failed to reach statistical significance ($p = 0.052$). However, the epidemiological analysis including all the study individuals supported the linear relationship between glucose control and MI. Each 1% decrease in $HbA_{1c}$ was associated with a 14% decrease in MI, a correlation that was statistically significant with a $p$ value $<0.0001$ (4).

Concomitant with our recognition of the increasing public health burden of type 2 diabetes has come the growing emphasis on glucose control as the cornerstone of the therapeutic approach to this disease. The American Diabetes Association (ADA) recommends an $HbA_{1c}$ goal of 7.0% (5). Several other organizations in the United States and internationally propose even lower goals of 6.5%, and a U.S. national trial is now underway to test the value of treating to a goal of ≤6.0% in type 2 diabetes.

Fortunately, many new oral medications with different mechanisms of action have become available to treat this disease (6). Progress has been made in moving our diabetes population toward the stated goals of glucose control. Yet, overall, we fail far too often. The focus must be on treating to goal.

The UKPDS helped clarify the progressive nature of type 2 diabetes. After 6 years of disease, only one-third of patients continued to have an $HbA_{1c}$ under 7.0% on their initially assigned treatment alone (7). Therefore, using 7.0% $HbA_{1c}$ as a measure of success, monotherapy failed at a rate of about 10% per year. Furthermore, this failure was shown to correlate with reduced β-cell function, or, more specifically, progressive insulin deficiency. It is clear that for many individuals with type 2 diabetes, insulin alone or in combination with oral agents will be required to treat the insulin deficiency. This will become an even greater issue in the years ahead as the number of individuals with long durations of type 2 diabetes increases. This expectation derives from the recognized relative increase in the number of younger adults being diagnosed with this form of diabetes as well as general increased longevity of our population (1).

## INDICATIONS FOR INSULIN THERAPY IN TYPE 2 DIABETES

Insulin therapy has multiple forms and applications in type 2 diabetes (Table 1). Some of these indications are temporary, such as during an acute illness, in pregnancy, and when those taking metformin are at risk for renal insufficiency or other factors predisposing to lactic acidosis. Insulin is also indicated as initial therapy when individuals present with severe hyperglycemia (fasting glucose over 300 mg/dl or random glucose values over 400 mg/dl) with significant symptoms such as severe polyuria, severe fatigue, and weight loss.

Obviously, insulin is often initiated as permanent therapy after a period of oral agent therapy when the insulin secretory defect has progressed to the point where insulin secretagogues are no longer able to supply adequate insulin to prevent severe hyperglycemia, even in the presence of complementary insulin sensitizers. At other times, insulin may be required earlier than normally expected because of intolerance or contraindications to one or more oral agents. For example, both metformin and thiazolidinediones are contraindicated in congestive heart failure, and insulin will be needed as soon as secretagogues alone fail to control glucose.

We have become increasingly aware of a diagnostic dilemma relevant to

TABLE 1   Indications for Insulin in Type 2 Diabetes

**Temporary insulin therapy**
At initial diagnosis if the patient has symptomatic severe hyperglycemia
Pregnancy
Acute intercurrent illness with glucose decompensation
During steroid therapy
Perioperatively
End-stage renal disease
Frequently during hospitalization
  During acute MI or CVA
When metformin is discontinued due to increased risk of lactic acidosis
    Fear of renal insufficiency due to intravenous dyes
    Hypoperfusion states such as sepsis or hypotension
    During parenteral or enteral alimentation
Ketosis or hyperosmolar state

**Permanent insulin therapy**
In CHF when metformin and thiazolidinediones are contraindicated and
    other agents fail to control glucose
When it is determined that patient may actually have latent autoimmune
    diabetes in adults (LADA) rather than type 2 diabetes
When oral combination therapy is not tolerated or fails to maintain $HbA_{1c}$
    under 7.0%

the differential diagnosis of the type of diabetes in adults. As opposed to the clinical presentation of type 1 diabetes in youth, adults may experience a more insidious onset and may respond to oral agents initially (8). This diagnosis is sometimes referred to as latent autoimmune diabetes of adults (LADA). This differentiation is generally made on clinical grounds. The diagnosis of type 1 diabetes should be considered when individuals have no family history of type 2 diabetes, are thin, and have an atypical treatment course. For example, if glucose levels are highly labile on oral agents or if there is failure of an oral therapy within a year, the diagnosis should be reconsidered.

There is no simple standardized laboratory method of differentiating these two main forms of diabetes. There is no standard for use of individual c-peptide levels in this setting, and stimulated c-peptide has been used only as a research test. The presence of anti-GAD (glutamic acid decarboxylase) antibodies or islet cell antibodies can be helpful, but the reliability of either test individually is only about 75% and it is not certain that commercial antibody tests are equivalent to those used in research.

## PATIENTS' AND PHYSICIANS' CONCERNS ABOUT INSULIN USE IN TYPE 2 DIABETES

There has been considerable controversy about the potential for exogenous insulin to promote macrovascular complications of diabetes. Much of this concern stems from evidence that insulin resistance is associated with increased rates of cardiovascular disease (9). Several studies have demonstrated a correlation between insulin levels and cardiovascular events. However, in these studies of a broad spectrum of individuals, it is likely that elevated endogenous insulin levels are simply a marker for the constellation of cardiovascular risk factors inherent in the insulin-resistance syndrome. It is quite clear from the UKPDS that individuals receiving insulin as their initial treatment did not experience increased cardiovascular complications (3). In fact, there was a trend toward reduced frequency of MI in insulin-treated patients. Evidence also exists that initiation of insulin therapy in the immediate post-MI period can reduce cardiovascular mortality at both 1 and 3 years (10). There is other evidence that insulin can reduce certain recognized risk markers for cardiovascular disease, such as c-reactive protein and small dense LDL (11,12). At this time the preponderance of evidence supports the cardiovascular safety of insulin therapy when it is required to control glucose. There is no good evidence that exogenous insulin administration advances cardiovascular disease.

Hypoglycemia is the primary adverse event associated with insulin therapy. However, this acute complication of therapy is much less frequent with type 2 diabetes than type 1 disease. Severe episodes occur in 0.5–2.0% of insulin-treated patients (3,13). Likewise, hypoglycemia is generally less severe with type 2 diabetes. Although insulin-induced hypoglycemia may influence the insulin doses and specific insulin regimen, it does not preclude safe and effective insulin therapy. In type 2 diabetes, the progression from an insulin regimen using one injection at bedtime to more complex regimens is associated with increased frequency of hypoglycemia. The most common precipitating factor for hypoglycemia is skipped meals (up to 80% of hypoglycemic events). Other significant factors are unusually heavy exercise and excess doses. When using insulin, more frequent home glucose monitoring is appropriate in order to identify hypoglycemia and to facilitate optimal insulin dosing.

Weight gain is frequently cited as a great concern with insulin therapy. The amount of weight gain is dependent on multiple factors, including the type of insulin regimen, the total dose, and the oral agents used concomitantly. We still lack clear information on the relative effects of various regimens of insulin dosing as well as the relative effects of the individual longer-acting insulins or insulin analogs. For example, there is some evidence that in individuals with type 2 diabetes, insulin glargine may result in less weight gain (14). Adding metformin to insulin alone or to combinations of insulin with other oral agents generally results in reduced weight gain as the $HbA_{1c}$ drops with therapy (15). However, the combination of insulin with thiozolidinediones (TZDs) appears to cause the greatest weight gain. This combination is also associated with more frequent peripheral edema and possibly with exacerbations of congestive heart failure in susceptible individuals. The degree of weight gain seen when insulin is combined with sulfonylureas is probably intermediate between that occurring with insulin–metformin and that with insulin–TZD combinations. However, there is preliminary evidence that glimepiride and glipizide GITS may be associated with less weight gain than other sulfonylureas such as glyburide. The amount of weight gain with insulin, alone or in combination, is usually modest, with the exception of occasional dramatic weight gain with an insulin–TZD combination. It appears that the weight gain seen with insulin therapy is insufficient to offset the benefit rendered by improved glucose control. Whenever possible, it is advantageous to accelerate exercise and improve the diet simultaneously with initiation of insulin therapy. Overtreatment with insulin must be avoided because hypoglycemia further stimulates appetite and may lead to unnecessary eating in order to prevent hypoglycemic episodes once the patient has had an emotionally traumatic experience with hypoglycemic reactions.

Finally, many patients have a predetermined aversion to injections and misconceptions about the ramifications of insulin therapy. There are also issues of convenience and the social stigma of giving injections in public. The ''needle phobia'' is almost always resolved after the initial several injections. Pen injection devices are one common means of addressing the convenience issue. Time spent with an experienced diabetes educator will facilitate the comfortable transition to injections and allay the patient's unfounded fears. Additionally, patient education on causes and treatment of hypoglycemia will be needed when initiating insulin therapy. In fact, this critical juncture in the continuum of diabetes management is an excellent opportunity to refresh patients' knowledge of their disease state by referring them to an updated diabetes education class or for needs assessment by a Certified Diabetes Educator.

Unfortunately, many physicians are reluctant to initiate insulin therapy in a timely fashion for the reasons noted above. This tendency may be compounded by the inconvenience of arranging safe insulin therapy and the extra time needed to communicate with patients as they begin to titrate the insulin doses. The primary-care physician, in particular, must come to appreciate the advantages of instituting insulin therapy at the appropriate time rather than leaving the patient uncontrolled and susceptible to the acceleration of chronic complications. Furthermore, delay will reduce the benefit that insulin may offer in preserving β-cell function that can contribute to more consistent glucose control.

## THE BENEFITS OF INSULIN THERAPY

Despite the reservations of many practitioners about initiating insulin therapy, there should be no question about the ability of insulin to help patients with type

2 diabetes reach therapeutic goals. A number of studies have documented the success of progressive treatment regimens that include graduated insulin therapy (16,17). Obviously, recognition of a progressive β-cell defect leads to the conclusion that exogenous insulin will be required when overall insulin secretion is inadequate to reach an $HbA_{1c}$ of 7.0%.

However, insulin has a number of other benefits that are important to understand. As blood glucose elevates due to failure of oral agent therapy or due to other factors such as an intercurrent illness, the elevated glucose levels create a vicious cycle often referred to as "glucotoxicity." This term applies to the ability of hyperglycemia to increase insulin resistance and to further inhibit β-cell function (18). Insulin therapy has proven to be the most predictable and rapid method of correcting the hyperglycemia and therefore overcoming the glucotoxicity. Accordingly, the doses of insulin required to attain the desired glucose reductions may be considerably higher than the doses required to maintain glucose goals later. In many cases in which insulin is used to control severe, symptomatic hyperglycemia at the time of diagnosis, oral agents can effectively replace insulin therapy after a period of glucose stabilization. Sometimes physicians ignore this possibility and patients remain on insulin indefinitely only because oral agent therapy was never attempted.

In type 2 diabetes, most obese patients experience significant elevations of fasting blood glucose. The postprandial glucose excursions are then added to this elevated baseline glucose. In many cases, early treatment with sulfonylureas will expose the tendency to maintain elevated fasting glucose levels despite the possibility of hypoglycemia at other times, such as before dinner. The underlying morning hyperglycemia is the result of excess hepatic glucose production during the night. Normally, insulin suppresses hepatic glucose production. In fact, exogenous insulin will reduce excess glucose production at doses that are significantly lower than those required to facilitate insulin-mediated glucose uptake in muscle tissue. Treatment with evening insulin is clearly the most targeted and effective method of reducing fasting blood glucose.

## COMBINATION THERAPY WITH ORAL AGENTS AND INSULIN

The addition of insulin to sulfonylureas became popularized over a decade ago as clinical researchers began to better understand the pathophysiology of type 2 diabetes and also recognized the reluctance of patients and physicians to proceed to insulin therapy when indicated. The concept of BIDS (bedtime insulin, daytime sulfonylurea) developed from the knowledge that bedtime intermediate insulin could effectively reduce nocturnal hepatic glucose production and reduce glucotoxicity. The improved morning blood glucose levels then promote the daytime effectiveness of the sulfonylureas, including reduced postprandial glucose excursions. The simplicity of this evening insulin strategy is also an excellent transition to later, more complex insulin therapy. Patients need take the bedtime dose of NPH insulin only when they enjoy relative privacy, and they need focus on morning blood glucose monitoring only initially, since the method will not be successful until the fasting glucose is controlled. Also, hypoglycemia is also relatively unlikely to occur with this method.

Compared with regimens consisting of morning NPH with sulfonylureas, Regular and NPH insulin twice daily, or a basal-prandial insulin regimen, the BIDS approach demonstrated equal efficacy with less weight gain (19). Combined insulin–sulfonylurea therapy has been followed by evening insulin combinations with subsequently released classes of oral agents, including metformin and TZDs. A carefully designed study comparing evening insulin combinations with metformin, glyburide, combined glyburide and metformin, or a second morning insulin dose demonstrated the ability of the metformin–insulin combination to maximize glucose reductions with minimum weight gain (20). Of course, various combinations of oral agents are routinely used with evening insulin in the normal progression of therapy. These various combinations have not been individually evaluated.

## INTENSIFIED INSULIN REGIMENS

Type 2 diabetes is not a homogeneous disease. For example, some individuals will have accelerated loss of insulin secretion and require multiple insulin injections within a few years. These patients are often of normal weight but have no evidence of type 1 diabetes. Nevertheless, their primary pathophysiological defect is related to insulin deficiency rather than insulin resistance. Many others will have a slowly progressive β-cell dysfunction that eventually results in severe insulin deficiency and the need for insulin. Because a larger number of individuals are developing type 2 diabetes at an early age, this latter segment of the population will also lead to the more frequent need for more complex insulin regimens. Twice-daily intermediate/Regular insulin dosing has been commonplace in treatment of type 2 diabetes. This regimen often implements premixed insulin twice daily for simplicity.

However, the trend now is toward more physiological insulin regimens, like those commonly used in type 1 diabetes. The most advanced scheme utilizing injectable insulin is frequently referred to as a ''basal-prandial'' or ''basal-bolus'' insulin regimen. These regimens are designed to simulate physiological insulin delivery as much as possible. They employ long-acting insulin in amounts necessary to suppress hepatic glucose production and provide the low levels of insulin needed during periods without food ingestion. Short-acting or very-short-acting insulins (analogs lispro and aspart) are then used to supply the insulin needed for food intake. If properly employed, this regimen offers increased lifestyle flexibility in addition to better consistency and possibly less hypoglycemia. Continuous subcutaneous insulin infusion (insulin pump) therapy is the most technologically advanced model of this approach but is not considered a standard option for type 2 diabetes at this time. Fortunately, after the struggle for many years with suboptimal long- and intermediate-acting "basal" insulins, the recent availability of the long-acting insulin analog glargine has greatly improved the practicality and simplicity of basal-prandial insulin therapy. Generally, the relative ratio of basal:prandial insulin is close to 1:1 (prandial doses combined comprise about 50% of total daily insulin). Historically, more complex insulin regimens have carried an increased risk of hypoglycemia. This is not necessarily true for glargine–lispro or glargine–aspart regimens. Glargine has a 24-hour duration and is more consistently absorbed than other basal insulin options. It is usually administered once daily, at bedtime. The dose is titrated to attain morning glucose values under 120 mg/dl.

## THE ROLE OF INSULIN IN TYPE 2 DIABETES TREATMENT PROGRESSION

Because type 2 diabetes is a progressive disease, the treatment strategy has evolved into a sequential intensification most often marked by addition of oral agents as needed to maintain glucose control goals. When appropriate combinations of oral agents fail, insulin is typically added. As shown in Table 2, unless initiated early because of severe hyperglycemia at diagnosis, insulin is most often introduced when two or three oral agents in combination have failed.

A significant decision point is noted at step 4 in the table. It is here that one must decide between adding a third oral agent, most often a TZD, or adding insulin. Although adding a TZD is reasonable, considering the role of insulin resistance in most cases of type 2 diabetes, this strategy is not as predictable as utilizing insulin in attempting to reach target glucose levels. When a TZD is added, one must be certain that an HbA$_{1c}$ of ≤7.0% is reached within 3 or 4 months. If this goal is not attained, one should change to insulin. Furthermore, the addition of insulin is generally more cost-effective in lowering blood glucose.

When adding evening NPH to a sulfonylurea and metformin, one should decrease the sulfonylurea to half the maximal dose (e.g., 4 mg glimepiride, 10 mg glipizide GITS, or 10 mg glyburide) if a larger dose had been used prior to this change. If glargine is used at bedtime, one should reduce the sulfonylurea to 25% of maximum dose. Because glargine will carry over a significant insulin effect before dinner, the sulfonylurea may require further reduction or may be eliminated.

Likewise, when triple oral agent therapy has been instituted but is no longer successful, insulin should be added to the three-drug regimen and the sulfonylurea

**TABLE 2** Typical Progression of Type 2 Diabetes Therapy (Goal HbA$_{1c}$ = 7.0%; therapeutic change point >7.0% × 2 (at 3-month intervals)

|  | Primary | Alternatives |
|---|---|---|
| Step 1 | **Lifestyle change** | |
| | Diet and exercise | If HbA$_{1c}$ ≤ 8.0% |
| | Go to Step 2 | If HbA$_{1c}$ 8–9.5% |
| | Go to Step 3 or 5 | If HbA$_{1c}$ > 9.5% |
| Step 2 | **Oral monotherapy** | Pioglitazone, rosiglitazone, |
| | Metformin or sulfonylurea | repaglinide, nateglinide |
| | | (acarbose, miglitol) |
| Step 3 | **Oral combination therapy** | Add acarbose or miglitol |
| | Add metformin, SU, TZD, Re-paglinide, or nateglinide | |
| Step 4 | **Three-agent therapy** | |
| | Add third drug with different mechanism | |
| | e.g., sulfonylurea + metfor-min + TZD | |
| | or | |
| | Add P.M. insulin to two-drug regimen | |
| | NPH or glargine at HS | |
| | 70/30 or Humalog Mix 75/25 before dinner | |
| Step 5 | **Insulin twice daily** | |
| | May add metformin or TZD if insulin dose is over 1 U/kg/d with suboptimal con-trol | |
| Step 6 | **Basal-bolus insulin regimen** | |
| | e.g., glargine at HS with lis-pro or aspart before each meal | |

decreased similarly. However, as control improves with the addition of insulin, one should attempt discontinuing at least one agent.

As an alternative to bedtime N or glargine, premixed insulin (70/30 or Humalog Mix 75/25) can be implemented before dinner if the patient is >150% ideal body weight (22). Humalog Mix contains rapid-acting lispro, which may provide added convenience because it can be given just before eating rather than 30 minutes prior, and specifically targets postprandial glucose reduction. How-

TABLE 3  Insulin Action Profiles

| Insulin type | Onset | Peak | Duration |
|---|---|---|---|
| Lispro/aspart | 5 min | 1 hr | 2–4 hr |
| Human Regular | 30–60 min | 2–3 hr | 3–6 hr |
| Human NPH | 2–4 hr | 4–10 hr | 10–16 hr |
| Human Lente | 3–4 hr | 4–12 hr | 12–18 hr |
| Human Ultralente | 6–10 hr | 12–16 hr | 18–20 hr |
| Insulin glargine | 1–2 hr | ? flat | About 24 hr |

ever, the cost is significantly greater than that of standard 70/30 human insulin. When glargine at bedtime is the first insulin used, as may be preferable for many patients, a premixed insulin can later be substituted or a second injection of lispro or aspart can be given before dinner if isolated hyperglycemia is noted after dinner.

When evening insulin strategy fails, one can easily transition to twice-daily insulin with premixed insulin or self-mixed NPH/Regular or NPH/rapid-acting insulin analog before breakfast and dinner. Table 3 shows the time–action relationships of the various insulin products (22). Exact insulin requirements are difficult to predict due to intraindividual variability in insulin sensitivity. Because the change has usually been motivated by poor glucose control, the initial b.i.d. dose can safely be determined by first calculating the total daily insulin dose as 1.5 times the previous evening insulin dose. This 24-hour dose is then delivered in two evenly divided doses before breakfast and dinner.

When twice-daily dosing is ineffective, is associated with nocturnal hypoglycemia, or is too inflexible for a patient's needs, he or she progresses to a basal-prandial insulin regimen. That transition is easiest if the patient was initially on glargine as part of a combined evening insulin–oral agent regimen and simply adds pre-meal insulin while stopping any insulin secretagogue. The initial pre-meal insulin doses can be estimated from the total glargine dose—a similar daily mealtime insulin requirement is divided into three doses according to the relative size of the three meals. Alternatively, advanced instruction in carbohydrate counting can be used to better determine individual meal requirements by establishing a ratio of rapid-acting insulin analog to grams of carbohydrate consumed. This practice also offers added flexibility in lifestyle. The basal-prandial insulin approach can more safely facilitate calorie restriction for weight loss as well.

Another alternative to this dual insulin regimen is the use of rapid-acting insulin analog to cover prandial excursions while an oral agent covers basal requirements (Table 4). In one study, this regimen, aimed at postprandial glucose control, reduced $HbA_{1c}$ more than metformin–glyburide and BIDS regimens.

TABLE 4  Typical Protocol for Adding Insulin to Oral Agent Therapy

Continue oral agents, but reduce the sulfonylurea to 50% maximum dose if using NPH at bedtime or premixed insulin at dinner or to 25% if using glargine at bedtime

Begin with a single dose of 10 units in the evening (or may go to 0.15 U/kg) in the evening:
NPH at bedtime
Glargine at bedtime
70/30 30 minutes before dinner
Humalog Mix 75/25 not more than 10 minutes before dinner

Measure the morning (fasting) blood glucose daily

Increase the insulin weekly by:
2 units if FBG is >120
4 units if FBG is >160

The goal is to have the morning glucose 90–130 mg/dl > 50% of the time if possible, with no symptomatic hypoglycemia

However, the study had some limitations, including poor success with the BIDS regimen aimed at reducing fasting blood glucose (23).

Any insulin regimen can benefit from the addition of insulin sensitizers when total insulin doses are high, i.e., 1 U/kg/day. Again, metformin is the preferred initial oral agent addition in this setting because it has a weight-reduction benefit. However, TZDs are very effective additions in patients who are highly insulin-resistant. As mentioned above, the prevalence of lower-extremity edema is higher when TZDs are used with insulin. However, many patients do not experience edema and weight gain, and fear of these complications should not preclude the use of these potentially highly effective agents if the patient is properly educated about possible problems. Both TZDs and metformin can be used with insulin simultaneously, but there is no reported experience with this practice. The cost would be significant if insulin doses are not significantly reduced by this approach.

## SUMMARY

Type 2 diabetes will become an ever-increasing part of most medical practices in the United States. Individuals are developing diabetes at an earlier age and will experience longer durations of disease with associated progressive insulin deficits. Insulin therapy will therefore become a common requirement in managing type 2 diabetes. New insulin products and regimens are changing the therapeutic approach. The combination of insulin with oral agents will remain an important first step in this form of diabetes, but many patients will progress to basal-prandial insulin regimens similar to those used in type 1 diabetes in recent years. The goal of therapy is to reach target $HbA_{1c}$ levels of $\leq 7.0\%$ without exposing the patient to adverse effects.

## REFERENCES

1.  Mokdad AH, Ford ES, Cowman BA, et al. Diabetes trends in the US: 1990–1998. Diabetes Care 23:1278–1283, 2000.
2.  American Diabetes Association. Economic consequences of diabetes mellitus in the U.S. in 1997. Diabetes Care 21: 296–309, 1998.
3.  UK Prospective Diabetes Study Group. Intensive blood-glucose control with sulphonylureas or insulin compared with conventional treatment and risk of complications in patients with type 2 diabetes (UKPDS 33). Lancet 352:837–853, 1998.
4.  Stratton IM, Adler AI, Neil HAW, et al. Association of glycemia with macrovascular and microvascular complications of type 2 diabetes (UKPDS 35): prospective observational study. Br Med J 321:405–412, 2000.
5.  American Diabetes Association. Standards of medical care for patients with diabetes mellitus. Diabetes Care 24(suppl 1):S33-S43, 2001.
6.  DeFronzo RA Pharmacologic therapy for type 2 diabetes mellitus. Ann Intern Med 131:281–303, 1999.
7.  Turner RC, Cull CA, Frighi V, Holman RR. Glycemic control with diet, sulfonylurea, metformin, or insulin in patients with type 2 diabetes mellitus: progressive requirement for multiple therapies (UKPDS 49). JAMA 281:2005–2012, 1999.
8.  Pozzilli P, DiMario U. Autoimmune diabetes not requiring insulin at diagnosis (latent autoimmune diabetes of the adult): definition, characterization, and potential prevention. Diabetes Care 24:146–167, 2001.
9.  Isomaa B, Almgren P, Tuomi T, et al. Cardiovascular morbidity and mortality associated with the metabolic syndrome. Diabetes Care 24:683, 2001.
10. Malmberg K for the DIGAMI Study Group. Prospective randomized study of intensive insulin treatment on long term survival after acute myocardial infarction in patients with diabetes mellitus. Br Med J 314:1512–1515, 1997.
11. Rivellese AA, Patti L, Romano G, et al. Effect of insulin and sulfonylurea therapy, at the same of level of blood glucose control, on low density lipoprotein subfractions in type 2 diabetic patients. J Clin Endo Metab 85:4188–4192, 2000.
12. Tudkin JS, Panahloo A, Stehouwer C, et al. The influence of improved glycaemic control with insulin and sulphonylureas on acute phase and endothelial markers in Type II diabetic subjects. Diabetologia 43:1099–1106, 2000.
13. Miller CD, Phillips LS, Ziemer DC, et al. Hypoglycemia in patients with type 2 diabetes mellitus. Arch Intern Med 161:1653–1659, 2001.
14. Rosenstock J, Schwartz SL, Clark CM, et al. Basal insulin therapy in type 2 diabetes: 28-week comparison of insulin glargine (HOE 901) and NPH insulin. Diabetes Care 24:631-636, 2001.

15. Yki-Jarvinen H. Combination therapies with insulin in type 2 diabetes. Diabetes Care 24:758–767, 2001.

16. Henry RR, Wallace P, Gumbiner B, et al. Intensive conventional insulin therapy for type II diabetes: metabolic effects during a 6-month outpatient trial. Diabetes Care 16:21–31, 1993.

17. Abraira C, Colwell, JA, Nuttall FQ, et al. Veterans affairs cooperative study on glycemic control and complications in type II diabetes (VA CSDM): results of the feasibility trial. Diabetes Care 18:1113–1123, 1995.

18. Rossetti L, Giaccari A, DeFronza RA. Glucose toxicity. Diabetes Care 13:610–616, 1990.

19. Yki-Jarvinen H, Kauppila M, Kujansuu E, et al. Comparison of insulin regimens in patients with non-insulin-dependent diabetes mellitus. N Engl J Med 327:1426–33, 1992.

20. Yki-Jarvinen H, Ryysy L, Nikkila K, et al. Comparison of bedtime insulin regimens in patients with type 2 diabetes mellitus: a randomized, controlled trial. Ann Intern Med 130:389–396.

21. Riddle MC, Hart J, Bingham R, et al. Combined therapy for obese type 2 diabetes: suppertime mixed insulin with daytime sulfonylurea. Am J Med Sci 303:151–156, 1992.

22. Owens DR, Zinman B, Bolli GB. Insulins today and beyond. Lancet 358:739–746, 2001.

23. Bastyr EJ. Stuart CA, Brodows RG, et al. Therapy focused on lowering postprandial glucose, not fasting glucose, may be superior for lowering HbA1c. Diabetes Care 23:1236–1241, 2000.

# 9

## Insulin Therapy in Children

**William V. Tamborlane**
**and JoAnn Ahern**
Yale School of Medicine, New Haven, Connecticut

### INTRODUCTION

Type 1 diabetes mellitus in childhood and adolescence presents special challenges to pediatric health-care providers. The combination of severe insulin deficiency and the physical and psychoemotional changes that accompany normal growth and development make day-to-day management of pediatric patients especially difficult. Moreover, the results of the Diabetes Control and Complications Trial (DCCT) have raised the bar considerably higher with respect to goals of treatment, since intensive treatment was shown to significantly reduce the risk of progression of retinopathy and the development of microalbuminuria (1–3). Current recommendations mandate that youths with type 1 diabetes should aim to achieve metabolic control as close to normal as possible and as early in the course of the disease as possible. Remarkably, a much greater proportion of young patients are meeting strict standards of care than ever imagined possible only a few years ago. Our approach to insulin replacement in children and adolescents with type 1 diabetes is discussed below.

## GOALS OF TREATMENT

The traditional goals of treatment of children and adolescents with diabetes were to use insulin, diet, and exercise to minimize symptoms of hypoglycemia and hyperglycemia, promote normal growth and development, and, using intensive education and psychosocial support, maximize independence and self-management in order to reduce the adverse psychosocial effects of this chronic disease. Since the results of the DCCT were published, additional primary aims of therapy are to lower blood glucose and glycosylated hemoglobin values to as close to normal as possible. In pediatric patients, achievement of such stringent treatment goals is best accomplished with a multidisciplinary team of clinicians to provide ongoing education and support of aggressive self-management efforts on the part of parents and patients. Matching the treatment to the patient (rather than vice versa) by taking a flexible and varied approach to insulin replacement, diet, and exercise is critically important.

It is recognized that intensive treatment places extra burdens on patients and families and that practical considerations, such as acceptability of and compliance with the treatment regimens, must be balanced appropriately to attain all these aims of therapy. Nevertheless, recent data suggest that an intensive approach to diabetes education and aggressive self-management by patients and families may reduce rather than increase the adverse psychosocial effects of this chronic illness (4).

## INSULIN REGIMENS

Initiation of insulin treatment can be accomplished in either the inpatient or outpatient setting. Many youngsters require hospital admission due to vomiting, dehydration, and/or moderate to severe ketoacidosis. In patients who are not ill at presentation, admission to the hospital may also provide the child and parent with a safe and supportive environment in which to adjust to the shock of the diagnosis. Outpatient management in a comprehensive day treatment program staffed by individuals knowledgeable in the care of children with diabetes can also provide a supportive environment in which to initiate therapy (5) and such programs are becoming more widely available.

Once so simple, the choice of types of insulin and insulin regimen has become much more complicated. To the standard human Regular, NPH, Lente, and Ultralente insulins have been added new insulin analogs. Lispro and aspart insulin are produced by amino acid substitutions near the C-terminal end of the B-chain. These substitutions do not affect the biological actions of insulin but result in more rapid absorption than Regular insulin following subcutaneous injection. The sharper peak and shorter duration of these insulins compared with Regular insulin may be of particular advantage in teenagers who require large pre-meal bolus doses of rapid-action insulin. There are fixed mixtures of both human insulin and human insulin analogs, and inhaled insulin preparations are currently under study (6). A sampling of the variety of conventional and unconventional insulin regimens is given in Table 1.

Although many clinicians start insulin treatment with three or more daily injections, we begin most newly-diagnosed patients on two injections of insulin per day using mixtures of human Lente (two-thirds) and lispro (one-third) insulins. The rationale for using two rather than three or more injections at onset of diabetes is that with aggressive control of blood levels, most children enter a "honeymoon" or partial remission period after a few weeks of therapy. This remission period is a result of increased insulin secretion by residual $\beta$-cells and improved insulin sensitivity with normalization of blood glucose levels (7). To achieve these effects, we start each patient on a total daily dose of at least one unit per kilogram body weight per day. Even more important, each component of the insulin regimen is adjusted on the basis of fingerstick blood glucose levels measured at least four times a day. The goal is to obtain pre-meal blood glucose values within the normal range, and this is achieved via daily telephone contact with the family for at least the first 3 weeks of treatment. The DCCT data indicate that strict control of diabetes also serves to prolong the period of residual $\beta$-cell function in patients with type 1 diabetes (8).

During the "honeymoon," insulin requirements rapidly decrease. Commonly, the doses of rapid-acting insulin are sharply reduced or discontinued during this time; many children are well managed with two injections of intermediate-acting insulin and some may not even require an evening injection. In the absence of symptomatic hypoglycemia, however, we try not to lower the total daily dose of insulin below 0.20–0.25 units per kilogram body weight per day, since these are doses that were safely employed even in prediabetic children in the DPT-1 study (9).

**TABLE 1** Sample Insulin Regimens

| Doses | Breakfast | Lunch/afternoon snack | Dinner | Bedtime |
|-------|-----------|----------------------|--------|---------|
| Two | R + I | | R + I | |
| | R + I + L | | R + I + L | |
| | I + L | | I + L | |
| Three | R + I ± L | | R | I ± R |
| | R + I | R | R + I ± L | |
| Four | R | R | I or L ± R | |

Types of insulin: R = rapid-acting (Regular, lispro, aspart) insulin; I = intermediate-acting (NPH, Lente) insulin; L = long-acting (Ultralente) insulin.

A major reason that the two-daily-injections regimen is effective during the honeymoon phase is that endogenous insulin secretion provides much of the overnight basal insulin requirements, leading to normal fasting blood glucose values. Thus, increased and more labile pre-breakfast glucose levels often herald the loss of the relatively small amount of residual endogenous insulin secretion that is required for overnight glucose control. When residual β-cell function wanes, problems with the two-injection regimen become apparent. One is that the peak of the pre-dinner intermediate-acting insulin may coincide with the time of minimal insulin requirements (i.e., midnight to 4 A.M.). Subsequently, insulin levels fall off when basal requirements are increasing (i.e., 4 to 8 A.M.). Increasing the pre-supper dose of intermediate-acting insulin to lower fasting glucose values often leads to hypoglycemia in the middle of the night without correcting hyperglycemia before breakfast. Patients are especially vulnerable to hypoglycemia in the middle of the night because the normal plasma epinephrine response to low blood glucose levels is markedly blunted during deep sleep (10). Another problem with the conventional two-injection regimen is high pre-supper glucose levels, despite normal or low pre-lunch and mid-afternoon values. This is due in part to eating an afternoon snack when the effects of the pre-breakfast dose of intermediate-acting insulin is waning.

One way to deal with these problems without increasing the number of injections is to add Ultralente insulin to the pre-breakfast and pre-supper mixtures of lispro and Lente. With this combination in the morning, lispro covers breakfast, Lente covers lunch, and Ultralente the late afternoon period. With the pre-supper dose, lispro covers supper, Lente covers the bedtime snack and part of the overnight period, and Ultralente helps limit the pre-breakfast rise in plasma glucose. However, when strict control cannot be achieved with two daily injections, we do not hesitate to switch to a regimen involving three or more daily injections. A common approach to the problem in the overnight period is to use a three-injection regimen: lispro and Lente at breakfast, lispro only at dinner, and Lente at bedtime. For youngsters who go to bed early, we recommend that parents give the third shot at their bedtime (i.e., 10:00–11:00 P.M.). Lispro can also be added to the bedtime dose, especially if glucose levels are elevated. For patients with elevated pre-supper glucose levels, a pre-lunch dose of Regular or a preafternoon-snack dose of lispro can be added. Such extra doses of insulin can be facilitated by the use of insulin pens, which are small, light, and easy to use. Only a small number of our patients are using a regimen of four or more injections of rapid-acting insulin before meals and intermediate insulin at bedtime.

Over the past few years, there has been a rediscovery of the effectiveness of insulin pump therapy in the management of young patients with diabetes (11). Indeed, we are much more likely to turn to this method of insulin replacement than to more frequent injections in preadolescents who are coming out of their honeymoon phase of diabetes.

With insulin pump treatment, small amounts of rapid-acting insulin are infused as a basal rate, and larger bolus doses are given at each meal or snack. Although it is not yet labeled by the FDA for use in pumps, lispro insulin appears to have advantages over Regular insulin in pump therapy (12). The pumps are battery-powered and about the size of a beeper. The "basal" rate can be programmed to change every half hour, but it is unusual to need more than five or six basal rates. Varying the basal rate can be particularly helpful in regulating overnight blood glucose levels, since it can be lowered for the early part of the night to prevent hypoglycemia and increased in the hours before dawn to keep glucose from rising. However, younger children seem to need a higher basal rate during the night, perhaps due to earlier nocturnal peaks of growth hormone in this age group. Bolus doses are given before meals based on glucose level, activity, and food intake. Pump treatment can be especially useful in infants and toddlers who are picky eaters. In this setting, part of the usual pre-meal bolus can be given prior to the meal and the rest at the end of the meal depending on the actual amount of carbohydrate intake. Indeed, most children and parents are encouraged to use carbohydrate counting (see below) as a means to adjust pre-meal bolus doses. Pump therapy also enhances flexibility in children with variable exercise and meal routines.

The pump employs a reservoir (syringe) to hold the insulin and the infusion set, which consists of tubing with a small plastic catheter at the end. The insertion site can be the abdomen or hip area, except in the young child in whom there may not be sufficient subcutaneous tissue in the abdomen. Our patients are encouraged to change their catheters every other day. Because only a rapid-acting insulin is used in this pump, the child and parent must understand that the insulin infusion should not be discontinued for more than 4 hours at a time.

## Case Study: A Child with Newly Diagnosed Diabetes

An 11-year-old girl who weighed 40 kg was diagnosed with diabetes in her pediatrician's office based on a fingerstick blood glucose level of greater than 300 mg/dl and glycosuria but no ketonuria. Since she was not ketotic, she was admitted directly to the hospital rather than being referred to the emergency department. The initial total daily dose was 40 units (1unit/kg body weight): 27 units before breakfast and 13 units before supper. Each of the doses was further divided as one-third lispro and two-thirds Lente insulin. Thus, the pre-breakfast dose was 9 units lispro and 18 units Lente and the pre-supper dose was 4 units lispro and 9 units Lente. These were just the starting doses, and they were adjusted every day based on blood glucose levels. After she went home, her mother was contacted daily by telephone at least once a day for about 4 weeks. By 2 weeks, insulin doses had to be decreased because of low blood glucose readings. By 4 weeks, blood glucose levels were much less labile and the family felt much more comfortable about making their own insulin dose adjustments.

## NEW INSULIN PREPARATIONS

Intermediate- and long-acting preparations of human insulin suffer from a number of pharmacological problems, not the least of which is the failure to uniformly mix these suspensions prior to injection. Human NPH insulin is a particularly poor choice for basal insulin replacement, since there is a substantial peak in insulin levels and insulin action 2–6 hours after subcutaneous injection. Even human Ultralente has a significant peak action 8–12 hours after injection and the dose-to-dose variability in absorption of all human insulin suspensions is substantial.

Glargine insulin (Aventis Pharmaceuticals) is an analog of human insulin with C-terminal elongation of the B-chain by two arginines and replacement of asparagine in position A21 by glycine. This molecule is soluble in the acidic solution in which it is packaged but relatively insoluble in the physiological pH of the extracellular fluid. Consequently, microprecipitates of glargine insulin are formed following subcutaneous injection, which markedly delays its absorption into the systemic circulation. Pharamacokinetic and pharmacodynamic studies have demonstrated that the insulin analog has a very flat and prolonged time-action profile. Results of a 6-month study of the efficacy and safety of glargine in adolescents and children with diabetes showed modestly lower fasting blood glucose levels and/or reduced risk of hypoglycemia with glargine than with human NPH insulin. Additional studies and more clinical experience need to be accumulated regarding use of this analog in youngsters with type 1 diabetes. Because glargine cannot be mixed with other insulins, it has to be given by separate injection, which might affect its acceptability to some youngsters.

Although there have been many failed attempts at finding alternatives to insulin injections (13), use of aerosolized preparations for inhaled insulin delivery is currently under active investigation. Preliminary studies in adults have been promising enough (6) that phase 3 studies are already underway in preadolescents as well as adolescents with type 1 diabetes. Like pump therapy, inhaled insulin allows the patients to take pre-meal boluses of insulin with each meal and snack without having to take extra insulin injections. However, one or more injections of intermediate- or long-acting insulin are still needed for basal insulin replacement.

## ADJUSTING INSULIN DOSES

Insulin replacement in children is a special challenge because insulin requirements increase as weight and calorie intake increase and as residual endogenous secretion declines. Regular self-monitoring of blood glucose (SMBG) allows the family and clinicians to keep up with the child's steadily increasing insulin needs. We request that blood glucose levels be checked at least four times per day (before each meal and at bedtime). The most important component of SMBG is the interpretation of the results. The parent or child must be taught the target value and the relationship among diet, exercise, and insulin. If the parent and/or child grasp these concepts, they will make accurate adjustments aimed at achieving target goals. If they are unable to make accurate adjustments, they should be given guidelines on when to call the diabetes service for help. Day-to-day adjustments in the doses of rapid-acting insulin can be made based on the pre-meal blood glucose value, amount of carbohydrate in the meal, and amount of anticipated exercise. In addition, patients and parents should be taught to look for repetitive patterns of hypo- or hyperglycemia, in order to make ongoing changes in the usual insulin doses. To facilitate identification of trends, families are encouraged to maintain either a handwritten or computer-generated record of glucose values in spreadsheet format.

Self-monitoring of blood glucose is subject to a variety of problems—for example, patients often make up false numbers (14). These issues must be addressed with the child and family. They must understand the reason for the tests and that they are used only to make proper adjustments to keep them healthy. Elevated glucose levels are not an indication that the diabetes is worsening or that patients have been cheating on their diet. Instead, we emphasize that the tests are being done primarily to determine when they have outgrown their current dose of insulin.

Even when performed correctly, four blood tests daily give only a limited glimpse of the wide fluctuations in blood glucose that occur during a 24-hour period in children with diabetes. Consequently, the recent introduction of continuous glucose monitoring systems has the potential to be the most important advance in assessing diabetes control in the past 20 years. In intensively treated children and adolescents with type 1 diabetes, preliminary results in a relatively small number of children suggest that continuous glucose monitoring will provide a wealth of data regarding postprandial glycemic excursions and asymptomatic nocturnal hypoglycemia that were unavailable from capillary blood glucose measurements (15). We anticipate that these technological breakthroughs will have a great impact on diabetes management over the next few years. Continuous monitoring of nocturnal glucose levels is likely to be particularly useful in programming overnight basal rates in pump-treated patients.

Measurements of glycosyolated hemoglobin ($HbA_{1c}$) provide the gold standard by which to judge the adequacy of the insulin regimen. A variety of methods are available for assaying glycosylated hemoglobin. A simple method that can be performed in the office in 6 minutes (Bayer DCA 2000) offers the opportunity to make immediate changes in the insulin regimen, while the patient is being seen. The goal of treatment is to achieve $HbA_{1c}$ levels as close to normal as possible. Based on DCCT results (2), our general goal of therapy is to try to keep all patients under 8.0%. $HbA_{1c}$ levels are determined at least every 3 months.

## MATCHING INSULIN TO FOOD INTAKE

Diet guidance for children with diabetes is best provided by a nutritionist who is an integral part of the treatment team and comfortable working with children. In addition to helping achieve optimal glucose levels and normal growth and development, nutritional management of diabetes is aimed at reducing the risk for other diseases such as obesity, high blood cholesterol, and high blood pressure. Underlying all these is the establishment of sound eating patterns that include balanced, nutritious foods and consistent timing of food intake (16).

The American Diabetes Association dietary guidelines are used for dietary counseling. In addition to incorporating sound nutritional principles concerning fat, fiber, and carbohydrate content, the importance of consistency in meal size and regularity in the timing of meals is emphasized. The prohibition of simple sugar in the diet has been de-emphasized, but it should still comprise no more than 10% of total carbohydrate intake. The success of the nutritional program may ultimately depend on the degree to which the meal planning is individualized and tailored to well-established eating patterns in the family. Moreover, flexibility can be enhanced if blood glucose monitoring results are used to evaluate the impact of change in dietary intake. As with other aspects of the treatment regimen, we preach consistency and teach how to adjust for deviations from the prescribed diet.

Carbohydrate counting, an increasingly popular way to increase flexibility in food intake, is commonly used by patients using insulin pumps or multiple daily injections. The amount of insulin that is needed for each gram or serving of carbohydrate is used to calculate the amount of Regular or lispro insulin to be taken depending on the amount of carbohydrate in the meal. With instructions on how to use nutritional labels on food packages, even children can become expert at counting carbohydrates. An even simpler method is to vary the dose of Regular or lispro by one or two units according to whether it is a small, regular, or large meal. Some foods—pizza, for example—that cause a prolonged increase in blood glucose levels may require an increase in the amount of intermediate-acting insulin or a temporary change in overnight basal rates in pump-treated patients.

## EXERCISE

Regular exercise and active participation in organized sports have positive implications for the psychosocial and physical well-being of our patients. Parents and patients should be advised that different types of exercise may have different effects on blood glucose levels. For example, sports that involve short bursts of intense exercise may increase rather than decrease blood glucose levels (17). On the other hand, long-distance running and other prolonged activities are more likely to lower blood glucose levels. Parents also need to be warned that a long bout of exercise during the day may lead to hypoglycemia while the child is sleeping during the night, which may require a reduction in the dose of intermediate- or long-acting insulin.

## OUTPATIENT CARE

Children and adolescents with type 1 diabetes should be routinely cared for by a diabetes center that uses a multidisciplinary team knowledgeable about and experienced in the management of young patients. Ideally, this team should consist of pediatric diabetologists, diabetes nurse specialists, nutritionists, and social workers or psychologists.

In newly diagnosed patients, the first few weeks are critically important in the process of teaching self-management skills to the parent and child. With this age group, the parent is usually in daily contact with the diabetes clinical nurse specialist. Glucose levels, adjustment to diabetes, diet, and exercise are reviewed. The timing of the phone calls should be prearranged and ideally made to the same clinician. After making the insulin adjustment for the day, the rationale should be explained to the parent. Usually within 3 weeks the parents are feeling more confident and many are ready to attempt to make their own adjustments.

Once glucose levels have been stabilized, regular follow-up visits every 2 or 3 months are recommended for most patients (18). The main purpose of these visits is to ensure that the patient is achieving primary treatment goals. In addition to serial measurements of height and weight, particular attention should be paid to monitoring of blood pressure and examinations of the optic fundus, thyroid, and subcutaneous injection sites. Routine outpatient visits provide an opportunity to review glucose monitoring, to adjust the treatment regimen, and to assess child and family adjustment. Follow-up advice and support should be given by the nutritionist, diabetes nurse specialist, and psychologist or social worker. Use of the telephone, fax, or email should be encouraged for adjustments in the treatment regimen between office visits.

## HYPOGLYCEMIA

Severe hypoglycemia is a common problem in patients striving for strict glycemic control with intensive treatment regimens. In the DCCT, the risk of severe hypoglycemia was threefold higher in intensively treated patients than in conventionally treated patients, and being an adolescent was an independent risk factor for a severe hypoglycemic event, as mentioned earlier (2). The majority of severe hypoglycemic events occur overnight due, in part, to sleep-induced defects in counterregulatory hormone responses to hypoglycemia (10).

Monitoring glucose is critical in order to detect asymptomatic hypoglycemia, especially in the young child with diabetes. The older child is usually aware of such symptoms as weakness, shakiness, hunger, or headache, and is encouraged to treat these symptoms as soon as they occur. The older child who can accurately recognize symptoms is taught to immediately treat with 15 grams of carbohydrate (e.g., three or four glucose tablets, 4 ounces of juice, or 15 grams of a glucose gel) without waiting to check a glucose level. Each episode should be assessed in order to make proper adjustments if a cause can be identified. Every family should have a glucagon emergency kit at home in order to treat severe hypoglycemia.

## SICK-DAY RULES

Children with intercurrent illnesses, such as infections or vomiting, should be closely monitored for elevations in blood glucose levels and ketonuria. On sick days, blood glucose levels should be checked every 2 hours and the urine should be checked for ketones with every void. Supplemental doses of short-acting insulin (0.1 to 0.3 units/kg) should be given every 2 to 4 hours for elevations in glucose and ketones. Because of its more rapid absorption, lispro will lower plasma glucose faster than Regular insulin. If the morning dose has not been given and the child has a modestly elevated glucose level (150 to 250 mg/dl), small doses of NPH can be given to avoid too rapid a fall in plasma glucose levels. This works especially well in young children whose glucose levels fall quickly with rapid-acting insulin. Adequate fluid intake is essential to prevent dehydration. Fluids such as flat soda, clear soups, popsicles, and gelatin water are recommended to provide some electrolyte and carbohydrate replacement. If vomiting is persistent and ketones remain moderate or high after several supplemental insulin doses, arrangements should be made for parenteral hydration and evaluation in the emergency department.

Children receiving Ultralente insulin seem to be prone to the development of hypoglycemia and ketonuria during episodes of gastroenteritis. If the child is unable to retain oral carbohydrate, then small doses of glucagon (i.e., 0.1–0.2 mg), given subcutaneously every 2 to 4 hours, can be used to maintain normal blood glucose levels.

Parents are told from the time of diagnosis that vomiting is a diabetes emergency and that they need to call for help after first checking blood glucose and urine ketone levels. This is especially true for children on pump therapy, since a catheter occlusion can throw the child into ketosis rapidly. If a pump-treated patient has elevated glucose and ketone levels, they are instructed to take a bolus injection of lispro insulin *by syringe*. The dose of insulin varies between 0.2 and 0.4 units per kilogram. They are then instructed to change their infusion set and to program a temporary basal rate at twice the usual basal rate for 4–5 hours.

Blood glucose and urine ketone levels are rechecked every hour, and additional bolus doses can be given as needed. Once vomiting ceases and ketones become negative, the basal rate is returned to its usual setting. If the patient is not improving with these measures, then the child should be evaluated by a physician.

## REFERENCES

1. DCCT Research Group. The effects of intensive diabetes treatment on the development and progression of long-term complications in insulin-dependent diabetes mellitus: the Diabetes Control and Complications Trial. N Engl J Med 329:977–986, 1993.
2. The DCCT Research Group. The effect of intensive diabetes treatment on the development and progression of long-term complications in adolescents with insulin-dependent diabetes mellitus: the Diabetes Control and Complications Trial. J Pediatr 125:177–188, 1994.
3. DCCT Research Group. Prolonged effect of intensive therapy on the risk of advanced complications in the Epidemiology of Diabetes Intervention and Complications (EDIC) follow-up of the DCCT cohort. N Engl J Med 342:381–389, 2000.
4. Grey M, Boland EA, Davidson M, Li J, Tamborlane W. Coping skills training for youth on intensive therapy has long lasting effects on metabolic control and quality of life. J Pediatr 137:107–114, 2000.
5. Dougherty G, Schiffrin A, White D, Soderstrom I, Sufrategui M. Home-based management can achieve intensification cost-effectively in type I diabetes. Pediatrics 103:122–128, 1999.
6. Patton JW, Bukar J, Nagarajan S. Inhaled insulin. Advanced Drug Deliv Rev 36: 235–247, 1999.
7. Yki-Jarvinen H, Koivisto VA. Natural course of insulin resistance in type I diabetes. N Engl J Med 315:224–230, 1986.
8. The DCCT Research Group. The effect of intensive diabetes treatment in the DCCT on residual insulin secretion in IDDM. Ann Intern Med 128:517–523, 1998.
9. Schatz DA, Rogers DG, Brouhard BH. Prevention of insulin-dependent diabetes mellitus: an overview of three trials [review]. Cleveland Clinic J Med 63:270–274, 1996.
10. Jones TW, Porter P, David EA, et al. Suppressed epinephrine responses during sleep: a contributing factor to the risk of nocturnal hypoglycemia in insulin-dependent diabetes. N Engl J Med 338:1657–1662, 1999.
11. Boland EA, Grey M, Fredrickson L, Tamborlane WV. CSII: a "new" way to achieve strict metabolic control, decrease severe hypoglycemia and enhance coping in adolescents with type I diabetes. Diabetes Care 22:1779–1894, 1999.
12. Zinman B, Tildesley H, Chiasson JL, Tsui E, Strack T. Insulin lispro in CSII: results of a double-blind crossover study. Diabetes 46(3):440–443, 1997. Erratum appears in Diabetes 46(7):1239, 1997.
13. Moses AC, Gordon GS, Carey MC, Flier JS. Insulin administration intranasally as an insulin-bile salt aerosol: effectiveness and reproducibility in normal and diabetic subjects. Diabetes 32:1040–1047, 1983.

14. Mazze RS, Shamoon H, Pasmantier R, et al. Reliability of blood glucose monitoring by patients with diabetes mellitus. Am J Med 77:211–217, 1984.

15. Boland EA, DeLucia M, Brandt C, Grey MJ, Tamborlane WV. Limitations of conventional methods of self blood glucose monitoring: lessons learned from three days of continuous glucose monitoring in pediatric patients with type I diabetes. Diabetes 49(suppl 1):A98, 2000.

16. Tamborlane WV, Held N. Diabetes. In: Tamborlane WV, ed. Yale Guide to Children's Nutrition. New Haven, CT: Yale University Press, pp 161–169, 1997.

17. Mitchell TH, Abraham G, Schiffrin A, Leiter LA, Marls EB. Hyperglycemia after intensive exercise in IDDM subjects during continuous subcutaneous insulin infusion. Diabetes Care 11:311–317, 1988.

18. American Diabetes Association: Clinical Practice Recommendations, 1992–1993. Diabetes Care 16(suppl 2):1–113, 1993.

# 10

## Insulin Therapy in Pregnancy

**Lois Jovanovic**

Sansum Medical Research Institute, Santa Barbara, California

## INTRODUCTION

Before the advent of insulin, few diabetic women lived to childbearing age. Before 1922, fewer than 100 pregnancies in diabetic women were reported; most likely these women had type 2 and not type 1 diabetes. Even with this assumption, these cases of diabetes and pregnancy were associated with a greater than 90% infant mortality rate and a 30% maternal mortality rate. As late as 1980, physicians were still counseling diabetic women to avoid pregnancy. This philosophy was justified because of the poor obstetric history in 30% to 50% of diabetic women. Infant mortality rates finally improved after 1980, when treatment strategies stressed better control of maternal plasma glucose levels, once self-blood glucose monitoring and hemoglobin $A_{1c}$ ($HbA_{1c}$) became available. As the pathophysiology of pregnancy complicated by diabetes has been elucidated and as management programs have achieved and maintained near-normal glycemia throughout pregnancy complicated by type 1 diabetes, perinatal mortality rates have decreased to levels seen in the general population. This review is intended to help clinicians understand the increasing insulin requirements of pregnancy and to design treatment protocols to achieve and maintain normoglycemia throughout pregnancy.

## GLUCOSE TOXICITY AND THE ROLE
## OF POSTPRANDIAL HYPERGLYCEMIA

If a mother has hyperglycemia, the fetus will be exposed to either sustained hyperglycemia or intermittent pulses of hyperglycemia. Both situations prematurely stimulate fetal insulin secretion. Fetal hyperinsulinemia may cause increased fetal body fat (macrosomia), and therefore a difficult delivery, or inhibition of pulmonary maturation of surfactant, and therefore respiratory distress of the neonate. The fetus may also have decreased serum potassium levels caused by the elevated insulin and glucose levels, which may lead to cardiac arrhythmias. Neonatal hypoglycemia may cause permanent neurological damage.

There is also a greater prevalence of congenital anomalies and spontaneous abortions among diabetic women who are in poor glycemic control during the period of fetal organogenesis, which is nearly complete by 7 weeks postconception. A woman may not even know she is pregnant at this time, so prepregnancy counseling and planning are essential in women of childbearing age who have diabetes. Because organogenesis is complete so early on, if a woman presents to her healthcare team and announces that she has missed her period by only a few days, there is still a chance to prevent cardiac anomalies by swiftly normalizing the glucose levels (although the neural tube defects are already "set in stone" by the time the first period has been missed). These findings emphasize the importance of glycemic control at the earliest stages of conception. Ideally, if a diabetic woman plans her pregnancy, then there is time to create algorithms of care that are individualized and a woman can be given choices. When a diabetic woman presents in her first few weeks of pregnancy, there is no time for individualization; rather rigid protocols must be urgently instituted to provide optimal control within 24–48 hours.

After the period of organogenesis, maternal hyperglycemia interferes with normal growth and development during the second and third trimesters. The maternal postprandial glucose level has been shown to be the most important variable in the subsequent risk of neonatal macrosomia. The fetus thus is "overnourished" by the peak postprandial. This peak response occurs in over 90% of woman 1 hour after beginning a meal. Therefore, the glucose level at that 1-hour point needs to be measured and treatment designed to maintain glucose in the normal range at that point. Studies have shown that when the postprandial glucose levels are maintained, from the second trimester onward, below 120 mg/dl 1 hour after beginning a meal, the risk of macrosomia is minimized.

## DIABETOGENIC FORCES OF NORMAL PREGNANCY
## INCREASE THE INSULIN REQUIREMENTS

Fetal demise associated with pregnancy complicated by type 1 diabetes seems to arise from glucose extremes. Elevated maternal plasma glucose levels should always be avoided, because of the association of maternal hyperglycemia with subsequent congenital malformation and spontaneous abortions. To achieve normoglycemia, a clear understanding of "normal" carbohydrate metabolism in pregnancy is paramount. Thus, the amount of insulin required to treat type 1 diabetic women throughout pregnancy needs to be sufficient to compensate for 1) increasing caloric needs, 2) increasing adiposity, 3) decreasing level of exercise, and 4) increasing anti-insulin or diabetogenic hormones of pregnancy.

The major diabetogenic hormones of the placenta are human chorionic somatomammotropin (hCS), previously referred to as human placental lactogen (hPL), estrogen, and progesterone. Also, serum maternal cortisol levels (both bound and free) are increased. In addition, at the elevated levels seen during gestation, prolactin has a diabetogenic effect.

The strongest insulin antagonist of pregnancy is hCS. This placental hormone appears in increasing concentration beginning at 10 weeks of gestation. By 20 weeks of gestation, plasma hCS levels are increased 300-fold, and by term, the turnover rate is about 1000 mg/dl. The mechanism of action whereby hCS raises plasma glucose levels is unclear, but probably originates from its growth-hormone-like properties. hCS also promotes free fatty-acid production by stimulating lipolysis, which promotes peripheral resistance to insulin.

Placental progesterone rises 10-fold above non-pregnancy levels and is associated with an insulin increase in normal healthy pregnant women by two- to fourfold.

Most of the marked rise of serum cortisol during pregnancy can be attributed to the increase of cortisol-binding globulin induced by estrogen. However, free cortisol levels are also increased. This increase potentiates the diurnal fluctuations of cortisol with the highest levels occurring in the early-morning hours.

The rising estrogen levels also trigger the rise in pituitary prolactin early in pregnancy. Prolactin's structure is similar to that of growth hormone, and at concentrations reached by the second trimester ($>200$ ng/ml) prolactin can affect glucose metabolism. Although no studies have examined prolactin alone as an insulin antagonist, there is indirect evidence that suppressing prolactin in gestational diabetic women with large doses of pyridoxine improves glucose tolerance.

In addition to the increasing anti-insulin hormones of pregnancy, there is also increased degradation of insulin in pregnancy caused by placental enzymes comparable to liver insulinases. The placenta also has membrane-associated insulin-degrading activity. Concomitant with the hormonally induced insulin resistance and increased insulin degradation, the rate of disposal of glucose slows. The normal pancreas can adapt to these factors by increasing the insulin secretory capacity. If the pancreas fails to respond adequately to these alterations, then gestational diabetes results. In a woman with type 1 diabetes, her insulin requirement will rise progressively. Failure to increase her insulin doses appropriately will result in increasing hyperglycemia.

## RATIONALE FOR THE USE OF HUMAN INSULIN DURING PREGNANCY

Maternal anti-insulin antibodies may contribute to hyperinsulinemia in utero and thus potentiate the metabolic aberrancy. Although insulin does not cross the placenta, antibodies to insulin do, and may bind fetal insulin; this necessitates the increased production of free insulin to re-establish normoglycemia. Thus, the anti-insulin antibodies may potentiate the effect of maternal hyperglycemia to produce fetal hyperinsulinemia. Human and highly purified insulins are significantly less immunogenic than mixed beef–pork insulins. Human insulin treatment has been reported to achieve improved pregnancy and infant outcome compared with the use of highly purified animal insulins. Recently the insulin analog lispro (which has the amino acid sequence in the β chain reversed at position B28, B29) has been reported to be more efficacious than human Regular insulin in normalizing blood glucose levels in gestational diabetic women. This insulin lowered the postprandial glucose levels, thereby decreasing the glycosylated hemoglobin levels, with fewer hypoglycemic episodes and without increasing the anti-insulin antibody levels. Although the safety and efficacy of insulin lispro in the treatment of type 1 and type 2 diabetic women throughout pregnancy have not yet been reported, there have been scattered case reports of infants born with congenital malformations. Regardless of the type of insulin used, the risk for severe malformations in infants of diabetic mothers is greater than that in infants of nondiabetic mothers: 5.2–16.8% versus 1.2–3.7%. This risk is drastically reduced, however, when the mother has excellent blood glucose control and maintains an $HbA_{1c}$ below 5%. Thus, the clinician needs to explain to the patient that there are no clinical trials in which insulin analogs have been proven to be without risk, but using the newer insulin analogs may facilitate better glucose control, and normalization of the glucose is paramount if congenital anomalies are to be prevented.

## INSULIN REQUIREMENTS

Type 1 diabetic women must increase their insulin dosage to compensate for the diabetogenic forces of normal pregnancy. However, the exact patterns of insulin-dosage increase are still controversial. Many observers have detected a decline in insulin requirement in the late first trimester of diabetic pregnancies. Jorgen Pedersen, the father of the study of diabetes in pregnancy, was among the first to write about first-trimester hypoglycemia as a symptom of pregnancy and noted that it had long been common knowledge among physicians. Pedersen wrote, ''Those physicians who manage diabetic women should be particularly alert for hypoglycemia in women who have recently become pregnant. About the 10th week of gestation there is an improvement in glucose tolerance manifesting itself as insulin coma, milder insulin reaction or an improvement in the degree of compensation. When a reduction in insulin dosage is called for it amounts to an average of 34%." Indeed, he even claimed, "Once in a while pregnancy may be diagnosed on account of inexplicable hypoglycemic attacks." In all 26 cases of insulin coma collected, he found that coma occurred in the first to fourth month, with the majority occurring at months 2 to 3. He also noted that by late gestation, regardless of the metabolic control and duration of diabetes, average daily insulin requirements increased twofold from earlier in pregnancy.

Early-first-trimester overinsulinization might explain a later-first-trimester drop in insulin requirement. One example of this effect may be the significantly greater weight gain seen in the first trimester by diabetic women compared with normal healthy women. Perhaps the drive to increase calorie intake to prevent hypoglycemia in the first trimester may have been the cause of the first-trimester excessive weight gain in the diabetic women.

On the other hand, others have not seen the first-trimester decrease in insulin requirement. There are also reports of rising insulin requirement in the first trimester. My colleagues and I have described the declining insulin requirements during pregnancy of a population of well-controlled type 1 diabetic women, possibly lending credence to the notion that first-trimester overinsulinization may be the cause of the hypoglycemia seen by some in the first trimester. Based on our studies of well-controlled diabetic women, we have created an algorithm for care and an insulin-requirement protocol based on gestational week and a woman's current pregnant body weight. The total daily dose of insulin in the first trimester (weeks 5–12) is 0.7 units/kg per day; in the second trimester (weeks 12–26), the total daily dose is 0.8 unit/kg per day; in the third trimester (weeks 26–36), it is 0.9 units/kg/day; and at term (weeks 36–40) the total daily dose of insulin is 1.0 units/kg/day (Table 1). The insulin needs to be divided throughout the day to provide the basal need (the dose of insulin that keeps levels normal in the fasting state) and the meal-related need.

The basal need—usually 50% of the total daily insulin dose (I)—may be delivered using a constant-infusion pump (Table 2) or by multiple doses of intermediate-acting insulin (Table 1). When using a constant-infusion pump, the basal need is calculated as an hourly rate and is delivered such that the calculated rate ($\frac{1}{2}$ I divided by 24) is given between 10 A.M. and midnight. The rate is cut in half ($\frac{1}{2}$ I divided by 24 × 0.5) from midnight to 4 A.M., and increased by another 50% ($\frac{1}{2}$ I divided by 24 × 1.5) to counteract the morning rise of cortisol levels that are potentiated during pregnancy.

When we use multiple insulin injections to provide the basal need, we prefer to use NPH insulin because it has a more predictable absorption pattern than Lente or Ultralente insulin. Also, the recently developed long-acting insulin analogs (insulin glargine or insulin detemir) have not yet been proven to be safe or efficacious in pregnancy.

**TABLE 1**  Initial Calculation of Insulin Therapy for Pregnancy

|  | Fraction of total daily insulin dose (I) | |
|---|---|---|
|  | NPH<br>(50% of I) | Regular/lispro/aspart<br>(50% of I) |
| Pre-breakfast | 1/6 | 4/20 (0.20) |
| Pre-lunch | — | 3/20 (0.15) |
| Pre-dinner | 1/6 | 3/20 (0.15) |
| Bedtime | 1/6 | — |

I = 0.7 units × present pregnant weight in kilograms for weeks 1–12; 0.8 units × present pregnant weight in kilograms for weeks 12–26; 0.9 units × present pregnant weight in kilograms for weeks 26–36; 1.0 units × present pregnant weight in kilograms for weeks 36–40.

Our preferred use of NPH is to give one-sixth of the total daily dose of insulin as morning, dinner, and bedtime injections (i.e., NPH dose equals 50% of daily dose divided into three equal injections of NPH given every 8 hours, or at 8 A.M., 4 P.M., and 12 midnight) (Table 1).

The other half of the total daily insulin dose should be a short-acting insulin (human Regular, insulin lispro, or insulin aspart) given before each meal to con-

**TABLE 2**  Basal Insulin-Pump Program Using Human Regular, Insulin Lispro, or Insulin Aspart (basal (B) = ½ total daily insulin dose (I); B/24 = hourly rate)

| Period | Basal requirement<br>(hourly infusion rate) | Rationale |
|---|---|---|
| 12:00–4:00 A.M. | 50% less basal<br>(B/24 × 0.5) | Maternal cortisol at nadir |
| 4:00–10:00 A.M. | 50% more basal<br>(B/24 × 1.5) | Highest level of maternal cortisol |
| 10:00 A.M.–12:00 A.M. | Basal<br>(B/24) | — |

To refine basal settings, have the patient perform SMBG at the end of each period to determine whether adjustments are needed. For instance, at the 4:00 A.M. test, blood glucose should be 60–90 mg/dl. If blood glucose is out of this range, dial up or down insulin in increments of 0.10 U/hr.

TABLE 3  Pre-Meal Sliding-Scale Dose Calculation Using
Rapid-Acting Insulin[a]

| Pre-meal BG (mg/dl) | Compensatory insulin |
|---|---|
| <60 | Meal-related insulin dose minus 3% of the total daily insulin dose |
| 61–90 | Meal-related insulin dose, no adjustment necessary |
| 91–120 | Meal-related insulin dose plus 3% of the total daily insulin dose |
| >121 | Meal-related insulin dose plus 6% of the total daily insulin dose |

[a] Human Regular insulin, insulin lispro, or insulin aspart.

trol postprandial glycemia (Table 1). This dose of short-acting insulin can be given using the insulin infusion pump or by multiple doses of subcutaneously injected insulin.

The meal-related insulin dose (one-half the total daily insulin requirement) is divided such that 40% of the meal-related dose is given to cover breakfast and the remaining 60% covers the lunch and dinner meals (Table 1). The exact division of this meal-related insulin dose depends on the size of the woman's lunch versus her dinner. Breakfast necessitates the majority of the meal-related dose because the diurnal variation in cortisol levels is potentiated by pregnancy.

Compensatory doses to adjust for high or low glucose levels are calculated as 3% of total daily insulin requirement (Table 3). Clinicians should note that hyperglycemia will occur if a patient uses only insulin lispro or insulin aspart for the meal-related needs and the woman goes a long time between meals. The dose of NPH insulin may not be sufficient to prevent an escape of the blood glucose before the next dose of insulin is given. To prevent this escape of blood glucose when longer than 3 hours elapses between injections of the rapid-acting insulin analogs of lispro or aspart, the patient should add 3% of her total daily insulin requirement as Regular human insulin to the lispro injection to extend the effectiveness of the short-acting component.

## DIETARY PRESCRIPTION

The goal of dietary management for the type 1 diabetic woman is to maintain normoglycemia. Moreover, in either the insulin-requiring gestational diabetic woman or the type 1 diabetic woman, the food and the insulin must match. The diet shown in Table 4 of frequent small feedings is designed to avoid postprandial

TABLE 4   Total Daily Dietary Calculations
for Pregnant Women

| Time | Meal | Fraction (kcal/24 hr) | % of daily carbohydrate allowed |
|------|------|------------------------|----------------------------------|
| 8:00 A.M. | Breakfast | 2/18 | 10 |
| 10:30 A.M. | Snack | 1/18 | 5 |
| 12:00 noon | Lunch | 5/18 | 30 |
| 3:00 P.M. | Snack | 2/18 | 10 |
| 5:00 P.M. | Dinner | 5/18 | 30 |
| 8:00 P.M. | Snack | 2/18 | 5 |
| 11:00 P.M. | Snack | 1/18 | 10 |

The total daily caloric need is calculated based on current pregnant weight to be 30 kcal/kg per day for a woman who is 80–120% of her ideal body weight, 24 kcal/kg per day for a woman 120–150% of her ideal body weight, 18 kcal/kg per day for a woman 150–200% of her ideal body weight, and 12 kcal/kg per day for a woman greater than 200% of her ideal body weight.

hyperglycemia and preprandial starvation ketosis, and to promote an average weight gain of 12.5 kg in accord with the Committee on Maternal Nutrition, National Academy of Sciences. In the obese type 1 diabetic woman, fewer calories per kilogram of total pregnant weight are needed to prevent ketosis yet provide sufficient nutrition for the fetus and mother (Table 4). Recently it has been reported that when overfeeding of the pregnant woman completely suppresses ketone production, there is an increased risk of macrosomia.

Each diabetic woman should have her diet prescribed and the monitoring protocol explained at the same visit. No matter how educated the pregestational woman is about managing her diabetes, metabolism is affected so greatly by pregnancy that reinforcement is necessary. Ideally, education to achieve and maintain normoglycemia should be before conception or as soon as the diagnosis of pregnancy has been made. Usually, it requires 5 to 7 days to teach the patient the requisite goals and skills to normalize her plasma glucose level throughout gestation through the use of insulin adjustments. The training process is best achieved in centers specialized for education of diabetes self-care.

## BLOOD GLUCOSE MONITORING

Because normal pregnant women have lower fasting glucose levels than nonpregnant people (fasting 60–90 mg/dl) and postprandial glucose levels should not exceed 120 mg/dl (or the risk of macrosomia increases exponentially), insulin doses should be adjusted upward if more than 2 days of glucose levels are above preprandial levels of 90 mg/dl or postprandial glucose levels are greater than 120 mg/dl. In order to titrate against the ever-increasing insulin requirements of pregnancy, the basal dose of insulin should be increased by 0.1 units per hour. This insulin increase will be heralded by a rise in the preprandial glucose levels. In addition, the increased insulin requirements are addressed by an increase in meal-related insulin dose. When the postprandial glucose levels are elevated (in 90% of women this peak is reached 1 hour after beginning a meal), the following day's corresponding pre-meal injection should be increased by an additional 3% of the total daily insulin.

This titration of insulin is based on frequent glucose monitoring and ensures a smooth increase of insulin as the pregnancy progresses to a higher insulin requirement of up to 1.0 unit/kg/day at term (Table 1). Twin gestations will cause an approximate doubling of the insulin requirement throughout pregnancy.

The outpatient visits should be frequent enough to provide the needed consultation, guidance, and emotional support to facilitate compliance. Moreover, tests and therapy should be appropriate for gestational age (Table 5). The healthcare delivery team should put forth an extra effort during pregnancy. Each patient should have telephone access to the team on a 24-hour basis for questions concerning therapy, and visits should be frequent (e.g., 2 weeks apart).

**TABLE 5** Important Tests for Monitoring Concomitant Diseases and Glucose During Pregnancies Complicated by Type 1 Diabetes

| Test | Frequency |
| --- | --- |
| Eye examination | Prior to conception and then once each trimester |
| Kidney function | Prior to conception and once each trimester |
| Thyroid function | Prior to conception and once each trimester |
| HbA$_{1c}$ | Prior to conception and once every 2–4 weeks |
| Self-blood glucose monitoring: target capillary whole blood glucose: Pre-meal <90 mg/dl Post-meal <120 mg/dl | Before meals and 1 hour after meals |
| Blood pressure and weight | Prior to conception and at each visit |

## GLYCOSYLATED HEMOGLOBIN DETERMINATIONS

Glycosylated hemoglobin levels are not sensitive enough to detect minor elevations of glucose and cannot be used as a screening tool for gestational diabetes;
however, the glycosylated hemoglobin levels can be used as a monitor of ''control.'' Serial determinations (once every 2 weeks) can reinforce the patient's records and are useful when the patient sees her own trends compared with her
starting glycosylated hemoglobin level. Treatment decisions should be based
solely on the self-monitored glucose levels, with double-checking of this value
with a laboratory standard.

The best way to use glycosylated hemoglobin in pregnancy is to create
''pregnancy norms.'' Because the mean plasma glucose level is about 20% lower
in pregnancy, the glycosylated hemoglobin levels in normal pregnancy are about
20% lower than nonpregnant levels. When a glycosylated hemoglobin level is
markedly elevated above the mean for a nondiabetic pregnant woman in the first
8 weeks of pregnancy, then the risk of a congenital anomaly in the infant rises
fourfold above the risk in the general population. Achieving a glycosylated hemoglobin level in the normal range of nondiabetic pregnant women decreases the
rates of retinopathy progression, spontaneous abortion, and birth defects to near
those in the general population.

## INSULIN AND GLUCOSE TREATMENT DURING LABOR

With improvement in antenatal care, intrapartum events play an increasingly crucial role in the outcome of pregnancy. The intravenous glucose and insulin may
be used to maintain normoglycemia during labor and delivery, but normoglycemia can be maintained easily by subcutaneous injections. Before active labor,
insulin is required, and glucose infusion is not necessary to maintain a blood
glucose level of 70 to 90 mg/dl. With the onset of active labor, insulin requirements decrease to zero and glucose requirements are relatively consistent at 2.5
mg/kg/min. From these data, a protocol for supplying the glucose needs of labor
has been developed.

The goal is to maintain maternal plasma glucose between 70 and 90 mg/dl.
In cases of the onset of active spontaneous labor, insulin is withheld and an
intravenous dextrose infusion is begun at a rate of 2.55 mg/kg/min. If labor is
latent, normal saline is usually sufficient to maintain normoglycemia until active
labor begins, at which time dextrose is infused at 2.55 mg/kg/min. Blood glucose
is then monitored hourly, and if it is below 60 mg/dl, the infusion rate is doubled
for the subsequent hour. If the blood glucose rises to more than 120 mg/dl, 2 to
4 units of Regular insulin is given intravenously each hour until the blood glucose
level is 70 to 90 mg/dl. In the case of an elective cesarean section, the bedtime
dose of NPH insulin is repeated at 8 A.M. on the day of surgery and every 8 hours

if the surgery is delayed. A dextrose infusion may be started if the plasma glucose level falls below 60 mg/dl, and 2 to 4 units of Regular insulin given intravenously every hour if the blood glucose rises to above 120 mg/dl.

## POSTPARTUM

Maternal insulin requirements usually drop precipitously postpartum, and these requirements may be decreased for 48 to 96 hours postpartum. Insulin requirements should be recalculated at 0.6 unit/kg based on the postpartum weight and should be started when the 1-hour postprandial plasma glucose value is above 150 mg/dl or the fasting glucose level is greater than 100 mg/dl. The postpartum caloric requirements are 25 kcal/kg/day, based on postpartum weight. For women who wish to breastfeed, the calculation is 27 kcal/kg/day and insulin requirements are 0.6 unit/kg/day. The insulin requirement during the night drops dramatically during lactation, owing to the glucose siphoning into the breast milk. Thus, the majority of the insulin requirement is needed during the daytime to cover the increased caloric needs of breastfeeding. Normoglycemia should especially be prescribed for nursing diabetic women, because hyperglycemia elevates milk glucose levels.

## NEONATAL CARE

If blood glucose concentration is normalized throughout pregnancy in a woman with diabetes, there is no evidence that excess attention need be paid to her offspring. However, if normal blood glucose level has not been documented throughout pregnancy, it is wise to monitor the neonate in an intensive-care situation for at least 24 hours postpartum. Blood glucose level should be monitored hourly for 6 hours. If the neonate shows no signs of respiratory distress, hypocalcemia, or hyperbilirubinemia at 24 hours after delivery, it is safe to discharge to the normal nursery.

## CONCLUSION

With the advent of tools and techniques to maintain normoglycemia before, during, and between all pregnancies complicated by diabetes, infants of diabetic mothers now have the same chances of good health as infants born to nondiabetic women. Animal and human studies clearly implicate glucose as the teratogen. These studies and others emphasize the need for preconceptional programs, and the need for support systems to facilitate the maintenance of normoglycemia throughout pregnancy. The morbidity and subsequent development of the infant of the diabetic mother are associated with hyperglycemia. Therefore, the goal of insulin therapy is to achieve and maintain normoglycemia before, during, and after all pregnancies complicated by diabetes.

## BIBLIOGRAPHY

Chew EY, Mills JL, Metzger BE, Remaley NA, Jovanovic L, Knopp RH, Conley M, Rand L, Simpson JL, Holms LB, Aarons JH, and The NICHD-DIEP. Metabolic control and progression of retinopathy. Diabetes Care 18:631–637, 1995.

Ilic S, Jovanovic L, Wollitzer AO. Is the paradoxical first trimester drop in insulin requirement due to an increase in C-peptide concentration in pregnant type 1 diabetic women? Diabetologia 43:1329–1330, 2000.

Jovanovic L, ed. Medical Management of Pregnancy Complicated by Diabetes. Alexandria, VA: American Diabetes Association, 1993, revised 1995 and 2000.

Jovanovic L. Editorial: retinopathy risk: what is responsible? Hormones, hyperglycemia, or Humalog? Diabetes Care 22:846–848, 1999.

Jovanovic L, section ed. Diabetes and pregnancy. Curr Diabetes Reports 1:69–86, 2001.

Jovanovic L. Editorial: what is so bad about a big baby? Diabetes Care 24:1317–1318, 2001.

Jovanovic L, Bierman J, Toohey B. The Diabetic Woman: All Your Questions Answered. 2nd ed. New York: GP Putman & Sons, 1996.

Jovanovic L, Druzin M, Peterson CM. The effect of euglycemia on the outcome of pregnancy in insulin-dependent diabetics as compared to normal controls. Am J Med 71:921-927, 1981.

Jovanovic L, Ilic S, Pettitt DJ, Hugo K, Gutierrez M, Bowsher RR, Bastyr EJ. Metabolic and immunologic effects of insulin lispro in gestational diabetes. Diabetes Care 22:1422–1427, 1999.

Jovanovic L, Kitzmiller JL, Peterson CM. Randomized trial of human versus animal species insulin in pregnancies complicated by diabetes. Am J Obstet Gynecol 167:1325–1330, 1992.

Jovanovic L, Metzger BE, Knopp RH, Conley MR, Park E, Lee YJ, Simpson JL, Holms L, Aarons JH, Mills JL and The NICHD–Diabetes in Early Pregnancy Study Group (DIEP). The Diabetes in Early Pregnancy Study: β-hydroxybutyrate levels in type 1 diabetic pregnancy compared with normal pregnancy. Diabetes Care 21:1978–1984, 1998.

Jovanovic L, Mills JL, Knopp RH, Metzger BE, Park E, Aarons JH, Holmes LB, Simpson JL, Brown Z, Conley MR, and the National Institute of Child Health and Human Development–Diabetes in Early Pregnancy Study Group. Declining insulin requirement in the late first trimester of diabetic pregnancy. Diabetes Care 24:1130–1136, 2001.

Jovanovic L, Peterson CM. Insulin and glucose requirements during the first stage of labor in insulin-dependent diabetic women. Am J Med 75:607–612, 1983.

Jovanovic L, Peterson, CM. Maternal milk and plasma glucose and insulin levels: studies in normal and diabetic subjects. J Am Coll Nutr 8:125–131, 1989.

Jovanovic L, Peterson CM. Editorial: sweet success, but an acid aftertaste? N Engl J Med 325:959–960, 1991.

Jovanovic L, Peterson CM, Reed GF, Metzger BE, Mills JL, Knopp RH, Aarons JH. Maternal postprandial glucose levels and infant birth weight: the Diabetes in Early Pregnancy Study. The National Institute of Child Health and Human Development–Diabetes in Early Pregnancy Study. Am J Obstet Gynecol 164:103–111, 1991.

Jovanovic L, Peterson CM, Saxena BB, Dawood MY, Saudek CD. Feasibility of maintaining euglycemia in insulin-dependent diabetic women. Am J Med 68:l05–112, 1980.

Kitzmiller JL, Gavin LA, Gin GD, Jovanovic L, Main EK, Zigrang WD: Preconceptional care of diabetes: glycemic control prevents congenital anomalies. JAMA 265:731–736, 1991.

Mills JL, Jovanovic L, Knopp R, Aarons J, Conley M, Park E, Lee Y, Holms L, Simpson J, Metzger B. Physiological reduction in fasting plasma glucose concentrations in the first trimester of normal pregnancy: the Diabetes in Early Pregnancy Study. Metabolism 47:1140–1144, 1998.

Mills JL, Simpson JL, Driscoll SG, Jovanovic L, et al., and The National Institutes of Child Health and Human Development–Diabetes in Early Pregnancy Study. Incidence of spontaneous abortion among normal women and insulin dependent diabetic women whose pregnancies were identified within 21 days of conception. N Engl J Med 319:1617–1623, 1988.

# 11

## Insulin Management of Hospitalized Diabetic Patients

**Muriel H. Nathan and Jack L. Leahy**
University of Vermont College of Medicine, Burlington, Vermont

### INTRODUCTION

Adults with diabetes mellitus are admitted to the hospital more frequently than nondiabetics, often for prolonged periods. Particularly common are admissions for hyperglycemic emergencies, local or systemic infections, unstable angina or myocardial infarction, stroke, and orthopedic injuries. One would hope that hospitalization would be a time to reinforce the principles of optimal diabetes care. Instead, glycemic control in the inpatient setting, especially in insulin-treated patients, is often unsuccessful. There are many reasons for this, some relating to glycemic effects of the underlying illness or the pharmaceuticals used to treat it; dietary changes are also a factor. More troubling is that hospital staffs are often poorly trained in insulin usage—''sliding-scale'' regimens are still standard medical practice despite the fact that they rarely allow stable glycemia even under ideal medical conditions (1). Further, there remains no consensus as to what constitutes optimal glycemic care for the inpatient. The past few years have seen the publication of many important studies proving the importance of rigorous outpatient glycemic control for the prevention of microvascular complications. In contrast, there is very little literature supporting benefits of aggressive glycemic control for inpatients in terms of lowered morbidity, mortality, or shorter hospitalization time. Rather, many practitioners consider prevention of hypoglycemia the dominant goal for inpatients, and aim to not let the blood glucose fall below 200 mg/dl. Thus, the average practitioner is unclear about the importance, or method, for blood glucose management in the hospital.

Not surprisingly, diabetes specialists have a different philosophy. They understand the difficulty of diabetes management for inpatients, but also advocate making every effort possible to optimize glucose control. Of concern are detrimental effects of hyperglycemia and insulin deficiency on mental alertness, volume status, wound healing, risk of infection, and nutritional status. Also, literature is beginning to appear showing benefits of aggressive diabetes control after myocardial infarction (2,3) and coronary bypass (4), with similar benefits assumed following stroke and in infected patients (5). [Recent information has shown intensive insulin therapy lowers morbidity and mortality in patients on mechanical ventilation in a surgical intensive care unit (5a).] The recommended approach is to establish a multidisciplinary team of experts in inpatient diabetes management—physicians, dietitians, nurse educators, and pharmacists—to care for complex patients. Several recent reviews explain how to provide optimal nutritional and metabolic care for insulin-taking inpatients (5–10).

## GENERAL PRINCIPLES

### Identify Patients with Diabetes

One complicating factor is that many patients are not known to have diabetes at admission. It is estimated that 50% of those with type 2 diabetes in the United States are undiagnosed. Also, as many as one-third of persons with hyperglycemia on admission have recent-onset diabetes from the acute illness or its therapy, such as steroids (11). Further confusing the issue, the diagnostic criteria for diabetes are based on blood glucose values in healthy ambulatory patients, and many physicians tend to discount newly recognized hyperglycemia in ill patients. Several years ago, a study of patients admitted with a myocardial infarction suggested that random glucose values of greater than 180 mg/dl predicted undiagnosed diabetes (12). A recent study used 200 mg/dl (10). *Hyperglycemia should be looked for in every patient admitted to the hospital whether or not there is a known diagnosis of diabetes. Finding hyperglycemia should lead to appropriate inpatient therapy as well as evaluation after the acute illness of the patient's glycemic status.*

### Type of Diabetes

It is useful to classify patients in terms of their type of diabetes. This is of greatest importance in the outpatient setting to ensure that insulin-deficient types of diabetes—type 1, pancreas damage, latent autoimmune diabetes in adults (LADA)—are identified and appropriately treated. Laboratory assessments of diabetes immune markers, such as glutamic acid decarboxylase (GAD) antibody or insulin secretion by c-peptide, may be needed, as it is now recognized that 10–15% of patients who are thought to have type 2 diabetes show presence of an autoimmune etiology (13). They are thinner on average than patients with type 2 diabetes, but phenotypic assessment alone is not able to discriminate type 2 diabetes from slow-onset type 1 diabetes in many of these patients.

Type of diabetes is less of an issue for the inpatient setting, since usage of oral hypoglycemics is generally discouraged for acutely ill patients. However, one benefit of knowing which patients have insulin deficiency is that it can be made sure that they receive 24-hour insulin coverage. Sliding-scale insulin orders are typically written to provide coverage for blood glucose values that are measured only during waking hours. Failing to give insulin during the night to insulin-deficient patients is guaranteed to cause nighttime and morning hyperglycemia, and may result in ketoacidosis. As described above, the pathogenesis of the diabetes is not always apparent from body phenotype or whether the patient was taking insulin on admission. Thus, a useful principle in the hospital is to *provide 24-hour coverage for all patients receiving insulin.*

## Nutritional Status and Required Caloric Support for the Patient

It is not possible to determine insulin coverage, in terms of either timing or dosage, without knowing your patient's schedule of nutrition. Caloric requirements for outpatients are typically 25–30 kcal/kg body weight. With illness or after surgery, caloric needs are usually higher; a useful rule of thumb is to add 25% to the above estimate if the illness is moderate and 50–100% if it is severe (9). Patients given only i.v. dextrose solutions (5%) receive far fewer calories than their estimated basal needs; an i.v. rate of 200 ml per hour provides less than 1000 kcal per day. Intravenous fluids are generally well tolerated for up to 72 hours, but after that patients who are unable to eat should receive enteral or parenteral nutrition. Because all these methods entail relatively constant 24-hour nutrient delivery, continuous insulin coverage is given using one of many protocols—i.v. infusion, 70/30 insulin every 8 hours, glargine at bedtime, Ultralente insulin every 12 hours, or Regular insulin every 4–6 hours—to attain a glucose level of 120–200 mg/dl. Our experience favors the first two methods of insulin coverage as providing the most stable around-the-clock glycemia, and in particular have found "q 8 hour 70/30 insulin" easy and effective in patients receiving i.v. glucose or continuous tube feeds who are otherwise medically stable.

Inpatients who are able to eat are ordered an ADA diet that usually provides three meals composed of 55% carbohydrates, 20% protein, and less than 30%

fat, along with a bedtime snack. Insulin coverage follows the outpatient method of combining short-acting and long-acting insulins to provide the basal and mealtime needs of the patient. Guidelines for glycemia in the hospital are generally looser (120–200 mg/dl) than for outpatients to avoid hypoglycemia. A particularly difficult situation is when a procedure or diagnostic test causes a meal to be delayed or missed in insulin-treated patients. The patient's caregivers need to be aware of the next day's schedule so that appropriate changes in insulin coverage can be planned. Also, it is important to emphasize to the nursing staff that the patient's mealtime insulin dosage should be based on the time of the meal (30 minutes prior for Regular, and when beginning eating for lispro or aspart). If there are unexpected changes in the time of eating, the staff should hold the short-acting insulin until the appropriate time.

## Inpatient Blood Glucose Monitoring

A routine part of outpatient diabetes care is self-monitoring of blood glucose to allow insulin dosage adjustments based on periodic reviews of the fingerstick data (''pattern analysis''). Inpatient units also collect bedside fingerstick data. Unfortunately, rather than being used to more precisely define insulin coverage for a patient, sliding-scale protocols generally entail one-time adjustments. It is thus common to find inpatients with blood glucose patterns over many days that show consistent periodic or persistently high blood glucose values who have had no adjustment in insulin orders. Contributing to this, many hospitals record the fingerstick data in a form that is hard to interpret, both in day-long sequence and over many days. A useful principle is to *keep at the bedside a chart that shows at least a week of glucose values and insulin doses in an easy-to-interpret, time-based pattern.*

Most of the currently available glucose meters report ''whole blood'' values, which are 10–15% lower than laboratory determinations of plasma glucose. This difference must be kept in mind when setting and monitoring glycemic goals. Also, accuracy of the results requires that the operator use correct technique and the meter be working properly. When bedside glucose readings are unexpectedly high or low, particularly if the patient is asymptomatic, it is prudent to confirm the finding with a laboratory measurement. Also, periodically testing the proficiency of those who do bedside testing and daily checking of glucose meters is mandatory.

For inpatients with known or recently identified diabetes, glucose monitoring should be performed at meals and bedtime. Also, it is useful to obtain a 2–3 A.M. value to monitor for nocturnal hypoglycemia, particularly if the patient is sedated or has a history of hypoglycemic unawareness. For patients who are not eating, optimal timing of bedside glucose monitoring is less well defined, but frequent measurements are important, especially if changes in medical condition are occurring that might affect glycemia.

## Glycemic Goals

Many outpatient studies show the importance of near-normoglycemia to prevent complications (refer to Chapter 1), but these studies are lacking for the inpatient setting. Poorly controlled hyperglycemia in inpatients can lead to dehydration, deterioration of mental status, electrolyte imbalances, delayed wound healing, and impaired immunological responses. Glucose concentrations above 200 mg/dl have been shown in numerous studies to decrease white-blood-cell chemotaxis, phagocytosis, and bacterial killing, and it has been inferred that a patient's ability to fight off and cure infection is similarly affected, although this has been harder to prove. Golden et al. (4) did a chart review of 411 patients who underwent coronary bypass (CABG) to evaluate the relationship of perioperative glucose control to the subsequent risk of infectious complications. Patients were divided into quartiles based on mean postoperative blood glucose values (insulin was given as a sliding scale, and glucose measured four times a day from 7 A.M. to 9 P.M.), with quartiles 2–4 (207–352 mg/dl) compared with quartile 1 (121–206 mg/dl). Hyperglycemia was found to be an independent predictor for short-term risk of infection independent of age, presence or absence of proteinuria, and comorbidities.

Also of great interest is the highly publicized observation that intensive insulin treatment following an acute myocardial infarction improves long-term survival in diabetics. Best known is the Diabetes Mellitus Insulin Glucose Infusion in Acute Myocardial Infarction (DIGAMI) study, which looked at patients with acute MI who had known diabetes or a blood glucose value on admission of greater than 200 mg/dl (2,3). Patients were randomized (about 300 in each group) to either a glucose-insulin infusion (see Appendix) for at least 24 hours followed by an intensive subcutaneous insulin program (four injections per day) for at least 3 months or standard practice. All patients received thrombolytic therapy followed by beta-blockade and aspirin. Admission glucose values in both groups averaged slightly more than 270 mg/dl. Glucose values in the control group averaged 210 mg/dl the day after admission and 160 mg/dl at discharge versus 173 mg/dl and 148 mg/dl, respectively, in the intensive-therapy group. One-year mortality was 30% lower in the intensive-therapy group. A recent meta-analysis supported an effect of hyperglycemia to increase in-hospital mortality following acute myocardial infarction in persons with and without known diabetes (14).

What are appropriate goals for glycemia in the hospital? Hirsch et al. (6) proposed pre-meal glucose values of 120–200 mg/dl to minimize the risk of hypoglycemia while preventing glucosuria and osmotic diuresis. These values are reasonable in patients with changing medical, surgical, or nutrition conditions. However, in stable patients, values within the upper half of this range can often be avoided. Also, certain kinds of patients, such as those who are infected or pregnant or have had a cardiovascular event or surgery, should receive intensive diabetes management using i.v. insulin and 1- to 2-hourly bedside blood glucose values to achieve as near-normal glycemia as is safely possible.

## WHY NOT SLIDING SCALES?

Hospitalized patients often have insulin orders written by "sliding scale." This regimen is popular because of the many factors that make glycemia unpredictable in inpatients, which make some practitioners uncomfortable about attempting to foresee their patients' insulin needs. Using a scale that provides insulin in response to blood glucose value seems more sensible. Unfortunately, many aspects of sliding-scale coverage cause it to work poorly in many patients: the same dosing scale is often used for patients with very different weight, illnesses, and nutrition and renal status; the dosing scale is rarely changed during the hospitalization regardless of the blood glucose values; insulin administration may be based on when the nurse measures a blood glucose value as opposed to when the patient eats; and blood glucose measurements, and thus insulin coverage, may be missed when the patient is off the floor getting a test or is otherwise not available, which causes patients with type 1 diabetes to go without insulin coverage for many hours, promoting hyperglycemia and catabolism. Another potential problem is the insulin's "running out" if the scale is written *not* to cover normal blood glucose values, causing glycemia to "see-saw." Thus, sliding scales often *promote* problems with glycemic control in the hospital.

### Historical Perspective on the Use of Sliding Scales

In 1970, MacMillan wrote a paper, "The Fallacy of Insulin Adjustment by Sliding Scale" (15), that criticized this method of insulin coverage because it ignored the amount and effect of corresponding doses on previous days and did not consider the anticipated needs over the next 6–8-hour period when the insulin would have its effects. His studies, conducted in children, were based on insulin coverage for degree of glycosuria. He observed a frequent pattern of giving too much, alternating with too little, insulin—excessive doses of insulin were given for 4+ glucosuria, and the next dose of insulin would be omitted because of aglycosuria. This omission of insulin would "almost invariably" result in recurrence of strong glucosuria, leading to "repetition of the cycle" (what many now call the "roller-coaster" or "see-saw" effect). In 1991, he again wrote that "the sliding scale method of insulin adjustment is seldom effective in establishing diabetic control because there is no anticipation of upcoming insulin needs and dosage changes are after-the-fact reactions to existing blood sugar levels'' (16). Further, he stated that control is impossible to establish with this regimen since no insulin is ordered if the patient is normoglycemic, which leads to marked hyperglycemia by the next scheduled testing. Also, nocturnal hypoglycemia may occur because the dose of insulin is determined by the level of hyperglycemia irrespective of whether it is before a meal, at bedtime, or during the night.

MacMillan's comments were made before routine bedside blood glucose testing, and it might be questioned whether today's therapy is more effective. Hanish (17) described two protocols from her hospital for sliding-scale regimens based on blood glucose testing. One gives 2 U of Regular insulin for a fingerstick of 151–200 mg/dl and then increases 2 U for every additional 50 mg/dl, up to 450 mg/dl. The physician is called if the glucose is under 80 mg/dl or over 450 mg/dl. The second uses a starting dose of 4 U of Regular insulin but is otherwise the same. This two-page report is surprisingly well known and quoted by house officers. However, it shows that her hospital developed these scales ''to decrease the possibility of transcription errors and to save physicians', nurses', and pharmacists' time.'' Nowhere is there any comment about how successful they were in controlling glycemia.

The effectiveness and safety of sliding scales were investigated by Queale et al. in 171 diabetic patients consecutively admitted for diabetes-unrelated reasons to cardiology or general medicine services in a large city hospital (1). Hypoglycemia was defined as ≤60 mg/dl, and hyperglycemia ≥300 mg/dl. Patients were followed for at least 4 days, and had to have at least four bedside fingerstick measurements daily. No uniform insulin scale was used in the study; coverage could start at 150 mg/dl (in 35%) or 200 mg/dl (in 52%), and typically increased 2 U for every 50 mg/dl. Hypoglycemia occurred in 23% of the patients (3.4/100 measurements) and hyperglycemia in 40% (9.8/100 measurements). Most telling, hyperglycemia was greatest (threefold increased risk) in the patients who received sliding-scale coverage without concomitant intermediate-acting insulin. The authors concluded that a sliding-scale regimen when used alone increased the risk of hyperglycemia, and when used in conjunction with a standing regimen provided no benefit over the standing regimen alone.

To summarize, the major (and perhaps only) advantage of a sliding-scale insulin regimen is that it is easy. More debatable are its effectiveness and safety. Sliding scales make sense when used in conjunction with a standard insulin regimen to compensate for inaccuracies in the basic insulin doses. Each day's supplement is used to adjust the next day's insulin dosage up or down if it is assumed there is an ongoing need for the change. Thus, the basic insulin program is ''fine-tuned'' until glycemia is as stable and close to the target range as can be achieved in the hospital. In contrast, sliding-scale therapy used on its own tends to oversimplify inpatient insulin usage. The worst form is the one-size-fits-all scale widely practiced by house officers, as it provides a false impression that the diabetes is being managed when, in reality, effectively no decisions about the diabetes management are made. Often, even the patient's caregivers do not know the blood glucose levels—the "don't ask, don't tell" approach to medical care.

## INSULIN ALGORITHMS: THE PREFERRED METHOD

The preferred approach is to provide insulin coverage based on the nutritional and medical characteristics of each patient. *Algorithms* are programs of insulin administration that are based on the nutrition pattern of the patient, and incorporate supplemental insulin dosing to attain a target range level of glycemia. Lilley and Levine (7) stated in their review of inpatient therapy for type 2 diabetes that "The algorithm takes into account the individual patient's insulin needs, caloric load and physical activity level, as well as the timing of insulin administration relative to caloric intake. Whereas the traditional sliding-scale insulin regimen is directed at lowering existing excessive blood glucose levels, supplements are given not only to correct hyperglycemia but also to control the anticipated effects of caloric intake and other factors that play a role in glycemia."

The first comprehensive paper on insulin algorithms for inpatients was published by Hirsch et al. (6) with the comment that "many of our recommendations are based on common sense or are extrapolations from other situations because the data examining nonsurgical inpatient diabetes therapy are limited." Multiple guidelines were suggested—for patients with type 1 or 2 diabetes, eating, or NPO. An i.v. insulin infusion was recommended for all patients who were not eating. Those eating standard meals were given twice-daily NPH and Regular insulin (0.5–1.0 U/kg) in the usual pattern of two-thirds of the total dose before breakfast as two-thirds NPH and one-third Regular, and the remainder before supper as half NPH and half Regular. There was also an algorithm for supplemental Regular insulin (0.075 U/kg for pre-meal glucose >200 mg/dl, 0.1 U/kg for pre-meal glucose >300 mg/dl). Lilley and Levine followed the suggestions of Hirsch, but recommended lispro over Regular insulin (7). These papers are mostly discussions of the principles of what to do, as opposed to giving formulas for inpatient insulin dosing that are proven to work. This is because correctly administering subcutaneous insulin to a hospitalized diabetic patient requires daily adjusting of the insulin program and dosing to get it right, as opposed to one-size-fits-all recommendations that rarely work.

In contrast, many studies of algorithms for i.v. insulin infusions have shown an ability to attain very good glycemic control. One example is by Watts et al. in postoperative patients (18). Their insulin infusion began at 1.5 U per hour, and was adjusted every 2 hours based on specific blood glucose cutoffs: <80 mg/dl, decrease by 0.5 U per hour and give 25 ml 50% dextrose; 80–119 mg/dl, decrease by 0.5 U per hour; 120–180 mg/dl, no change; 181–240 mg/dl, increase by 0.5 U per hour; >240 mg/dl, increase by 0.5 U per hour and give 8 U i.v. Regular insulin. The patients given the insulin infusion reached the target glycemia level within 8 hours, and 12–24 hours after surgery had a mean glucose of 136 mg/dl (range 120–180), whereas those on subcutaneous insulin had a mean of 208 mg/dl (range 30–306). Also striking was an absence of hypoglycemia in the i.v. insulin group.

   *In summary, successful inpatient diabetes management requires designing an insulin program based on the special needs of that patient, followed by blood glucose monitoring and daily adjustments of the insulin doses, all in an attempt to attain glycemia that maximizes the well-being, nutritional status, and medical outcome of the patient while minimizing his or her risk of hypoglycemia.*

## INPATIENT INSULIN PROGRAMS

### Subcutaneous Insulin for the Patient Who Is Eating

The recommended approach in type 1 and insulin-requiring type 2 diabetes patients who are eating is shown in Table 1. For those with type 2 diabetes who were taking oral agents on admission, as a general principle it is safest to discontinue oral hypoglycemics and substitute insulin in patients undergoing surgery or with major illness of any kind. The recommended program is 0.5 U/kg glargine

TABLE 1   Subcutaneous Insulin Program for Inpatients Who Are Eating

**Calculate starting insulin doses.**
   Glargine 0.5 U/kg at bedtime (0.3 U/kg for conditions with concern over risk of hypoglycemia; 0.7 U/kg for those with type 2 diabetes, obesity, infections, or open wounds, or those receiving steroids or post-CABG).
   Humalog 0.1 U/kg each meal (adjust downward or give after meal for inconsistent eating habits)
**Bedside glucose measurements at mealtimes and bedtime—supplemental lispro.**
   200–299 mg/dl—give extra 0.075 U/kg lispro
   >300 mg dl—give extra 0.1 U/kg lispro
**Adjust glargine doses to attain fasting blood glucose 120–200 mg/dl.**
   **Once attained, adjust lispro to achieve pre-meal and bedtime blood glucose 120–200 mg/dl.**

The suggested starting doses are for an "average" patient, and variation is common based on the unique medical circumstances of each patient.
Suggested starting program if NPH or Ultralente is used instead of glargine: 0.25 U/kg NPH or Ultralente at breakfast and bedtime (0.15 U/kg twice daily for conditions with concern about hypoglycemia, and 0.35 U/kg for conditions with increased basal insulin needs) and 0.1 U/kg Humalog at meals.

at bedtime for basal coverage and mealtime lispro (0.1 U/kg at each meal). However, it must be emphasized that these are "average" starting doses. We frequently vary them because of many factors that affect the patient's insulin needs. For example, inconsistent eating of the delivered food is a major issue, especially in the elderly or persons who are slowly advancing their diet following abdominal surgery or an illness such as pancreatitis. Using lispro as opposed to Regular allows the nurse to give the insulin toward the end of the meal, after seeing how much has been eaten; guidelines for meal dosing based on the amount of the meal or carbohydrate consumed can be very helpful. Also, a variety of illnesses cause concern for hypoglycemia from the injected insulin because of impaired glucose production from the liver, defective nutrient influx through the bowel, or slowed insulin metabolism. Examples are renal dysfunction, poor renal perfusion from cardiac failure or volume depletion, hepatic disease, malabsorption from bowel or pancreatic disease, and hypothyroidism or adrenal insufficiency. In those cases, we tend to lower the starting dosage of glargine to 0.3 U/kg. Alternatively, basal insulin needs are higher than 0.5 U/kg in many patients, in particular those with type 2 diabetes, obesity, infections, or open wounds, or those post-CABG or receiving steroids. We prefer not to go much higher than 0.7 U/kg as a starting dose, but advance their doses quickly.

Along with these starting doses, lispro supplements are written using a scale that starts at 200 mg/dl (Table 1) to compensate for substantial hyperglycemia if the patient's insulin needs far exceed the calculated starting doses. It is important to appreciate that the supplemental doses are there as a backup. The goal is to fine-tune the standard program so that within a day or two target glycemia is achieved without the need for supplements. This is accomplished by adjusting the glargine to achieve a fasting glucose value of 120–200 mg/dl, and then the lispro doses so that pre-meal and bedtime glucose values are in the same range (2-hour post-meal values sometimes are needed to adjust the lispro). Then, each day's insulin doses are adjusted as needed based on the prior day's glucose values, insulin doses and supplements, as well as the next day's planned nutrition schedule.

NPH or Ultralente has traditionally been used to provide basal coverage, and recommended starting doses for NPH or Ultralente are listed in Table 1. However, neither is an ideal "basal" insulin because of their slow "on–off" effect, which causes peaks and valleys in insulin action that tend to bring about swings in glycemia. This is worsened by the unforeseen changes in medical condition or meal schedule that frequently occur during a hospitalization. It is thus common to underdose these insulins to avoid hypoglycemia. The "peakless" nature of glargine's action has a significant advantage in this regard. Also advantageous are its more consistent day-to-day absorption compared with Ultralente and NPH and the fact that it is given at bedtime, which avoids the problem with

NPH or Ultralente of an occasional missed injection because the patient is away from the floor for a test or procedure.

## Intravenous Insulin Infusions

A continuous i.v. insulin infusion is very useful in acutely ill patients, in the postoperative period, and in those with generalized edema or dermatological disease. Also, patients who are not eating, or are getting around-the-clock nutrition by TPN or tube feeds, do very well with an insulin infusion, although methods that are less intensive in terms of nursing care are more often used. A protocol recommended by Gebhart (9) (Table 2) is based on the study of Watts et al. (18) but uses lowered glucose cutoff values that better match the whole blood method of most bedside meters. We generally start with 1.5 U per hour, analogous to Watts and colleagues' study (18). However, considerably more insulin is needed in patients who are obese, infected, or on steroids. Insulin requirements are often particularly high post-CABG in otherwise uncomplicated patients. Under these circumstances, we start a higher infusion rate of 2–3 U per hour. Although glycemia is easily and safely controlled with this algorithm in most patients, it requires that bedside glucose monitoring be performed frequently—every 1–2 hours after starting the infusion until steady-state glycemia within the target range is achieved, and thereafter no less then every 4 hours in stable patients and every 2 hours in less stable patients. This is because changes in a patient's medical

---

**TABLE 2**  Algorithm for Continuous Intravenous Insulin Infusion

---

Start continuous dextrose infusion (D5/W) at 100 ml per hour
Start Regular insulin 125 U in 250 ml 0.9% saline infused by syringe pump
   (1 U = 2 ml)
Glucose checks every 1–2 hours
Algorithm—begin at 1.5 U per hour (up to 3 U per hour in patients who
   are obese, infected, on steroids, post-CABG):
   <80 mg/dl—Decrease rate by 1 U per hour and give 25 ml 50% dextrose
   i.v.
   80–110 mg/dl—Decrease rate 1 U per hour
   110–160 mg/dl—No change in rate
   161–220 mg/dl—Increase rate 0.5 U per hour
   >220 mg/dl—give 8 U Regular insulin i.v. push and increase 0.5 U per
   hour
Physician to be notified if <80 mg/dl or >220 mg/dl on two consecutive
   checks

---

*Source*: Adapted from Ref. 9.

condition will typically alter his or her insulin need/glycemia level on the infusion, so continued glucose monitoring is essential to ensure safety and effectiveness. In most institutions insulin infusions thus pose a difficult challenge outside intensive care units.

One note of caution is that the algorithm is *not to be used in markedly hyperglycemic patients*. An insulin infusion rate that is appropriately active as evidenced by hourly lowering of glycemia by 50–100 mg/dl may take several hours to bring the patient's glucose level to where upward adjustments in the infusion rate are no longer mandated. The insulin infusion rate is now well in excess of the patient's need for steady-state glycemia, and he or she goes on to become seriously hypoglycemic. Instead, the hyperglycemia should be aggressively treated first (see Chapter 12), and then the algorithm employed to maintain glycemia in the target range.

A common problem is how to switch a patient from an insulin infusion to subcutaneous insulin. If the medical condition has not changed, the infusion rate gives a good idea of the patient's basal insulin needs. *The key principle when switching to subcutaneous insulin is to make sure there is no interruption of insulin delivery*. The half-life of i.v. insulin is only a few minutes. In a patient with type 1 diabetes, being withdrawn from insulin for a surprisingly short time causes the diabetes to get out of control. This is seen in studies in which subcutaneous insulin pumps are turned off to mimic what happens when outpatient insulin pump therapy is inadvertently interrupted; hyperglycemia and ketosis develop within a few hours (19). *When switching from i.v. to subcutaneous insulin, a plan must be in place that links stopping of the i.v. infusion to starting the subcutaneous insulin*. We generally give the first dose of subcutaneous insulin 30–60 minutes *before* stopping the infusion, usually with breakfast so that both short-acting and long-acting insulins are given. This avoids what sometimes happens in the hospital—the infusion is turned off and the nurse is called away elsewhere so the subcutaneous insulin is not given for some time. Caution should be taken in patients who have undergone a procedure such as abdominal surgery that may prevent their tolerating normal meals. Also problematic are patients with known gastroparesis, or those receiving narcotics that can disrupt bowel motility. In these patients, it is preferable to continue the insulin infusion for a day or two after the patient starts eating, with lispro for meal coverage, until it is confirmed the meals are tolerated.

## The Patient Who Is Receiving Enteral Nutrition

For patients receiving continuous tube feeds, an i.v. insulin infusion as described above can be used, generally with great success. Its advantage is the ability to stop the insulin should the tube feeds be acutely discontinued because the tube has become dislodged or for another reason. Most tube feed preparations provide

12–16 grams of carbohydrate per hour when given at a rate of 100 ml per hour, which corresponds to about 1 carbohydrate exchange per hour, calling for 1 U of insulin per hour (20). Thus, if an NPO patient had glycemic control on an insulin infusion at 2 U per hour, adding tube feeds would cause the rate to be increased to 3 U per hour.

However, because an i.v. insulin infusion places considerable demands on floor nurses, a subcutaneous regimen is most often used. Using the formula in Table 1, combining the mealtime and basal coverage—i.e., 0.8 U/kg can be given over a 24-hour period. That estimate is adjusted as needed, as described previously under "Subcutaneous Insulin for the Patient Who Is Eating." For instance, it is lowered 0.2 U/kg for renal, cardiac, or hepatic dysfunction, in the elderly, and when tube feeds are beginning and being advanced slowly. It is adjusted upward to 1 U/kg in those who are obese or have open wounds or infections, or are receiving steroids. Tube feeds are generally not recommended in patients with gastroparesis, since jejunal feeding is usually more successful (10).

We have had great success with 70/30 insulin given every 8 hours (Table 3) in patients on continuous tube feeds. For instance, a 75-kg male with type 1 diabetes moved out of the ICU post-pneumonia who is tolerating tube feeds would be given 20 U 70/30 insulin every 8 hours (75 kg × 0.8 U/kg divided by three doses of 70/30 insulin). Fingerstick glucose values are taken every 4–6 hours, and the 70/30 doses adjusted to attain glycemia of 120–200 mg/dl. We also include in the order sheet instructions for close monitoring of glycemia and starting of i.v. glucose if needed should the tube feeds be unexpectedly discon-

---

**TABLE 3** 70/30 Insulin Every 8 Hours for Continuous 24-Hour Nutrition

Calculate starting insulin doses
   Total daily dosage 0.8 U/kg (0.6 U/kg for renal, cardiac, or hepatic dysfunction, in the elderly, and when tube feeds are just beginning and are being advanced slowly; 1 U/kg in obesity, or those with open wounds or infections, or receiving steroids)
   Divide by 3 to get 70/30 dose to be given every 8 hours
Bedside glucose measurements every 4–6 hours around the clock
Adjust 70/30 insulin doses to attain blood glucose 120–200 mg/dl
Continue blood glucose monitoring while the patient is receiving tube feeds, and make daily adjustments in the 70/30 insulin doses as needed
If the tube feeds are unexpectedly discontinued, glycemia is closely monitored (every 1–2 hours), and i.v. glucose started if needed (blood glucose <100 mg/dl)

---

Tube feeds are generally not recommended in patients with gastroparesis, because jejunal feeding is usually more successful.

tinued. It is likely that glargine would be equally effective, although the three-time-a-day dosing of the 70/30 insulin provides added flexibility to alter the insulin dose if the tube feed amount is lowered or stopped.

## The Patient Who Is Receiving Parenteral Nutrition

The concept behind insulin coverage in TPN-receiving patients is similar to that with tube feedings. However, the amount of insulin required is often greater—it may exceed 100 U per day. The carbohydrate content of TPN is higher than for tube feeds, generally 25 grams per hour if infused at a rate of 100 ml per hour. Also, giving the nutrients directly into the vascular system bypasses the gut, which normally plays a crucial role in glucose homeostasis since food in the gut releases hormones from the small bowel that are potent stimulants of insulin secretion (''incretin hormones'') (21). Thus, TPN in patients with type 2 diabetes causes the loss of a key regulator for meal-related insulin secretion. Not surprisingly, patients who are not known to have diabetes sometimes develop hyperglycemia when started on TPN (22).

The TPN bag provides a convenient mechanism for delivery of insulin, usually 1 U for every 10 grams of carbohydrates (10). Should the TPN be discontinued, the insulin also stops, which provides an important safety feature. After the TPN has started, the insulin dosage in the bag is adjusted daily, based on the bedside glucose values, to attain a target range of 120–200 mg/dl. Some practitioners prefer to place only part (or none) of the insulin in the bag, and to also provide small doses of subcutaneous insulin to provide a little more flexibility for adjusting the insulin dosage. For instance, 5 U 70/30 insulin every 8 hours or 5 U Regular every 6 hours is given and the insulin in the bag lowered proportionately. Caveat—in such cases, avoidance of hypoglycemia should the flow of TPN be interrupted or halted must be considered.

## The Patient Who Will Undergo Ambulatory Surgery or a Procedure That Does Not Require General Anesthesia

It is common to be called by patients who are scheduled for an outpatient procedure or test that requires them to be NPO after midnight. Their concern is about how to manage their diabetes medications. This issue was discussed in a recent review of perioperative management of diabetes (8). Table 4 shows a suggested protocol.

Oral diabetes medications are held the morning of the procedure, and generally restarted once the patient is tolerating food after the procedure, although with dye-based studies the patient must wait 48 hours to restart metformin. It is safest to have a glucose-containing i.v. (D5/W) running during the procedure at ≈100 ml per hour. Blood glucose should be measured before and after the procedure, and supplements of Regular insulin (5–10 U) given for glucose values above 120 mg/dl. This is done by the hospital or office nursing staff in the periop-

TABLE 4   Diabetes Management for Outpatient Surgery or Procedure that Requires NPO

**Patients taking oral agents**

Preprocedure: hold oral hypoglycemics morning of procedure
Blood glucose is measured prior to procedure—5 U Regular insulin > 120 mg/dl
D5/W at 100 ml per hour during procedure
Postprocedure
  Measure blood glucose: >120 mg/dl, 5 U Regular; >200 mg/dl, 10 U Regular
  Eat breakfast to show tolerance of normal food intake
  Restart orals at next scheduled dose (wait 48 hours to restart metformin if dye-based study)
  Four-times-per-day blood glucose measurements for next 2 days to ensure that glycemia is controlled as usual

**Patients taking insulin**

Preprocedure: take half usual long-acting insulin and no short acting-insulin
Blood glucose is measured prior to procedure—> 120 mg/dl, 5 U Regular insulin
D5/W at 100 ml per hour during procedure
Postprocedure
  Measure blood glucose: >200 mg/dl, 5 U additional short-acting insulin
  Take remainder of morning long-acting insulin, also usual short-acting insulin if not nauseated or vomiting
  Eat breakfast to show tolerance of normal food intake
  Restart usual insulin schedule
  Four-times-per-day blood glucose measurements for next 2 days to ensure that glycemia is controlled as usual

erative period. If insulin is likely to be needed after the procedure, it is important to teach the patient or a family member injection technique ahead of time, and to ensure that they have Regular insulin as well as injection equipment at home. Prefilled insulin pens are particularly convenient for this purpose.

For patients who take insulin, it is recommended that the procedure or test be is scheduled for early morning. Generally, the usual dosage of long-acting insulin is taken the night before, but it can be lowered 10–20% if food intake at supper is less than normal or patient is using glargine. The morning of the procedure, the patient takes half of his or her usual morning dose of long-acting insulin, but *no* short-acting insulin. A blood glucose value is measured prior to the procedure, and a small dosage of Regular insulin (3–5 U) given if more than 120 mg/dl. A D5/W i.v. should be started and run at 100 ml per hour. Once the procedure is finished, and if the patient is not experiencing nausea or vomiting, he or she takes the remainder of his or her morning long-acting insulin and all of the short-acting insulin, is fed, and goes back to his or her usual schedule. Blood glucose should be measured frequently over the next day or two to make sure that glycemia is controlled as usual. On the other hand, if the patient is nauseated after the procedure, the remainder of the long-acting insulin is taken but no short-acting insulin, and it is seen whether the patient tolerates eating without vomiting. If not, Regular insulin is taken every 4–6 hours to keep glycemia below 200 mg/dl until eating habits return to normal.

## The Patient Who Will Undergo Prolonged Surgery That Requires General Anesthesia

Ideal management of the patient who will undergo major surgery is to use an i.v. insulin infusion. In hospitalized patients, it is started the night before and continued through the postsurgery period. For those admitted the day of surgery, the infusion should be started at least 2–3 hours prior to the surgery to allow titration of the infusion to the desired glucose goal. The patient should not be given any subcutaneous insulin during this time because it would obscure the effect of the infusion. Bedside glucose values are performed every hour during the titration and through the surgery to make sure the patient is not hypoglycemic, and to adjust the rate of the infusion to keep the blood glucose in the desired range. The insulin infusion is continued postoperatively until the patient is eating, and then he or she is converted to subcutaneous insulin.

The algorithm in Table 2 works well for this purpose, with some minor variations. The suggested starting infusion rate in Table 2 (1.5 U per hour and up) is for postsurgical or otherwise medically stressed patients. Preoperative needs are generally less. Also, you may not have several hours to determine the steady-state infusion rate. One shortcut is to use the patient's insulin doses from home as a guide to his or her basal needs by taking one-half of the usual total daily insulin dose divided by 24. This is when the $HbA_{1c}$ of the patient is reasonably good (arbitrarily, $<8.5\%$). For example, a patient taking 5–8 units of lispro at meals and 12 units of NPH at breakfast and 8 units of NPH at bedtime with $HbA_{1c}$ of 7.5% would be started at 0.8 U per hour (half of the total dose of $\approx 40$ units divided by 24). In patients with a higher $HbA_{1c}$, it is prudent to increase 25% for $HbA_{1c} < 10\%$, and 50% for $HbA_{1c} \geq 10\%$. In the patient described above but with an $HbA_{1c}$ of 10.2%, the starting infusion rate would be 1.2 U per hour. Blood glucose values are measured hourly (including during the surgery), and the infusion adjusted up or down to keep glycemia at 120–200 mg/dl. If the glucose value drops below 120 mg/dl, the infusion is stopped and the blood glucose measured every 15 minutes until glycemia rises above 120 mg/dl, and then the infusion is restarted at a lower infusion rate. If glycemia falls below 80 mg/dl, 25 ml of 50% dextrose should also be given intravenously.

## CONCLUSIONS

Optimal care of hospitalized individuals with diabetes cannot, and should not, ignore control of their glycemia. Hyperglycemia and insulin deficiency can slow the patient's recovery through dehydration, electrolyte abnormalities, and inducing a catabolic state. Also, mental status, wound healing, gastric emptying, and ability to fight infection can all be impaired. Too often, individuals who as outpatients strive to attain near-normal glycemia through intensive insulin regimens and optimal lifestyle practices are not consulted about their inpatient management. Their blood glucose status may not even be discussed with them. Patients may not understand what is being done, leading to miscommunication with caregivers and a general feeling of mistrust. This can be avoided by discussing with patients ahead of time what effects the surgery, medications, or other aspects of the hospitalization will have on their blood glucose level. Also, reasonable glucose goals for the hospitalization, and plans for diabetes management, should be outlined. Patients are reassured if it is clear that glucose values will be carefully monitored and action taken if the target range is not achieved within a reasonable time period.

Standardized algorithms for subcutaneous and intravenous insulin usage are preferred over sliding-scale coverage, as they are based on titrating the bedside glucose value to a target range believed to provide optimal glycemic control for a successful outcome to the medical problem that caused that patient to be hospitalized. It is time for institutions to move away from sliding scales; they don't work, and too often cause patients to needlessly suffer hypoglycemia or hyperglycemia that may negatively impact their recovery. Their use should be discouraged, and their propagation among medical students and residents stopped.

With critically ill patients with multiple-organ dysfunction, it is understandable that glycemic management may be forgotten. This can be avoided by setting blood glucose goals at the start of the hospitalization that are known by all the patient's caregivers—nurses, dieticians and physicians. Also needed is a system for recording the bedside glucose data in a way that is visible and easy to interpret. Effective communication between services and floors is essential. This is particularly true when transferring patients with diabetes to another service or floor; a fail-safe mechanism must be in place that prevents a prolonged omission of insulin because of failure by the new caregivers to expeditiously implement the insulin program.

Most institutions have access to inpatient diabetes consultants. They should be consulted if the blood glucose target goals are not attained within 48 hours of hospitalization, or if a patient experiences a severe hypoglycemic reaction or hyperglycemic event.

## APPENDIX: INSULIN INFUSION PROTOCOL FROM THE DIGAMI STUDY*

1.  80 U Regular insulin in 500 ml D5/W ($\approx$1 U per 6 ml). Start infusion at 5 U (30 ml) per hour.
2.  Check blood glucose after 1 hour. Adjust infusion rate according to protocol:
    *   270 mg/dl—give 8 units insulin as i.v. bolus and increase infusion by 1 U (6 ml) per hour.
    *   200–269 mg/dl—increase infusion by 0.5 U (3 ml) per hour.
    *   126–199 mg/dl—leave infusion rate unchanged.
    *   72–125 mg/dl—decrease infusion rate by 1 U (6 ml) per hour.
    *   <72 mg/dl—stop infusion for 15 minutes. Test blood glucose and continue testing every 15 minutes until glucose >72 mg/dl. If symptomatic from hypoglycemia, give 20 ml of 30% glucose i.v. The infusion is restarted with a infusion rate decreased by 1 U (6 ml) per hour when glucose $\geq$72 mg/dl.
    *   If fall in blood glucose exceeds 30% but blood glucose is above 200 mg/dl, leave infusion unchanged; if blood glucose is 126–199 mg/dl, decrease infusion rate by 1 U (6 ml) per hour.
3.  Check blood glucose after 1 hour if infusion is changed, otherwise every 2 hours.
4.  If blood glucose is stable at 199 mg/dl after 10 P.M., reduce infusion rate by 50% during the night.

## REFERENCES

1.  Queale WS, Seidler AJ, Brancati FL. Glycemic control and sliding scale insulin use in medical inpatients with diabetes mellitus. Arch Intern Med 157:545–552, 1997.
2.  Malmberg K. DIGAMI (Diabetes Mellitus, Insulin Glucose Infusion in Acute Myocardial Infarction) Study Group. Prospective randomised study of intensive insulin treatment on long term survival after acute myocardial infarction in patients with diabetes mellitus. Br Med J 314:1512–1515, 1997.
3.  Malmberg K, Norhammar A, Wedel H, Ryden L. Glycometabolic state at admission: important risk marker of mortality in conventionally treated patients with diabetes

---

\* From Malmberg KA, Ryden LE, Efendic S. Feasibility of insulin-glucose infusion in diabetic patients with acute myocardial infarction. Diabetes Care 17:1007–1014, 1994.

mellitus and acute myocardial infarction: long-term results from the Diabetes and Insulin-Glucose Infusion in Acute Myocardial Infarction (DIGAMI) study. Circulation 99:2626–2632, 1999.

4. Golden SH, Peart-Vigilance C, Kao WH, Brancati FL. Perioperative glycemic control and the risk of infectious complications in a cohort of adults with diabetes. Diabetes Care 22:1408–1414, 1999.

5. Levetan CS, Magee MF. Hospital management of diabetes. Endocrinol Metab Clin North Am 29:745–770, 2000.

5a. Van Der Berghe G, et al. Intensive insulin therapy in critically ill patients. N Engl J Med 345:1359–1367, 2001.

6. Hirsch IB, Paauw DS, Brunzell J. Inpatient management of adults with diabetes. Diabetes Care 18:870–878, 1995.

7. Lilley SH, Levine GI. Management of hospitalized patients with type 2 diabetes mellitus. Am Fam Physician 57:1079–1088, 1998.

8. Jacober SJ, Sowers JR. An update on perioperative management of diabetes. Arch Intern Med 159:2405–2411, 1999.

9. Gebhart SSP. Inpatient management of diabetes. In: Leahy JL, Clark NG, Cefalu WT, eds. Medical Management of Diabetes Mellitus. New York: Marcel Dekker, pp 615–630, 2000.

10. McMahon MM. Nutritional support in the diabetic patient. In: Leahy JL, Clark NG, Cefalu WT, eds. Medical Management of Diabetes Mellitus. New York: Marcel Dekker, pp 641–654, 2000.

11. Levetan CS, Passaro M, Jablonski K, Kass M, Ratner RE. Unrecognized diabetes among hospitalized patients. Diabetes Care 21:246–249, 1998.

12. Husband DJ, Alberti KG, Julian DG. ''Stress'' hyperglycaemia during acute myocardial infarction: an indicator of pre-existing diabetes? Lancet ii:179–181, 1983.

13. Zimmet P, Turner R, McCarty D, Rowley M, Mackay I. Crucial points at diagnosis: type 2 diabetes or slow type 1 diabetes. Diabetes Care 22(suppl 2):B59–B64, 1999.

14. Capes SE, Hunt D, Malmberg K, Gerstein HC. Stress hyperglycaemia and increased risk of death after myocardial infarction in patients with and without diabetes: a systematic overview. Lancet 355:773–778, 2000.

15. MacMillan DR. The fallacy of insulin adjustment by the sliding scale. J Ky Med Assoc 68:577–579, 1970.

16. MacMillan DR. Insulin adjustment by the sliding scale method—a straw man who won't stay down? J Ky Med Assoc 89:211–212, 1991.

17. Hanish LR. Standardizing regimens for sliding-scale insulin. Am J Health Syst Pharm 54:1046–1047, 1997.

18. Watts NB, Gebhart SP, Clark RV, Phillips LS. Postoperative management of diabetes mellitus: steady-state glucose control with bedside algorithm for insulin adjustment. Diabetes Care 10:722–728, 1987.

19. Scheen A, Castillo M, Jandrain B, Krzentowski G, Henrivaux P, Luyckx AS, Lefebvre PJ. Metabolic alterations after a two-hour nocturnal interruption of a continuous subcutaneous insulin infusion. Diabetes Care 7:338–342, 1984.

20. Gavin LA. Perioperative management of the diabetic patient. Endocrinol Metab Clin North Am 21:457–475, 1992.

21. Fehmann HC, Goke R, Goke B. Cell and molecular biology of the incretin hormones

glucagon-like peptide-I and glucose-dependent insulin releasing polypeptide. Endocr Rev 16:390–410, 1995.

22.   Rosmarin DK, Wardlaw GM, Mirtallo J. Hyperglycemia associated with high, continuous infusion rates of total parenteral nutrition dextrose. Nutr Clin Pract 11:151–156, 1996.

# 12

## Hyperglycemic Emergencies
Diabetic Ketoacidosis and Nonketotic
Hyperosmolar Syndrome

**Muriel H. Nathan**

University of Vermont College of Medicine, Burlington, Vermont

### INTRODUCTION

Ketoacidosis and nonketotic hyperosmolar syndrome are the two most serious hyperglycemic emergencies of diabetes mellitus. Insulin-deficient states most typically lead to diabetic ketoacidosis in those with autoimmune diabetes (type 1) or pancreatic disease, while the hyperglycemic hyperosmolar nonketotic syndrome occurs in the setting of relative, but not absolute, insulin deficiency (type 2 diabetes).

Diabetic ketoacidosis (DKA) is characterized by a high blood glucose level, ketonemia and ketonuria, and metabolic acidosis. The hyperosmolar syndrome entails hyperglycemia and profound dehydration without significant ketoacidosis. The most common term in general use for this syndrome is nonketotic hyperosmolar coma. However, since few patients actually present in coma (<10%), most experts prefer to call this entity nonketotic hyperosmolar syndrome (NKH).

## INCIDENCE AND MORTALITY

### Diabetic Ketoacidosis (1–4)

In 1987, hospital admissions in the United States with a primary diagnosis of DKA were 12.5/1000 and mortality was 0.25/1000 (≈2%) (5). In a European study, 8.6% of 3250 patients with type 1 diabetes had been admitted to the hospital for DKA one or more times in the previous year (6). In 1995, the incidence of DKA in the United States was 4.6–8 episodes/1000 diabetic patients (7). However, surveys of hospital admissions probably underestimate the incidence of DKA because most mild cases are treated in emergency rooms or ambulatory care centers. Although most episodes of DKA occur in children or young adults with type I diabetes, DKA is increasingly being found in children in nonwhite populations with a high incidence of type 2 diabetes, as well as in adults with a prior diagnosis of type 2 diabetes (8,9).

Deaths during episodes of DKA are rarely due to the hyperglycemia and metabolic changes associated with poorly controlled diabetes *per se*, but rather because of associated catastrophic illnesses such as sepsis or cardiovascular events. Patients older than 65 have a much higher risk of death in DKA; their mortality rate is 20% compared with less than 2% in younger individuals (10). A rare but often fatal complication of DKA in children and young adults is cerebral edema, which occurs in 0.7–1% of DKA episodes (11). *In summary, all persons above 65 years of age or those younger than age 5 with DKA should be considered high-risk patients. Furthermore, during treatment of DKA, careful bedside assessment at regular intervals is mandatory since deterioration in mental status is viewed as a medical emergency.*

### Nonketotic Hyperosmolar Syndrome (12)

In comparison with DKA, most surveys show fewer episodes of NKH although it may be underreported because of difficulties in recognizing this syndrome. In one survey of nearly 5000 adult urban blacks hospitalized for diabetes between 1993 and 1994, 156 patients met the criteria for moderate or severe DKA and 23 had NKH (8). Another urban center reported a frequency of 17.5/100,000 person-years for NKH while DKA was 14/100,000 person-years (13). Because DKA and NKH represent a continuum of hyperglycemic decompensation, patients can present with a mixture of the two; a review of admissions to a large city hospital found pure NKH in 32% of patients with uncontrolled diabetes, and mixed hyperosmolarity and ketoacidosis in another 18% (14).

The reported mean age of patients with NKH is 57–69 years. Newly diagnosed diabetes is present in 33–60%. NKH can occur during hospitalization for other illnesses, and in one study 18% of cases were transferred from skilled nursing facilities (15). *To increase recognition and reporting of this diabetic emer-*

*gency, clinicians should think of it when evaluating any elderly patient with men-*
*tal-status changes or obtundation.*

The reported mortality rate in NKH varies from 10 to 60%; reviews done
in the past 15 years report a rate of 10–17% (16,17). Because the syndrome may
go unrecognized, mortality from NKH is likely underreported; instead, death may
be attributed to a complication of the syndrome such as thromboembolism or cardiovascular failure. The risk of death is higher with a serum osmolarity of greater
than 340 mOsm/kg. Death within the first 72 hours of treatment is mostly because
of progressive shock or cardiovascular failure; later mortality is usually due to
thromboembolic events. The risk of thromboembolism is increased in the presence
of dehydration, increased blood viscosity, and coagulation abnormalities.

## PATHOGENESIS

Tissues in the body can be classified according to whether they take up glucose
through insulin-mediated (''insulin-sensitive'') or insulin-independent (''insulin-
insensitive'') mechanisms. Figure 1 depicts the metabolism of glucose, amino
acids, and fatty acids in the major insulin-sensitive tissues (liver, muscle, and
fat) in the fed state, during fasting, and during DKA. Also shown is brain, which
is insulin-insensitive. Glucose is an essential fuel for the brain. Having a glucose-
uptake system that is unregulated by insulin means constant fuel availability
whether in feast or famine, which is mandatory for survival. In contrast, states
of fuel deprivation, such as prolonged fasting, require the other tissues' fuel needs
to be met from endogenous sources, e.g., the adipose tissue. This is accomplished
through hormonal shifts—a fall in the circulating insulin level and increases in
the counterregulatory hormones catecholamines, glucagon, and cortisol —that
promote lipolysis, and also alter intermediary metabolism in the insulin-sensitive
tissues to fat metabolism. Additional effects of the counterregulatory hormones
are to increase glycogenolysis and gluconeogenesis by the liver (increased glucose production), inhibit glucose uptake into muscle (decreased peripheral utilization), and cause the liver to metabolize the liberated fatty acids to ketones (become ketogenic). This array of effects is normally kept in perfect balance by
feedback loops in which ketones and hyperglycemia are potent stimuli for insulin
secretion. Consequently, during fasting exactly enough insulin is produced so
that glucose production is enhanced and glucose utilization is lowered to preserve
normoglycemia—i.e., not too little, causing hypoglycemia, or too much so that
hyperglycemia occurs. Also, the production of ketones is controlled so that ''starvation ketonuria,'' not ketoacidosis, is observed.

In DKA, the profound insulin deficiency of type 1 diabetes allows the system to spiral out of control. Hyperglycemia occurs, causing an osmotic diuresis
and eventual dehydration, which further raises the levels of the catecholamine
hormones. The results are:

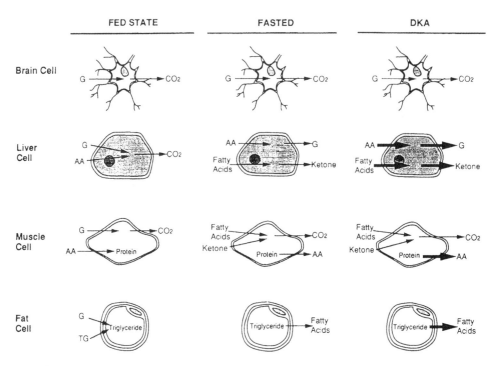

FIGURE 1   Metabolism of glucose, amino acids, and fatty acids in the fed state, during fasting, and during DKA. Insulin-insensitive tissue (brain) is compared with insulin-sensitive tissues (liver, muscle, and fat). G = glucose; AA = amino acids; TG = triglycerides. (Adapted from Cahill GF. Pathophysiology of diabetes. In: Hamwi GJ, Danowski TS, eds. Diabetes Mellitus: Diagnosis and Treatment. New York: American Diabetes Association, pp 1–6, 1967.)

- Hyperglycemia—primarily from enhanced gluconeogenesis, but also increased glycogen breakdown in the liver and lack of glucose uptake/metabolism by muscle and fat
- Dehydration—from the osmotic diuresis, which leads to progressive loss of fluid and electrolytes
- Ketoacidosis/ketonuria—the increased lipolysis results in increased liberation of free fatty acids, which are converted by the liver to ketones because of the raised counterregulatory hormones and lowered insulin that make the liver ketogenic

In NKH, insulin is deficient but less so than in DKA (relative insulin deficiency). Also, the counterregulatory hormones are increased, but not as much as in DKA (12). Normally the circulating levels of insulin required to control glucose production and utilization are much higher than those needed to inhibit lipolysis. Thus, the net result of this hormonal milieu is hyperglycemia without fatty-acid conversion to ketones. Because it is ketoacidosis-related symptoms in DKA (abdominal pain, vomiting, perceived shortness of breath, large ketones on their home urinary measurements) that often cause patients to seek medical help, the lack of significant ketonemia in NKH means the typical presentation is:

- Severe dehydration—because of the absence of ketonemia symptoms, the clinical picture is more subtle than that of DKA so the prodromal period is typically longer than in DKA. The lengthy duration of the osmotic diuresis results in severe dehydration. Further, lack of access to water, such as by bedbound nursing home patients, often exacerbates this problem.
- Profound hyperglycemia—the mechanisms for hyperglycemia are the same as in DKA: the relative insulin deficiency and excess counterregulatory hormones. However, the glycemia levels in NKH are typically higher than in DKA because of the profound dehydration, which diminishes or eliminates glycosuria, after which glycemia rises rapidly.
- Hyperosmolarity—a consequence of the profound dehydration and greater hyperglycemia is a markedly raised serum osmolarity, which may cause mental-status changes or coma.

## CLINICAL FEATURES

### Dehydration and Electrolyte Losses

The cause of dehydration in both DKA and NKH is the osmotic diuresis that is brought about by the excess serum glucose being excreted in the urine. Excess sodium, chloride, and potassium are lost from the polyuria. Fluid and electrolyte deficits per kilogram of body weight in DKA are typically 100 ml water, 7–10 mEq $Na^+$, 3–5 mEq $K^+$, and 5–7 mEq $Cl^-$ (see Table 1); this is equivalent to a 10% loss of body weight. In the later stages, if volume depletion is sufficient to lower the glomerular filtration rate, and consequently glycosuria, the blood glucose level rises precipitously—this effect is especially pronounced in NKH.

**TABLE 1** Fluid and Electrolyte Deficits

|                     | DKA     | NKH     |
|---------------------|---------|---------|
| Water (ml/kg)       | 100     | 100–200 |
| Sodium (mEq/kg)     | 7–10    | 5–13    |
| Potassium (mEq/kg)  | 3–5     | 5–15    |
| Chloride (mEq/kg)   | 3–5     | 3–7     |
| Phosphorus (mM/kg)  | 1–1.5   | 1–2     |

## Relatively Preserved Intravascular Volume

The average fluid deficit in DKA of 100 ml/kg exceeds the normal intravascular volume. The loss may be even greater in NKH. However, patients rarely present in cardiovascular collapse. This is because the intravascular glucose osmotically pulls water from the intracellular compartment, thereby preserving intravascular volume. Thus, the clinical volume status of the patient underrepresents his or her true level of hydration. *A key point in the management of DKA and NKH is that vascular collapse can occur if therapy is given to correct the hyperglycemia (insulin) without aggressive expansion of the intravascular space with fluid.*

## Hyponatremia

The osmotic activity of the intravascular glucose in DKA and NKH expands the intravascular compartment with intracellular fluid that is rich in $K^+$ and low in $Na^+$ so the plasma sodium is diluted. The following formula is used to correct for this dilution: for every 100-mg/dl rise in plasma glucose above the normal 100 mg/dl, serum sodium decreases by 1.6 mEq/L. For example, a plasma glucose of 700 mg/dl with a serum sodium of 128 mEq/L implies a ''true'' sodium of 138 mEq/L.

## Potassium Depletion

In DKA and NKH, potassium loss is usually 5 mEq/kg body weight and can be as high as 10 mEq/kg. One cause is the osmotic drag of the potassium-rich intracellular fluid into the vascular space, coupled with the relative or absolute lack of insulin to shift potassium back intracellularly. An additional effect in DKA is the acidosis-mediated exchange of intravascular hydrogen ions with intracellular potassium, which further increases the flux of potassium out of cells into the vascular space. Urinary excretion of the potassium leads to whole-body potassium depletion. Thus, in DKA, the serum potassium level is not an accurate indicator of body potassium stores. A useful formula to correct for the pH-related exchange of vascular $H^+$ and cellular $K^+$ is: for every 0.1 change in pH from 7.4, serum potassium changes in the opposite direction by 0.8 mEq/L. For example, a blood sample with a pH of 7.1 and a serum potassium of 5.0 mEq/L implies a ''true'' potassium of 2.6 mEq/L.

## Metabolic Acidosis: Increased Anion Gap

In DKA, acidosis evolves when there is inadequate buffering of the ketoacids. The $H^+$ ions are first buffered by intravacular (mostly bicarbonate) and intracellular anions. Ketones are also eliminated in the urine, although this diminishes as dehydration causes the glomerular filtration to fall. When the buffering capacity is outpaced by the ketogenesis, metabolic acidosis occurs. The excess ketoacids (β-hydroxybutyrate and acetoacetate) in the serum cause the anion gap to increase, which is calculated by subtracting the sum of the serum chloride ($Cl^-$) and bicarbonate ($HCO_3^-$) from the sodium ($Na^+$) concentration. The normal anion gap is $12 \pm 2$ mEq/L, which represents the normal quantity of unmeasured anions.

## Hypertonicity

Effective osmolarity (effective Osm = 2 (Na + K) + glucose/18) rather than total osmolarity (total Osm = 2 (Na + K) + glucose/18 + BUN/2.8) is most important in regulating cell volume, and consequently the brain-cell shrinkage that underlies the confusion and obtundation in NKH. The osmotically active substances in the body include those that freely pass through cell membranes such as urea and alcohols, and those that are impermeable and require transport mechanisms such as $Na^+$, $K^+$, glucose, and mannitol. Excess osmotic substances that are freely permeable—e.g., urea—do not cause shifts of intracellular volume out of brain cells because of the lack of an osmotic gradient across the cell membrane. Hence, renal failure elevates serum osmolarity without changing the mental state of the patient. In contrast, rises in serum tonicity (also called "effective osmolarity") from increased levels of impermeable substances such as $Na^+$, $K^+$, and glucose shift intracellular volume out of brain cells, and in extreme form cause confusion, obtundation, or coma.

It is important to understand that, while uncontrolled diabetes causes hypertonicity, very large elevations in glucose are needed to cause the degree of hypertonicity required for clinically evident alterations in brain function (340 mOsm/L). This is because the osmotic contribution of glucose is only 5.5 mOsm/L for every 100-mg/dl elevation in glucose. In comparison, sodium adds 2 mOsm/L for every 1-mEq/L increase. Thus, blood glucose levels of more than 1000 mg/dl are typically required for the hyperosmolar syndrome. Also, in many patients, dehydration is a major contributory factor through relative or absolute increases in the serum sodium.

## DIAGNOSIS AND INITIAL EVALUATION

### Diabetic Ketoacidosis

Precipitants of DKA include new onset of disease, pneumonia or urinary-tract or other infections, omission of insulin in patients with poor access to medical care or supplies, or those lacking in diabetes education about "sick-day rules," and occasionally psychological factors such as fear of weight gain or hypoglycemia (18). Presenting features of DKA (Table 2) are polyuria, polydipsia, nausea and vomiting, hyperventilation, and abdominal pain. Despite the common usage some years ago of the term diabetic coma for DKA, profound mental-status

TABLE 2  Signs and Symptoms of DKA

Polyuria, polydipsia, and polyphagia
Weight loss
Abdominal pain, nausea, and vomiting
Drowsiness or profound lethargy; coma is rare
Rapid, deep respirations (Kussmaul)
Fruity breath, poor skin turgor, dry mucous
  membranes
Tachycardia and hypotension
Blood glucose is usually 400–500 mg/dl

changes are unusual. The ketonemia is likely responsible for the abdominal pain
and nausea, but hypokalemia can also worsen gastroparesis and cause an ileus.
Clinical findings include dehydration and orthostatic or overt hypotension, Kussmaul respiration (deep, sighing hyperventilation), tachycardia, warm skin, and
occasionally confusion or coma. Hyperventilation, which is more obvious when
the pH is less than 7.2, is a respiratory compensation for the metabolic acidosis.
There may be symptoms and signs of sepsis and shock.

The definitive diagnosis of DKA consists of: 1) hyperglycemia (>250 mg/
dl), 2) low serum bicarbonate (<15 mEq/L), and 3) low pH (<7.3) with 4) ketonemia (positive minimally at 1:2 dilution). Urinary ketones are more variable,
as discussed below. Virtually all patients have an increased anion gap. Many
patients will have a high white-blood-cell count, usually with a left shift, but
typically less than 25,000/mm$^3$ unless there is a coexistent bacterial infection.
The presence of pneumonia may be difficult to confirm until the patient is better
hydrated. Also, serum amylase is often transiently elevated, and serum BUN and
creatinine are usually raised because of the dehydration.

Initial evaluation consists of blood chemistries, glucose by fingerstick,
blood and urine ketones by nitroprusside reaction, complete blood cell counts
with differential, arterial blood gases, and urinalysis. Patients with DKA often
have low serum sodium (osmotic-induced dilution) and normal to high potassium
($H^+$–$K^+$ exchange) levels. It is important to note that the diagnosis of DKA is
not dependent on finding a serum glucose of 400 mg/dl or higher, a common
misconception of many clinicians. Glycemia levels are often lower in pregnant
women or in those who have been unable to eat, have been vomiting, or took
insulin in the prodromal phase. A careful physical examination is performed,
looking for evidence of infection. This is followed by infusion of a liter of 0.9%
NaCl while the bacterial cultures, when appropriate, and EKG are obtained to
evaluate possible precipitating factors. Transferring the patient before stabilization for noninvasive or invasive procedures should be avoided if possible. Treat-

TABLE 3   Treatment Stages of DKA and NKH

Volume restoration (hours 0–12)
   Improve circulating volume and tissue perfusion
   Correct electrolyte abnormalities, particularly potassium
   Lower blood glucose by promoting glucosuria and by giving insulin
Treatment of underlying cause (hours 12–48)
   Restoration of tonicity to normal
   Correction of acid–base imbalance
   Avoid hypoglycemia by supplying glucose when blood sugar is around
     250 mg/dl
Excretion and metabolism of excessive ketoacids with replacement of wa-
   ter and electrolytes
   Start subcutaneous insulin regimen, meeting the basal and meal require-
    ments
   Avoid hypoglycemia and recurrence of hyperglycemia or ketoacidosis
   Emphasize outpatient "sick-day rules" to avoid hyperglycemic emergen-
    cies

ment goals for DKA are to: 1) improve circulatory volume and tissue perfusion, 2) correct electrolyte abnormalities, 3) decrease serum glucose, and 4) excrete or metabolize the excess serum ketoacids (see Table 3).

## Measurement of Urinary Ketones

The ketone bodies acetoacetate, acetone, and β-hydroxybutyrate are formed during periods of insulin deficiency by hepatic fatty-acid oxidation. Bedside measurements of urinary or blood ketones are usually done by the nitroprusside method, which detects acetoacetate and acetone, but *not* β-hydroxybutyrate. The ratio of β-hydroxybutyrate to acetoacetate is elevated by coexisting lactic acidosis—possible causes are sepsis, tissue necrosis, or other catastrophic causes for the DKA, but mostly the dehydration of DKA alone is causative—which makes the urinary ketone measurement by test strip underrepresent the degree of ketosis, i.e., 1+ or 2+ positive when profound ketoacidosis is present. A few drops of hydrogen peroxide can be added to the urine to convert "unmeasurable" β-hydroxybutyrate to the measurable acetoacetate. This concept also underlies the common clinical confusion of an apparent worsening of a patient's ketosis based on urinary ketone measurements when by all other clinical parameters the patient is improving. This is most frequently seen after starting aggressive volume repletion. The explanation is reversal of the dehydration-induced lactic acidosis which converts β-hydroxybutyrate to acetoacetate, causing a seemingly "paradoxical" increase in the measured ketones by the nitroprusside reaction. Thus, venous pH, serum glucose, and bicarbonate levels are evaluated during therapy. Ketones are measured initially to confirm the diagnosis of DKA, and at the end of therapy to confirm that the patient is relatively free of ketonuria and ready to be put back on subcutaneous insulin.

## Nonketotic Hyperosmolar Syndrome

In contrast to the onset of DKA, NKH is often insidious and typically entails several days of polyuria, deteriorating glycemic control, and eventual lethargy. Common precipitants are infection, myocardial infarction or stroke, medications (e.g., diuretics, beta-blockers, phenytoin, or glucocorticoids), initiation of hyper-alimentation, and alcohol or cocaine abuse (4,12).

Signs of NKH are those of profound dehydration. Patients have dry mucous membranes, absent sweating, and poor skin turgor, as well as postural or overt hypotension. Cardiac and respiratory examinations are typically normal in the absence of pneumonia. Tachypnea, hypotension or fever may indicate a gram-negative infection. The gastroparesis that is often present is due to the hypertonic state; thus, nausea and vomiting may not necessarily mean that an underlying gastrointestinal illness precipitated the event.

Neurological symptoms are common and can consist of focal findings that mimic a cerebrovascular accident to frank coma. The cause of coma is not known, but it is postulated that dehydration, loss of brain-cell volume, changes in neuro-transmitter levels, and microvascular ischemia are all operative (12). Lethargy and confusion are more common than frank coma, which usually does not occur unless the plasma osmolarity is 340 mOsm/L or greater. Most patients with coma have a relative or absolute increase in serum sodium along with their hyperglyce-mia, causing the increased osmolarity. If focal or diffuse mental-status changes persist after hydration, CNS lesions or infection should be suspected. Seizures occur in 25% of patients and can be focal. NKH-related seizures may be resistant to anticonvulsant therapy. Phenytoin should be used with caution as it may exac-erbate hyperglycemia by inhibiting insulin release. Cerebral edema is rare and is almost always due to rapid overcorrection of blood glucose or large amounts of insulin being given with large amounts of hypotonic fluids.

NKH is characterized by extreme fluid and electrolyte depletion with total body water losses of 22–25% (i.e., considerably in excess of those in DKA). The more profound water loss in NKH is due to a longer prodromal period and limited access to water for many of the patients. Osmotic diuresis leads to hypotonic fluid loss, with electrolyte losses equivalent to roughly one-half of the water loss. Remember to correct the serum $Na^+$ for the osmotic effect of the hyperglycemia (1.6-mEq/L change for each 100-mg/dl increase in glucose). Thus, a patient with severe hyperglycemia from NKH with a normal or elevated serum sodium at diagnosis has had massive water loss. Also, $K^+$ loss may be exacerbated by diuretic use. A mild metabolic acidosis may be present (pH >7.3), owing to the accumulation of lactate from hypoperfusion or uremic acids from dehydration which initially can be confused for DKA (lack of ketones in the blood and urine helps to differentiate these). A mixed ketoacidosis and NKH (pH <7.3, strongly positive serum acetone, and effective osmolarity >320 mOsm/L) may occur in as many as 33% of patients with uncontrolled diabetes.

Other serum markers may be abnormal during NKH, including liver transaminases, LDH, and CPK-MM; these changes are transient and due to dehydration. Hypercholesterolemia and hypertriglyceridemia are usually present. There may be mild elevations of the albumin, amylase, bilirubin, calcium, total protein, SGOT, SGPT, and BUN. Leukocytosis with elevated granulocytes is common, and may not imply infection but rather is a response to stress and dehydration, with white-blood-cell counts usually 12,000–15,000. Hemoglobin and hematocrit are also elevated because of dehydration.

## Differential Diagnosis

It is usually not difficult to differentiate among the different causes of diabetic coma. Whereas acidosis causes a negative inotropic effect and peripheral vasodilatation such that patients in DKA often have warm skin, those in NKH have normal skin temperature, higher blood glucose levels, and more profound dehydration, with no or trace ketones in the blood. Alternatively, hypoglycemic coma can be distinguished by the lower blood glucose (usually less than 50 mg/dl) and the presence of cold and clammy extremities. If there is any doubt as to the cause of coma, 20 ml of 50% glucose can be given intravenously. Other causes of acidosis with an increased anion gap include lactic acidosis, uremia, and ingestion of salicylates or methanol. However, these are generally easily differentiated from DKA by the serum glycemia and serum/urine ketones being minimally elevated, if at all.

## TREATMENT (1–4,12,18)

### Hydration

*DKA*

- 1 liter of 0.9% saline in the first hour. Continue this rate for an additional hour if hypotension is not corrected or urine flow is less than 50–100 ml/hr.
- Subsequent fluid therapy is 0.45% NaCl at 250–500 ml/hr, adjusting the rate for renal losses, plasma sodium, and clinical response.

*NKH*

- 1 liter of 0.9% saline per hour until blood pressure, pulse, and urine output improve.
- Subsequent fluid therapy is 0.45% NaCl at 250–500 ml/hr, adjusting the rate for renal losses, plasma sodium, and clinical response. Replace one-half of the free water deficit in the first 12 hours and the remainder over the next 24 hours.
- Central vein pressure measurement, cardiovascular monitoring, and/or dialysis as clinically indicated.

Numerous studies have demonstrated the safety and efficacy of giving hydration therapy in the treatment of DKA and NKH before initiation of insulin therapy. This chapter has also emphasized the importance of early rehydration to avoid vascular collapse when the excess blood glucose is excreted or moves intracellularly. Fluids are administered to restore normal circulatory volume and consequently tissue perfusion, reverse lactic acidosis, augment urinary glucose excretion, and decrease concentrations of the counterregulatory hormones. Indeed, much of the lowering of blood glucose that occurs during the first few hours of therapy is from urinary glucose excretion, not cellular uptake.

Initial fluid therapy should be isotonic saline because this fluid more rapidly corrects plasma volume than hypotonic fluid does. For most patients with DKA, 10% dehydration is common, and 1 liter of 0.9% saline is given in the first hour. This rate is continued for an additional hour if hypotension is not corrected or urine flow is less than 50–100 ml/hr. If the patient is in shock, colloids can also be used, as these are retained in the intravascular space. Dehydration is judged by the physical examination (postural blood-pressure changes, tachycardia, poor skin turgor, lack of sweating, dry mucous membranes), corrected sodium concentration, and the calculated effective plasma osmolarity. Corrected sodium concentrations of greater than 140 mEq/L or calculated osmolalities of greater than 340 mOsm/kg are associated with the largest fluid deficits.

In NKH, 0.9% saline is also used at 1 liter per hour until blood pressure, pulse, and urine output improve. Patients with coexisting cardiac or renal disease or those requiring large fluid volumes may need central vein pressure measurements to avoid under- or overhydration.

After hypotension has been corrected by the use of isotonic saline and vital signs are stable, subsequent fluid therapy is given as hypotonic saline (0.45% NaCl) at 250–500 ml/hr, adjusting the rate for renal losses, plasma sodium, and clinical response. Remember that the osmotic diuresis will continue until the hyperglycemia is reversed. This combined with the substantial initial fluid deficit means that large amounts of fluid are typically given for many hours.

The greatest danger to the patient with NKH is hypovolemia causing progressive shock or thromboembolism. Volume restoration is essential. Initial fluid replacement is 1–2 liters in the first 2 hours of treatment, then 7–9 liters over the next 2–3 days since the fluid deficit is usually 20–25% of body stores. Isotonic fluid replacement is generally recommended because rapid correction of hypernatremia can lead to diffuse myelinolysis and death. Once the effective arterial blood volume has been restored, as reflected by reversal of orthostasis and good urine output, the intravenous fluid is changed to 0.45% saline; one-half of the free water deficit is replaced in the first 12 hours and the remainder over the next 24 hours. Colloids are not recommended as they can contribute to elevated plasma viscosity. Many of these patients have a prior history of renal insufficiency, and there is always concern that anuria or oliguria during the aggressive fluid resuscitation will cause congestive heart failure or adult respiratory distress syndrome. In most cases, cardiovascular monitoring and dialysis may be necessary. On the other hand, a prior history of coronary or renal disease does not obviate the need for substantial fluid replacement in most patients.

## Insulin

### DKA and NKH

- 10–20 units Regular insulin i.v. push
- Continuous intravenous infusion 0.1 U/kg/hr Regular insulin, which in adults is 6–10 U/hr. If no improvement in anion gap, pH, and hyperglycemia is noted within 2 hours, the hourly insulin dosage is doubled each hour until clinical effect is seen.
- If necessary, can substitute s.q. injections 0.3–0.4 U/kg of Regular or lispro insulin, followed by 5–10 units each hour.

While fluids restore organ perfusion, reverse dehydration, and allow a fall in blood glucose by promoting urinary excretion, insulin is required to correct the metabolic derangement of DKA and reverse the acidosis and ketone production. For moderate to severe DKA (bicarbonate less than 10), Regular insulin is given intravenously as a continuous infusion of 0.1 U/kg/hr; 6–10 U/hr is generally given. If the anion gap and venous pH have not improved within 2 hours, the dose is doubled every hour until clinical improvement occurs. It is often suggested that a minimum hourly decrement in the blood glucose level of 60–90 mg/dl is the parameter to follow in order to show adequate response to therapy. However, it must be remembered that fluid therapy alone can cause a rapid decline in glycemia, so seeing an improvement in the anion gap and pH are more important clinical indicators of successful therapy. In situations in which intravenous insulin cannot be given, s.q. injections of 0.3–0.4 U/kg of Regular or lispro insulin can be given, followed by 5–10 units each hour (19). Experts differ on whether to use a loading dose before starting continuous i.v. insulin infusion. Our practice is to give 10–20 units Regular insulin i.v. push, which allows up to an hour before starting the continuous infusion for transfer to the ward, diagnostic tests, etc.

These recommended dosages of $\approx 10$ U/hr have been referred to as low-dose therapy, as opposed to the 50–100 U/1–2 hours (high-dose therapy) that were routinely given until the mid-1980s. In comparative studies, low-dose insulin therapy led to less hypokalemia and hypoglycemia (20,21), and is standard practice today.

There is more confusion among practitioners over insulin therapy for NKH. Many believe the absence of ketosis indicates that less insulin is needed to reverse the hyperglycemia, and that the standard doses of insulin used in DKA are dangerous in NKH. In reality, large insulin doses are generally needed because most of the patients have type 2 diabetes (and have pre-existing insulin resistance), and the common precipitating factors of infection, myocardial infection, and sepsis require large insulin doses. Most experts recommend the same insulin doses for DKA and NKH.

## Potassium

### DKA

- If serum $K^+$ is less than 3.5 mEq/L and pH is less than 7.3 initially, place 20–40 mEq KCl in the first liter i.v. fluids to be administered with cardiac monitoring. Otherwise begin intravenous KCl in second i.v. bag.
- Start oral potassium repletion as soon as the patient is tolerating oral fluids. Diuretic users and alcohol abusers may also need magnesium replacement.
- Check serum potassium every 1–2 hours, and add 20–40 mEq KCl to each liter of i.v. fluids if it is less than 5.5 mEq/L and the patient is urinating.

### NKH

- Start oral potassium repletion as soon as the patient is tolerating oral fluids. Diuretic users and alcohol abusers may also need magnesium replacement.
- Check serum potassium every 1–2 hours, and add 20–40 mEq KCl to each liter of i.v. fluids if it is less than 5.5 mEq/L and the patient is urinating.

After starting hydration and insulin treatment in DKA, there is a rapid decline in potassium—particularly in the first 3 hours—which can be life-threatening if not aggressively managed. Most of the decline is due to the increase in pH that reverses the exchange of serum $H^+$ for intracellular $K^+$, and the beginning of insulin-mediated re-entry of potassium with glucose into the intracellular compartment. Nonetheless, potassium is typically not added to the first liter of 0.9% saline that is given within the first hour unless the patient is hypokalemic, because most patients are normokalemic or even hyperkalemic secondary to the acidosis. Replacing potassium when the fluid is being rapidly administered may dangerously increase serum potassium and precipitate cardiac arrhythmias. With subsequent fluid therapy, serum potassium is checked every 1–2 hours, and if it is less than 5.5 mEq/L and the patient is urinating, 20–40 mEq $K^+$ given as KCl is added to each liter. Occasionally potassium phosphate is used in one of the i.v. bags, as discussed below. The goal is to maintain the $K^+$ between 4.0 and 5.0 mEq/L.

Patients who present in DKA with low or normal $K^+$ levels in the face of acidosis have the greatest total body potassium deficit and should be viewed as being at high risk. Insulin therapy without aggressive potassium replacement can lead to profound hypokalemia as the acidosis reverses, which can induce life-threatening arrhythmias, respiratory muscle weakness, and cardiovascular collapse. These patients should receive potassium in the first liter of fluid, with the rate of intravenous administration never to exceed 40 mEq/hr, and cardiac monitoring. Patients who are not nauseated and are able to drink fluids can receive potassium supplements orally.

Total body potassium losses in NKH are also large. However, the absence of acidosis means that acute falls in serum potassium during the first few hours of therapy are less likely than in DKA. Also, the possibility of concomitant renal or cardiovascular disease in these patients requires a more conservative approach to potassium repletion, relying heavily on oral replacement as well as intravenous replacement.

## Bicarbonate

### DKA

- If serum pH is less than 6.9, give 2 ampoules bicarbonate (88 mEq).
- If serum pH is 6.9–7.0, give 1 ampoule bicarbonate (44 mEq).
- Otherwise, bicarbonate is not recommended.

Bicarbonate is generally not recommended for DKA unless there is life-threatening acidosis. Retrospective and prospective studies have shown no benefit in clinical outcomes such as time to correction of hyperglycemia, morbidity, or mortality with bicarbonate therapy (22–24). Instead, the use of alkali may be counterproductive because it can acutely cause hypokalemia as well as paradoxical central nervous system acidosis.

Most authors suggest using bicarbonate in the treatment of DKA if the pH is under 7.0. For pH 6.9–7.0, 44 mEq of sodium bicarbonate is recommended; when the pH is less than 6.9, 88 mEq sodium bicarbonate is used. These amounts are intended not to fully correct the acidosis but to stabilize the patient from immediate life-threatening effects of the acidosis until the fluid and insulin therapy can be started. Indeed, during therapy the metabolism of ketones regenerates bicarbonate. Previous usage of exogenous bicarbonate can result in an overcorrected pH and alkalosis once the ketoacidosis has been fully corrected, which underlies the caution to use it only if needed, and in small amounts. It is also recommended that 15 mEq KCl be given with each ampoule (44 mEq) of bicarbonate to avoid hypokalemia.

## Phosphorus

### DKA

- With severe hypophosphatemia ($<1.0$ mg/dl), replace one-third of potassium deficit as potassium phosphate.
- Otherwise, use is optional. Many experts recommend 30 mmol of potassium phosphate (44 mEq $K^+$) instead of KCl in one of the i.v. bags for adults.
- Not indicated without severe hypophosphatemia.

Phosphate is an intracellular ion that shifts to the extracellular compartment during DKA, so serum levels initially are usually normal or increased. Phosphate, like glucose and potassium, re-enters the intracellular compartment during insulin therapy, resulting in a rather dramatic fall 6–12 hours after beginning therapy. Arguments have been made for the replacement of phosphorus during DKA based on the known effects of severe hypophosphatemia: respiratory depression, skeletal muscle weakness, hemolytic anemia, and cardiac dysfunction. A further concern is depletion of 2,3-diphosphoglycerate (2,3-DPG) altering the $O_2$ dissociation curve such that tissue oxygen delivery is impaired. Counterarguments are that the loss of phosphorus during DKA represents only a small portion of the body stores, plus case reports, mostly in small children with DKA, that show a risk of hypocalcemia, tetany, and soft-tissue calcification with phosphate replacement (25). Furthermore, clinical studies have generally shown no clinical benefit of phosphorus replacement in DKA (26,27). Regardless, many experts recommend 30 mmol of potassium phosphate (44 mEq $K^+$) instead of KCl in one of the i.v. bags for adults to prevent the marked hypophosphatemia that is sometimes seen in DKA. In contrast, there is little indication for its use in NKH in the absence of severe hypophosphatemia.

## GENERAL MANAGEMENT

Clinical monitoring during treatment of DKA and NKH involves taking postural blood pressure and pulse, tracking urine flow, jugular-vein distention, and auscultation of heart and lungs for signs of fluid overload. Nasogastric intubation may be needed for those with nausea and vomiting or obtundation. It is recommended that the clinical and laboratory data be properly recorded in a flowsheet and logged into the medical chart for easy access. Blood glucose determinations should be done hourly, especially to detect the unusual patients who do not respond to 0.1 U/kg/hr. Once the acute situation has passed, fingerstick glucose measurements are continued at least every 4 hours until full recovery and the patient is back on subcutaneous insulin. Similar guidelines are followed for electrolytes, particularly potassium. Electrolytes are checked every 2 hours until the emergent situation has passed, then every 4–6 hours until full recovery. After the initial arterial blood gas, venous blood can be used to follow the pH because it is easier to obtain, and less painful for the patient. Venous pH is about 0.03 lower than the arterial pH.

Intravenous fluid is generally hypotonic after the initial first liter of 0.9% NaCl. The average amount of fluid given during the first 6–8 hours is about 5 liters. Overzealous hydration can lead to edema, congestive heart failure, or adult respiratory distress syndrome. Antibiotics are often used because many cases of NKH and DKA are precipitated by infections, although their use should not be considered routine. Low-grade fever is often seen in NKH, and leukocytosis is common in both DKA and NKH. Thus, it is appropriate to look for clear evidence of infection before beginning antibiotic coverage. It is also prudent to withhold anticoagulation for the first 1–2 days to allow gastroparesis to remit (when present, it increases the risk of GI bleeding with heparin). Prophylactic heparin given subcutaneously (5000 units every 12 hours) should be used if prolonged bed rest is likely.

The range of time needed for the reversal of DKA depends to a large extent on the initial degree of metabolic derangement. Recovery is defined as blood glucose under 200 mg/dl, bicarbonate over 15 mEq/L, pH greater than 7.3, and ketonemia negative at 1:2 dilution. For a patient with an initial glucose of 800 mg/dl, bicarbonate less than 10 mEq/L, and pH under 7.1, it should take about 7.5 hours for the blood glucose to reach 200–250 mg/dl as the insulin therapy generally lowers the blood glucose at a rate of 80 mg/dl/hr. It takes longer for bicarbonate and pH to reach their recovery levels—often twice the time, or about 15 hours. It is thus necessary to continue the insulin infusion for several hours after reaching the target glucose level (200–250 mg/dl), albeit at a lower dose (0.05 U/kg/hr) to ensure full correction of the excess ketoacid production and acidosis. This is done by substituting D5-0.9% NaCl or D5-0.45% NaCl for the intravenous saline solution to prevent hypoglycemia.

In NKH, obtunded or comatose patients usually have a serum osmolality greater than 340 mOsm/kg. Thus, an obtunded patient with an osmolality less than 340 mOsm/kg should be evaluated for CNS lesions, drug intoxication, sepsis, hypercalcemia, or other coexisting illnesses to account for the change in mental status. A patient with obtundation due to DKA needs at least as much time to fully clear the sensorium as for normalization of serum bicarbonate.

The half-life of insulin given intravenously is only 5–10 minutes, so any interruption in insulin delivered by this method can lead to recurrence of DKA.

Often this occurs when the patient is changed from intravenous insulin to subcutaneous insulin, because of delays either in writing the orders during transfer from the intensive care setting to the general ward or in getting the doses, or because of underdosing, in particular when long-acting insulin preparations like NPH make up the majority of the subcutaneous insulin. To prevent recurrence of hyperglycemia and ketoacidosis, it is best to switch from intravenous to subcutaneous insulin before a meal so that the patient can go back (or start) his or her usual insulin program. Zero to thirty minutes before the meal (depending on whether a short-acting analog or Regular insulin is to be used), the subcutaneous insulin(s) determined by the patient's program is given. Fifteen to thirty minutes later, the intravenous insulin drip is stopped. The patient is monitored for the next 6–12 hours by 1–2-hourly urinary ketones and blood glucose measurements, and electrolytes are measured at the end of that period to prove no recurrence of an elevated anion gap and/or lowered bicarbonate level.

## APPENDIX: PROTOCOL FOR MANAGEMENT OF DIABETIC KETOACIDOSIS*

- Careful history and physical exam with attention to mental state, cardiovascular and renal status, sources of infection, and hydration.
- Initial biochemical evaluation: blood ketones, fingerstick glucose, urine ketones, serum glucose, arterial blood gases and pH, serum electrolytes, BUN, amylase, CBC, urinalysis. Chest x-ray, EKG, and bacterial cultures if appropriate.
- Administer 1 liter 0.9% NaCl rapidly (within the first hour or faster if frank hypotension), then 0.45% NaCl at 250–500 ml/hr unless there is concern about cardiac or renal dysfunction. Monitor urine output, blood pressure, and pulse rate. Central vein pressure measurement and/or cardiovascular monitoring as clinically indicated.
- If the initial serum $K^+$ is less than 3.5 mEq/L, 40 mEq/L KCl is placed in each of the i.v. bags. For $K^+$ 3.5–5.5 mEq/L, 20–30 mEq KCl is added after the first liter of 0.9% NaCl if urinary output is adequate. Give no $K^+$ supplements if $K^+$ is above 5.5 mEq/L, but measure serum potassium every 1–2 hours. Oral potassium supplements can also be given if the patient is not nauseated or vomiting.
- No bicarbonate is given for pH $>7.0$, 1 ampoule (44 mEq) for pH 6.9–7.0, and 2 ampoules (88 mEq) for pH $<6.9$. Each ampoule is given over 30 minutes with 15 mEq KCl.
- Give 10–20 units Regular insulin i.v. as a loading dose. Start continuous

---

* Adapted from Ref. 18.

intravenous infusion 0.1 U/kg/hr Regular insulin, which in adults is 6–10 U/hr (as soon after loading dose as possible but can wait up to 1 hour). If no improvement in anion gap, pH, and hyperglycemia within 2 hours, double the hourly insulin dosage each hour until clinical effect is noted.

- When plasma glucose reaches 250 mg/dl, change to 100–300 ml/hr D5-0.45% NaCl (KCl is added depending on the serum potassium level). Substitute D5-0.9% NaCl if the serum sodium is <135 mEq/L. Decrease the i.v. insulin infusion to 0.05 U/kg/hr and adjust the infusion every 2 hours based on blood glucose:

| | |
|---|---|
| <60 mg/dl | Decrease 2 U/hr and give 25 ml 50% dextrose |
| 60–100 mg/dl | Decrease 1 U/hr |
| 100–160 mg/dl | No change |
| 161–220 mg/dl | Increase 1 U/hr |
| 221–280 mg/dl | Increase 2 U/hr |
| >280 mg/dl | Give 8 units i.v. bolus and increase 3 U/hr |

- When DKA has been controlled (serum glucose <200 mg/dl, bicarbonate > 15 mEq/L, pH >7.3, and serum ketone negative at 1:2 dilution), patient is changed to subcutaneous insulin.

## REFERENCES

1.  Kitabchi AE, Wall BM. Diabetic ketoacidosis. Med Clin North Am 79:9–37, 1995.
2.  Lebovitz HE. Diabetic ketoacidosis. Lancet 345:767–772, 1995.
3.  Umpierrez GE, Khajavi M, Kitabchi AE. Review: diabetic ketoacidosis and hyperglycemic hyperosmolar nonketotic syndrome. Am J Med Sci 311:225–233, 1996.
4.  Delaney MF, Zisman A, Kettyle WM. Diabetic ketoacidosis and hyperglycemic hyperosmolar nonketotic syndrome. Endocrinol Metab Clin North Am 29:683–705, 2000.
5.  Wetterhall SF, Olson DR, DeStefano F, Stevenson JM, Ford ES, German RR, Will JC, Newman JM, Sepe SJ, Vinicor F. Trends in diabetes and diabetic complications, 1980–1987. Diabetes Care 15:960–967, 1992.
6.  EURODIAB Study Group. Microvascular and acute complications in IDDM patients: the EURODIAB IDDM complications study. Diabetologia 37:278–285, 1994.
7.  Fishbein H, Palumbo PJ. Acute metabolic complications in diabetes. In: Diabetes in America (National Diabetes Data Group). Publication 95-1468. Bethesda, MD: National Institutes of Health, pp 283–291, 1995.
8.  Umpierrez GE, Kelly JP, Navarrete JE, Casals MM, Kitabchi AE. Hyperglycemic crises in urban blacks. Arch Intern Med 157:669–675, 1997.
9.  Sellers EA, Dean HJ. Diabetic ketoacidosis: a complication of type 2 diabetes in Canadian aboriginal youth. Diabetes Care 23:1202–1204, 2000.
10. Malone ML, Gennis V, Goodwin JS. Characteristics of diabetic ketoacidosis in older versus younger adults. J Am Geriatr Soc 40:1100–1104, 1992.

11. Glaser N, Barnett P, McCaslin I, Nelson D, Trainor J, Louie J, Kaufman F, Quayle K, Roback M, Malley R, Kuppermann N. The Pediatric Emergency Medicine Collaborative Research Committee of the American Academy of Pediatrics. Risk factors for cerebral edema in children with diabetic ketoacidosis. N Engl J Med 344:264–269, 2001.

12. Lorber D. Nonketotic hypertonicity in diabetes mellitus. Med Clin North Am 79: 39–52, 1995.

13. Wachtel TJ, Tetu-Mouradjian LM, Goldman DL, Ellis SE, O'Sullivan PS. Hyperosmolarity and acidosis in diabetes mellitus: a three-year experience in Rhode Island. J Gen Intern Med 6:495–502, 1991.

14. Arieff AI, Carroll HJ. Nonketotic hyperosmolar coma with hyperglycemia: clinical features, pathophysiology, renal function, acid-base balance, plasma-cerebrospinal fluid equilibria and the effects of therapy in 37 cases. Medicine 51:73–94, 1972.

15. Wachtel TJ, Silliman RA, Lamberton P. Predisposing factors for the diabetic hyperosmolar state. Arch Intern Med 148:747, 1988

16. Wachtel TJ, Silliman RA, Lamberton P. Prognostic factors in the diabetic hyperosmolar state. J Am Geriatr Soc 35:737–741, 1987.

17. Carroll P, Matz R. Uncontrolled diabetes mellitus in adults: experience in treating diabetic ketoacidosis and hyperosmolar nonketotic coma with low-dose insulin and a uniform treatment regimen. Diabetes Care 6:579–585, 1983.

18. Kitabchi AE, Umpierrez GE, Murphy MB, Barrett EJ, Kreisberg RA, Malone JI, Wall BM. Management of hyperglycemic crises in patients with diabetes. Diabetes Care 24:131–153, 2001.

19. Fisher JN, Shahshahani MN, Kitabchi AE. Diabetic ketoacidosis: low-dose insulin therapy by various routes. N Engl J Med 297:238–241, 1977.

20. Kitabchi AE, Ayyagari V, Guerra SM. The efficacy of low-dose versus conventional therapy of insulin for treatment of diabetic ketoacidosis. Ann Intern Med 84:633–638, 1976.

21. Piters KM, Kumar D, Pei E, Bessman AN. Comparison of continuous and intermittent intravenous insulin therapies for diabetic ketoacidosis. Diabetologia 13:317–321, 1977.

22. Lever E, Jaspan JB. Sodium bicarbonate therapy in severe diabetic ketoacidosis. Am J Med 75:263–268, 1983.

23. Hale PJ, Crase J, Nattrass M. Metabolic effects of bicarbonate in the treatment of diabetic ketoacidosis. Br Med J (Clin Res Ed) 289:1035–1038, 1984.

24. Morris LR, Murphy MB, Kitabchi AE. Bicarbonate therapy in severe diabetic ketoacidosis. Ann Intern Med 105:836–840, 1986.

25. Zipf WB, Bacon GE, Spencer ML, Kelch RP, Hopwood NJ, Hawker CD. Hypocalcemia, hypomagnesemia, and transient hypoparathyroidism during therapy with potassium phosphate in diabetic ketoacidosis. Diabetes Care 2:265–268, 1979.

26. Wilson HK, Keuer SP, Lea AS, Boyd AE 3rd, Eknoyan G. Phosphate therapy in diabetic ketoacidosis. Arch Intern Med 142:517–520, 1982.

27. Fisher JN, Kitabchi AE. A randomized study of phosphate therapy in the treatment of diabetic ketoacidosis. J Clin Endocrinol Metab 57:177–180, 1983.

# 13

## Insulin Therapy and Hypoglycemia

**Anthony L. McCall**

University of Virginia Health System, Charlottesville, Virginia

## INTRODUCTION

Hypoglycemia impedes attainment of optimal glycemia. The benefits of excellent glycemia in reducing diabetes complications are clearer than ever. Despite this, those wishing to decrease the risk of microvascular complications through glycemic control inevitably face an increased risk of hypoglycemia, often without warning symptoms and potentially with severe consequences. This is especially true for those with type 1 diabetes mellitus, but also for some with type 2 diabetes mellitus (see Figure 1).

Optimal glycemia is defined as $HbA_{1c}$ of less than 7% (Table 1), as recommended by the American Diabetes Association (ADA) (1). This goal is based on evidence from studies in both type 1 and type 2 diabetes mellitus, such as the Diabetes Control and Complications Trial (DCCT) (2) and the United Kingdom Prospective Diabetes Study (UKPDS) (3,4). Moreover, such control is more possible than ever with the panoply of therapies available. Newer insulins and strategies for their use in type 1 diabetes mellitus and use of drugs combined with insulin that enhance insulin sensitivity in type 2 diabetes mellitus make excellent control achievable.

The pathophysiology of hypoglycemia unawareness (inability to recognize hypoglycemia) and defective insulin counterregulation (weakened hormone de-

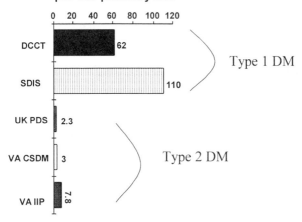

Severe insulin reactions
per 100 patient-years

**FIGURE 1**  Severe hypoglycemia type 1 versus type 2 diabetes mellitus. Studies of glycemic control and diabetes complications indicate that severe hypoglycemia is less common with tight glycemic control in type 2 than type 1 diabetes mellitus. Two studies of type 1, the DCCT and Stockholm Diabetes Intervention Study, found that severe insulin reactions occur at a rate of more than 60 per 100 patient-years and have a threefold increased risk compared with conventional therapy. In contrast, the UKPDS and two VA cooperative studies of type 2 diabetes found a risk of severe hypoglycemia with tight glycemic control that was an order of magnitude less.

**TABLE 1**  Goals for Glycemic Control Recommended by the ADA

| Biochemical index | Normal | Goal | Additional action suggested |
|---|---|---|---|
| Whole blood values | | | |
|   Avg. preprandial (mg/dl) | <100 | 80–120 | <80 or >140 |
|   Avg. bedtime glucose | <110 | 100–140 | <100 or >160 |
| Plasma values | | | |
|   Avg. preprandial | <110 | 90–130 | <90 or >150 |
|   Avg. bedtime | <120 | 110–150 | <110 or >170 |
| HbA$_{1c}$ (%) (normal 4–6%) | <6 | <7 | >8 |

Note that self-monitored blood glucose (SMBG) values are about 10–15% higher in glucose meters using plasma-referenced testing. As a result, glycemic goals are adjusted upward in plasma referenced systems. The values above are appropriate for relatively healthy patients who have no identified increased risk of severe hypoglycemia.
*Source*: American Diabetes Association, 2001.

fenses against hypoglycemia) is under active investigation. The importance of hypoglycemia as a barrier to safe therapy is confirmed in recent studies. Risk factors for severe hypoglycemia include: 1) prior severe hypoglycemia, 2) hypoglycemia unawareness, 3) defective insulin counterregulation, 4) age under 5 years, and 5) being elderly. New noninvasive and minimally invasive monitoring of glycemia in addition to self-monitoring of blood glucose (SMBG) with fingerstick testing hold the promise of better information to attain safe control. Eventually, these monitoring methods may be successfully linked with delivery devices to create an artificial $\beta$ cell. As providers and patients increasingly strive for excellent glycemic control, treatment strategies need to focus on reducing the frequency of hypoglycemia. This chapter first reviews the risks of hypoglycemia and then explains how to reduce that risk. These sections can be read separately. Readers wishing more information on these subjects are referred to two excellent books (5,6) for in-depth information.

## THE IMPORTANCE OF HYPOGLYCEMIA IN TYPE 1 DIABETES MELLITUS

Hypoglycemia is an inevitable consequence of insulin therapy and the main barrier to safe attainment of optimal glycemia in type 1 diabetes mellitus. Most well-controlled patients average symptomatic hypoglycemic reactions twice a week, and asymptomatic hypoglycemia is more common than that. Historically, about 25% of those with type 1 diabetes mellitus experience a temporarily disabling hypoglycemic episode each year. Heightened awareness of hypoglycemia's importance arose from studies of glycemic control and diabetic complications in type 1 diabetes mellitus, such as the DCCT (2). Hypoglycemia may also cause the weight gain with intensive treatment (7). In the DCCT improvement in HgbA$_{1c}$ of 2% over 6.5 years reduced chronic diabetes microvascular and neuropathic complications by 50% or more (Table 2 summarizes its benefits and risks).

### The DCCT

In the DCCT, despite dramatic benefits of tight control, a threefold excess of severe hypoglycemia—defined as requiring another person's assistance to recover—accompanied intensive therapy (8). During follow up of the 1441 patients, there were 3788 episodes of severe hypoglycemia. Of these, 1027 were associated with coma and/or seizure. Overall, 65% of patients in the intensive group and 35% of patients in the conventional group had at least one episode of severe hypoglycemia during the study. Several subgroups had a particularly high risk of severe hypoglycemia. They included: 1) males, 2) adolescents, 3) those without residual C-peptide, and 4) those with prior severe hypoglycemia. Glycemic goals need adjustment for safety in such high-risk patients. Similar to the

**TABLE 2**  Benefits and Risks of Glycemic Control in the DCCT

| Reduction of risk (2) | Increased risk (8) |
|---|---|
| Primary prevention<br>   Retinopathy 76% (62–85% CI) | Hypoglycemia<br>Serious hypoglycemia<br>RR of 3.28 |
| Secondary prevention<br>   Retinopathy 54% (39–66% CI) | Coma and seizures<br>RR of 3.02 |
| Combined cohorts<br>   Severe retinopathy 47% (14–67% CI) | Hospitalization for hypoglycemia<br>RR 1.5 (54 vs. 36 hospitalizations) |
|    Microalbuminuria (>40 mg/d) | Weight gain (4.6 kg > controls at 5 years) |
| 39% (21–52% CI) | RR of 1.33 for >120% of ideal body weight |
|    Albuminuria (>300 mg/d)<br>   54% (19–74% CI) | |
| Clinical neuropathy by 60%<br>   (38–74% CI) | Weight-related metabolic abnormalities (7) |

The increase or decrease in risk for intensive insulin therapy is given for several parameters based on data from the DCCT.
CI = confidence intervals; RR = relative risk.
*Source*: Adapted from Refs. 2, 7, and 8.

DCCT, the Stockholm Diabetes Intervention Study (SDIS) (9) reported reduced risk for microvascular complications and increased risk of hypoglycemia with intensive glycemic control. There were 1.1 episodes of serious hypoglycemia with intensive treatment versus 0.4 episodes per patient per year with conventional treatment (10). The clinical question raised by these trials is how to recognize and reduce the risk of hypoglycemia.

## Recognizing Hypoglycemia: Common Clinical Manifestations

Symptoms of hypoglycemia are usually divided into two main categories: 1) autonomic (sometimes called neurogenic or sympathoadrenal) and 2) neuroglycopenic, which means related to deprivation of glucose as fuel to the brain (Table 3). Typically, autonomic symptoms precede neuroglycopenic symptoms; that is, patients become shaky and sweaty before confusion sets in. A reversal of this usual sequence manifest as loss of early autonomic symptoms occurs in patients with hypoglycemia unawareness. For example, some patients will sweat when markedly hypoglycemic after only an hour or two of mental slowing. Retraining

TABLE 3  Common Symptoms
of Hypoglycemia

| Autonomic | Neuroglycopenic |
|---|---|
| Cold sweats | Confusion or slow mentation |
| Paresthesias | Blurred vision or diplopia |
| Fine tremor | General fatigue or weakness |
| Hunger | Faint or dizzy feeling |
| Palpitations | Mood disturbance |
| Anxiety | Feeling of warmth |

Autonomic = associated with hypoglycemia awareness; neuroglycopenic = related to fuel deprivation of
the brain symptoms.

patients and families to recognize changing symptoms (blood glucose awareness training) is a focus for research and shows promise as a potential aspect of treatment for patients with problematic hypoglycemia (11,12).

Potential harm to the brain exists with repeated or severe hypoglycemia. The common symptoms from moderate hypoglycemia that are caused by fuel deprivation to the brain are confusion, visual disturbances, generalized fatigue, feeling of faintness, mood disturbances, and a feeling of warmth (Table 3). Full neurocognitive recovery after severe hypoglycemia may take as much as a day and a half (19) even though patients may state that they are back to normal function and superficially appear to be recovered when glucose has returned to normal levels.

When more severe, acute hypoglycemia may have clinical manifestations that are less well recognized clinically, such as acute hemiparesis. Some of these less common neurological manifestations of severe hypoglycemia are summarized in Table 4.

TABLE 4  Neurological Manifestations of Acute Hypoglycemia

| | |
|---|---|
| Decortication | Locked-in syndrome |
| Decerebration | Amnesia |
| Hemiplegia (transient) | Stroke |
| Choreoathetosis | Cortical atrophy |
| Ataxia | Peripheral neuropathy |
| Convulsions (generalized or focal) | Other focal neurological abnormalities (pons, visual pathways) |

## Hypoglycemia Unawareness

Hypoglycemia unawareness is associated with more profound cognitive dysfunction during hypoglycemia, as shown by Gold et al. (20). Moreover, recovery of intellectual function is delayed significantly in those with hypoglycemia unawareness.

## Brain Vulnerability to Hypoglycemia

Repeated bouts of severe hypoglycemia may impair cognitive function or damage the brain. Deary et al. (13) found that patients with type 1 diabetes mellitus and a history of severe hypoglycemia had a slight but significant decline in IQ scores compared with a matched control group. Using MRI imaging, Perros et al. (14) compared 11 subjects with type 1 diabetes mellitus with no history of severe hypoglycemia to 11 type 1 diabetes mellitus patients with a history of five or more episodes of severe hypoglycemia and found cortical atrophy in nearly half of those with a history of severe hypoglycemia ($p < 0.05$). CT and MRI have been used to show that the basal ganglia, cerebral cortex, substantia nigra, and hippocampus are vulnerable brain areas after profound, but sublethal, hypoglycemia (15). Hypoglycemia with seizures predicts cognitive dysfunction in diabetic children (16,17); early onset (<5 years old) of diabetes also portends cognitive problems (18). The clinical concern raised by such findings is that repeated hypoglycemia may interfere with the complex task of managing insulin therapy in type 1 diabetes mellitus. This may result in a vicious circle in which subtle neurocognitive dysfunction increases the risk of subsequent hypoglycemia.

## Hypoglycemia and Sudden Death

While it is emphasized that the brain is at risk from hypoglycemia, other organs, including the heart may be affected, perhaps to a greater degree in type 2 diabetes mellitus. Consequences of hypoglycemia include possible alterations in cardiac ventricular repolarization that could underlie sudden death (21). Hypoglycemia creates a prothrombotic state (22) and may predispose to acute ischemia, in either the coronary or cerebral circulation. This may be more common for type 2 diabetes patients or those with longstanding type 1 diabetes because of underlying atherosclerosis. Surprisingly few reports of such events occur in the literature (23,24), although they do occasionally occur in practice, with an acute hypoglycemic event appearing to trigger a myocardial infarction or a thrombotic stroke. One of the most feared consequences of hypoglycemia is the ''dead-in-bed'' syndrome (25,26).

## HYPOGLYCEMIA IN TYPE 2 DIABETES MELLITUS

Generally, hypoglycemia is less frequent and less severe in type 2 diabetes mellitus than in type 1 diabetes mellitus. This may reflect a relative resistance to insulin action in type 2 diabetes mellitus, greater retention of β-cell function, and better preserved hormonal counterregulation at below-normal glucose levels (27). For example, in the DCCT-like Kumamoto study of glycemic control and complications in those with type 2 diabetes mellitus (28), no severe hypoglycemia occurred and mild hypoglycemia was only slightly increased with intensive insulin therapy. In the UKPDS, symptomatic hypoglycemia occurred in about 30% with intensive therapy, but severe hypoglycemia in only about 2% (3). Figure 1 shows that rates of severe hypoglycemia in studies of type 1 diabetes mellitus (top two bars) are an order of magnitude greater than in type 2 diabetes mellitus (bottom three bars).

## Hypoglycemia and the Elderly

Despite these apparently reassuring findings, hypoglycemia in the elderly and certain others with type 2 diabetes mellitus may be a serious concern. Matyka et al. (28) compared counterregulatory hormones and symptoms with controlled hypoglycemia in younger versus older subjects. Hormonal responses were similar, but hypoglycemic symptoms began at higher glucose levels in the younger men and were more intense, permitting recognition and self-treatment. Neurological function, such as reaction time, deteriorated earlier and to a greater degree in the older men. Most importantly, the normal difference between the glucose levels for awareness of hypoglycemia and the onset of cognitive dysfunction was lost in the older men. This means that older subjects were less likely to experience autonomic warning symptoms. Thus, reduced warning of hypoglycemia characterizes normal aging. In the United States, some 6.3 million people above age 65 have diabetes; many eventually will need insulin therapy and thus may be at greater risk for significant hypoglycemia.

## Risk Factors for Serious Hypoglycemia in Type 2 Diabetes Mellitus

Certain factors may predispose to serious hypoglycemia in type 2 diabetes mellitus. In a large study of Medicaid enrollees aged 65 years or older who used insulin or sulfonylureas from 1985 through 1989, Shorr et al. (30) found that the rates of serious hypoglycemia were 2.76 per 100 person-years among insulin users. Predictors of subsequent hypoglycemia included: 1) recent hospitalization (the strongest predictor)—relative risk of serious hypoglycemia was 4.5 from 1 to 30 days after discharge, 2) advanced age (1.8 relative risk), 3) black race (2.0 relative risk), and 4) use of five or more concomitant medications (1.3 relative risk).

## Awareness and Defenses in Type 2 Diabetes Mellitus

Counterregulation and hypoglycemia unawareness have been much less studied in type 2 diabetes mellitus than in type 1 diabetes mellitus (31). Bolli and colleagues (32) reported deficient hypoglycemia-induced glucagon, growth hormone, and cortisol responses, but normal epinephrine responses and increased norepinephrine release in type 2 diabetes mellitus. Enhanced suppression of glucose utilization contributed more to restoration of euglycemia than did increased glucose production by the liver. Similarly, Shamoon et al. (33) found decreased glucagon but increased epinephrine responses to hypoglycemia in type 2 diabetes mellitus. Spyer et al. (27) recently reported that counterregulation occurs at higher glucose levels in well-controlled (HgbA$_{1c}$ 7.4%) type 2 diabetes mellitus than in nondiabetic individuals. In a study comparing those with and without hypoglycemia unawareness and type 2 diabetes mellitus, Ohno et al. (34) found indirect evidence to suggest autonomic neuropathy in those with hypoglycemia unawareness. Importantly, Hepburn and colleagues (35) found that when type 1 and type 2 diabetes mellitus patients are matched for insulin therapy and glycemic control, there is not a significant difference in hypoglycemia frequency. Thus, while hypoglycemia may be less frequent overall in type 2 than type 1 diabetes mellitus, the underlying pathophysiology seems similar, and when matched for insulin therapy the risk may also be similar.

## REVERSIBLE HYPOGLYCEMIC DISORDERS

Reversible physiological abnormalities are often an important feature in patients who experience serious hypoglycemia. The following discussion indicates their important features for the clinician.

### The HAAF Syndromes

Cryer (37) coined the term hypoglycemia-associated autonomic failure (HAAF) to indicate a constellation of abnormalities that are largely reversible, are induced by prior hypoglycemia, and affect protective body responses to hypoglycemia. Reduced glucagon and epinephrine responses to hypoglycemia appear to be especially important. The etiology of these syndromes, which include hypoglycemia unawareness and defective insulin counterregulation, is incompletely understood. Altered transport of glucose into the brain may underlie ineffective hypoglycemia defenses (38–40). Excessive glucocorticoid secretion in response to hypoglycemia could be an important aspect of defective awareness and counterregulation, as proposed by Davis and colleagues (41,42). Recently, the possibility has been raised that beta-adrenergic receptor down-regulation may be important in hypoglycemia unawareness and defective counterregulation (43,44). Whether these mechanisms are complementary, overlapping, or independent is unknown. One of the most important aspects of the HAAF syndromes is that they appear to be directly linked to prior episodes of hypoglycemia and can reverse in days to weeks (see Table 5 on management of hypoglycemia unawareness) following

TABLE 5   Management of Patients with Hypoglycemia Unawareness
(Mnemonic: Rule of Threes)

Test SMBG more than three times a day (typically, four to seven needed)
May need up to three times usual Rx to go over 100 mg/dl (i.e., usual 15
    grams may be increased temporarily to up to 45 grams of dextrose)
First goal is to avoid all hypo for 3 days—this is when pattern begins to
    emerge of therapy response (reduction of insulin resistance from prior
    hypoglycemia)
Next goal is to avoid hypoglycemia for 3 weeks, which is associated with
    recovery of hypoglycemia awareness and/or counterregulation for those
    without DAN
Need 3 to 6 months to improve awareness in DAN patients

DAN = chronic diabetic autonomic neuropathy, which differs from HAAF (hypoglycemia-associated autonomic failure) in that the former is seldom significantly reversible.

cessation of hypoglycemia. The clinical take-home point is this: *when confronted
with a patient who is experiencing frequent hypoglycemia, do whatever is necessary to prevent recurrence of hypoglycemia.* If this is done, the problem may
rapidly resolve itself.

## Reversibility of HAAF Syndromes

Recovery from hypoglycemia unawareness (often coupled with improving hormonal counterregulation) may begin within 2–3 days (Table 5) if hypoglycemia
is strictly avoided (36,45). It is not necessary, however, to reduce insulin doses
so markedly that severe hyperglycemia results (46). This may be reassuring to
patients who might otherwise resist dose reduction for fear of the (long-term)
consequences of hyperglycemia and intolerance of symptoms related to hyperglycemia. With avoidance of hypoglycemia over 2–3 weeks, recovery of symptom
awareness and insulin counterregulation may be substantial in type 1 diabetes
mellitus patients without autonomic neuropathy (36). In patients with severe diabetic autonomic neuropathy, 6 months may be needed and recovery is typically
less complete (47).

## Nocturnal Hypoglycemia

The frequency and importance of nocturnal hypoglycemia are critical to recognize. Nocturnal hypoglycemia can induce hypoglycemia unawareness and reduced insulin counterregulatory defenses (48). Routine bedtime snacks protect
poorly against nocturnal hypoglycemia (49). Some have recommended the use
of uncooked corn starch (50). Children were found in one study to have nocturnal
hypoglycemia half of nights studied, and half of the hypoglycemia was asymp-

tomatic (51). Matyka et al. (52) have suggested that children with nocturnal hypoglycemia have prolonged episodes due to defective insulin counterregulation. Since awareness of hypoglycemia is normally reduced during sleep, nighttime (2 to 3 A.M.) home glucose monitoring may help detect such events.

## MANAGING PATIENTS WITH HYPOGLYCEMIA ON INSULIN THERAPY: IDENTIFY RISK

How can one prevent serious hypoglycemia in patients taking insulin? The first step is to recognize those who are at increased risk. Table 6 depicts the known risk factors that impair hypoglycemia defenses. Another important early step is to set appropriate glycemic goals for patients and individualize them according to the risk of hypoglycemia. The American Diabetes Association (1) suggests the glycemic goals listed in Table 1.

### Adjust Glycemic Goals

In practice, one needs to adjust glucose goals upward, at least temporarily, until hypoglycemia unawareness reverses in patients at clearly increased risk of serious hypoglycemia. A standard approach is to raise glucose targets in elderly, chronically ill, or debilitated patients, including those with severe cardiac or cerebral ischemia or other known risk factors for severe adverse consequences of hypoglycemia. Increasing $HbA_{1c}$ by about 1% is usually all that is needed to reverse hypoglycemia unawareness and improve counterregulation (36). This correlates

TABLE 6   Common Factors Impairing Hypoglycemia Defenses

| | |
|---|---|
| Antecedent hypoglycemia | Hormonal environment |
| Diabetic autonomic neuropathy | Adrenocortical insufficiency |
| Defective insulin counterregulation | Hypopituitarism |
| Hypoglycemia unawareness | Pregnancy |
| Nutritional factors | Hypothyroidism |
| Gastroparesis | Glucocorticoid excess |
| Alcohol intake | Extremes of age |
| Fasting and skipped meals | Renal and hepatic insufficiency |
| Low-carbohydrate fad diets | Sliding-scale insulin therapy |
| Malnutrition | Erratic schedules |
| | Exercise |

Antecedent hypoglycemia itself is perhaps the most important precursor to significant later hypoglycemia. Prior hypoglycemia may occur during the daytime and often occurs at night. It need not be very severe to be important in reducing hypoglycemia defenses. A history of severe hypoglycemia, however, is an important predictor of recurring severe hypoglycemia.

TABLE 7 Overview of Strategies to Reduce Hypoglycemia Risk

1. Learn to copy normal β-cell physiological responses with insulin therapy.
2. Teach patients to adjust their lives to their insulin therapy or, preferably, their insulin therapy to their lifestyles.
3. Ensure safety by providing all patients (and their families or colleagues) with adequate remedies for hypoglycemia.
4. Set appropriate glycemic goals. Modify goals if patients have history of severe hypoglycemia, hypoglycemia unawareness or defective counterregulation, or other risk factors that predispose to severe hypoglycemia.
5. Recognize signs of overtreatment early, including nocturnal hypoglycemia, to minimize the risk of severe hypoglycemia.
6. Provide alternative insulin strategies for patients not doing well on current strategies (see Table 8).
7. If frustration or lack of success ensues, seek consultation with a diabetes specialist.

with an average increase of fasting and preprandial blood glucose of about 30 mg/dl.

Elsewhere in this book are chapters dealing with other aspects of insulin therapy. Some overlap is unavoidable; the presentation below suggests strategies that are particularly tied to reducing hypoglycemic risks in patients with problematic hypoglycemia. Tables 7 and 8 provide an overview and summarize the strategies for reducing hypoglycemic risk in treatment of diabetes.

## TREATMENT OF HYPOGLYCEMIA (A TREATMENT, NOT A TREAT)

Urgent situations dictate use of any available sugar source to remedy acute hypoglycemia. However, it is preferable to use a measured, standard amount of pure dextrose when possible. This has several advantages. Most importantly, dextrose is rapidly absorbed and will quickly correct hypoglycemia. Hypoglycemia should not be treated with a candy bar or other sugar source that contains unwanted saturated fat, which slows sugar absorption, delays hypoglycemic recovery, and may adversely affect hyperlipidemia and caloric balance. Hypoglycemia-unaware patients often undertreat themselves, probably because hypoglycemia is less unpleasant when there are few or no distressing autonomic symptoms. Typically ~15–20 g of dextrose will restore euglycemia in adults; children should base doses on weight. Depending on the initial SMBG value, patients may need as little as one-half (for mild symptoms and blood glucose a little less than 100 mg/

**TABLE 8** Detailed Strategies to Reduce Hypoglycemia by Improving Insulin Therapy

---

Switch from sliding-scale insulin to pattern management.

Change fixed ratio insulins to individual doses (e.g., switch 70/30 insulin to 70% NPH and 30% Regular to permit individual dose adjustment).

Move NPH to bedtime but leave Regular (or other bolus insulin) at dinnertime.

Use a correction bolus (1500 rule for Regular, 1800 rule for lispro) but also minimize overlap with other short-acting insulin doses and avoid near bedtime.

Reduce hypoglycemia before addressing hyperglycemia.

Ensure that hypoglycemia is fully treated (not just symptom improvement) by checking SMBG 15 minutes after treatment.

Provide adequate carbohydrate snacks for increased activity.

If patient varies dose, check total daily dose to ensure that there is not too much variation.

Check balance of long-acting and short-acting insulin: overreliance on long-acting insulin causes late delayed hypoglycemia; overreliance on short-acting insulin causes postprandial hypoglycemia.

Manipulate the timing of short-acting insulin injection relative to meals (lag time).

Decrease lag time with hypoglycemia or take insulin after meals; increase with hyperglycemia.

Discourage use of short-acting insulins (Regular, lispro, aspart) at bedtime.

Switch from NPH- or Lente-based regimen to basal-bolus strategy (Ultralente b.i.d., glargine q.d.).

Switch from Regular insulin-based regimen to lispro-based regimen (or insulin aspart).

Dose short-acting (meal bolus) insulins based on carbohydrate counting.

Add a shot of short-acting insulin at noon.

Reduce overall insulin doses ~20% when going from a simple to a more complex regimen (multiple injections, insulin pumps) if adequate overall control exists.

Use insulin pumps in appropriately trained and motivated patients.

---

dl) or as much as double this amount (for profound symptoms or blood glucose of <40 mg/dl) of dextrose to start. Table 9 gives common and preferred sources of dextrose or other carbohydrates for the treatment of hypoglycemia. Once hypoglycemia has been fully treated, either a meal or at least a snack containing protein and carbohydrate should be eaten.

**Retest and Re-treat**

It is very important to have patients retest glucose values 15 minutes after dextrose treatment for hypoglycemia; some patients require two or three treatments

TABLE 9  Therapies to Reverse Hypoglycemia

**First choice (dextrose-based, easily dosed)**
Four dextrose tablets (e.g., DEX4): 16 grams of dextrose
One tube of glucose gel (small tube is ⅓ of a large tube): 15 grams of dextrose
**Second choice (dextrose-based)**
Nine Sweet Tarts: 15.4 grams of dextrose
Three rolls of Smarties: 15 grams of dextrose
Nine Spree candies: 15.4 grams of dextrose
**Third choice (all contain 15–20 grams of carbohydrate)**
½ cup of fruit juice
6 oz Kool-Aid or lemonade
½ can non-diet soda (6 oz)
Six or seven Lifesavers
Six or seven jelly beans
Three pieces of hard candy (e.g., butterscotch, peppermint)
8 oz of a sport drink
1 heaping tablespoon (3–4 teaspoons) of table sugar
**If patient cannot swallow**
0.5 to 1 mg s.q. or i.m. glucagon (caution: vomiting can occur)
**Other safety issues**
ID bracelet or necklace needed for any with prior severe hypoglycemia or hypoglycemia unawareness
Glucagon instruction of friends, relatives, or co-workers may be needed
Difficulty reversing hypoglycemia or need for glucagon indicates need for emergency-room evaluation

Treatments, in our suggested order of preference, that will reverse hypoglycemia (i.e., increase SMBG to 100 mg/dl or more). It is important to remember that one treatment may not reverse hypoglycemia. *All patients, particularly those who are hypoglycemic unaware, should retest 15 minutes after 15 grams of dextrose treatment and re-treat if SMBG is not >100 mg/dl (the 15/15 rule for hypoglycemia treatment).* Patients can also be asked to read food labels if the above choices are not available and look for 15 grams of carbohydrate in foods that are free of protein, fat, and fiber.

to raise plasma glucose above 100 mg/dl, the minimum goal. For safety, all patients with increased hypoglycemia risk need a Medic Alert or other ID bracelet and glucagon kits with instruction given to friends and relatives on their use.

## β-CELL MIMICRY AS AN INSULIN STRATEGY TO REDUCE HYPOGLYCEMIA

Mimicking the pancreatic β cell with insulin treatment is an important strategy for attaining successful glycemic control while reducing the risk of hypoglycemia. Evidence of this is the growing use of insulin pumps in the management of type

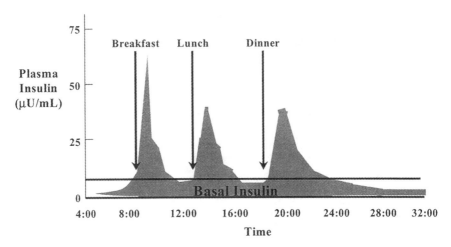

FIGURE 2   The pattern of normal peripheral plasma insulin levels throughout the day in a normal-weight nondiabetic individual. (Adapted from Ref. 66.)

1 and even type 2 diabetes. Physiologically, the β cell has two components of insulin output (see Figure 2). The first is a relatively constant level of insulin secretion between meals and at night to maintain euglycemia. This is the *basal insulin*. It represents half or a little less of normal insulin secretion. There is a diurnal rhythm in basal insulin needs—insulin sensitivity is reduced in the early hours of the morning, mandating increased insulin secretion in some patients, especially younger ones. This early-morning rise of basal insulin secretion/requirement has been termed the dawn phenomenon. The second component is adequate meal-related insulin secretion. This is the *bolus insulin*.

### Newer Insulins Mimic Basal and Bolus Better than NPH and Regular

The two components are matched better with some insulin strategies than with others. Currently, most physicians primarily use NPH and Regular. These two insulins can sometimes be successfully combined to achieve excellent control, but they are generally less likely to provide a physiological mimicry than alternative strategies. The newer "designer" insulins (which have a modified amino acid structure) may better mimic pancreatic basal and bolus insulin replacement. They are playing an increasingly important role in intensive insulin therapy programs that are designed to provide physiological insulin replacement while minimizing hypoglycemic risk. These insulin analogs include the very quick-onset and quick-acting lispro and aspart and the long-acting basal insulin glargine (see Figure 3).

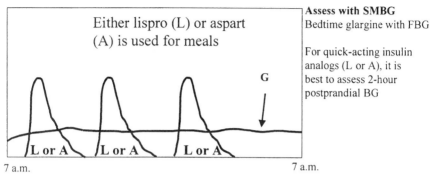

0/L - 0/L - G/L - 0/0   B-L-D-Hs
0:1 - 0:1 - 3:1 - 0:0   A basal-bolus strategy

Either lispro (L) or aspart (A) is used for meals

G

**Assess with SMBG**
Bedtime glargine with FBG

For quick-acting insulin analogs (L or A), it is best to assess 2-hour postprandial BG

L or A   L or A   L or A

7 a.m.                                          7 a.m.

May be useful for erratic lifestyle
Need to dose quick-acting insulin based on carbohydrates

FIGURE 3   A basal-bolus strategy for insulin administration may reduce risk of hypoglycemia in those with erratic schedules or in whom diabetes is more labile because of greater insulin deficiency, such as in type 1 or late-type 2 diabetes mellitus. Insulin glargine (G) once daily may offer a reduced risk of hypoglycemia and more consistent levels than NPH or Ultralente insulin given twice daily. Usually, quick-acting, physiological insulin replacement at meals is provided by insulin analogs such as lispro (L) or insulin aspart (A). The timing and relative dose (divided initially into six parts distributed as illustrated) are given for glargine and the quick-acting insulin analogs at breakfast (B), lunch (L), dinnertime (D), and bedtime (Hs).

## Reducing Insulin with Exercise

Another issue that commonly arises in physiological replacement of insulin, particularly in younger patients, is the adjusting of therapy for increased physical activity. Exercise enhances insulin sensitivity during the activity and up to 12 hours afterward (causing delayed hypoglycemia) while repletion of depleted glucose stores (glycogen) in muscle occurs. For example, lively activity in the evening (e.g., dancing) can enhance the risk of nocturnal hypoglycemia 4 to 8 hours later and generally calls for a reduction of the bedtime insulin dosage. Exercise after meals, of modest intensity (25% $VO_{2\,max}$) for an hour or of moderate intensity (50% $VO_{2\,max}$) for 30 minutes, requires a 50% reduction in bolus insulin doses (53). More vigorous or longer-duration exercise requires a 75% or greater reduction in bolus insulin. Recognition of hypoglycemia is reduced with exercise partly because of catecholamine depletion.

## MONITORING OF DIABETES TO ADJUST INSULIN THERAPY

SMBG is crucial to successful and safe insulin therapy. The frequency required should be individualized, but generally should be frequent in those with an increased risk of hypoglycemia, particularly hypoglycemia unawareness—in general, routinely before meals and at bedtime. Occasional tests in the middle of the night (typically 2–3 A.M.) can be helpful to identify nocturnal hypoglycemia. Testing before driving and when working with dangerous machinery is often also indicated. Testing at times of anticipated peak insulin action (e.g., ~2 hours postprandial with lispro or aspart) is sometimes needed. With hypoglycemia unawareness, patients may be surprised to find that they are hypoglycemic much more frequently than they suspect.

### Problems with Sliding Scales

Adjusting insulin therapy based on monitoring can be done in several ways. Many patients base their insulin adjustments primarily on the current blood glucose concentrations, an approach similar to sliding-scale insulin therapy, which is often used in the hospital setting. This can increase hypoglycemia risk, particularly if long-acting doses are adjusted in this manner. In ambulatory care, as in the hospital, sliding-scale insulin is usually a relatively poor choice, often resulting in erratic control with unpredictable hypoglycemia (54,55) (see Table 10). An alternative strategy to supplement insulin, called a correction bolus, is illustrated in Table 11.

### Pattern Management

A better means for adjusting insulin therapy is sometimes called *pattern management* (56), which typically examines the pattern and consistency of therapy re-

**TABLE 10** Problems with Sliding-Scale Insulin

| |
|---|
| Attempts to make insulin work backward |
| Doses insulin based on a single glucose value |
| Ignores pattern of therapy response |
| Does not lead to stability of regimen |
| Requires hyperglycemia to initiate therapy if given without basal insulin |

Sliding-scale insulin works poorly to match insulin needs and timing. It removes context from interpretation of SMBG testing (e.g., rebound hyperglycemia). Although supplemental insulin may be important, particularly on sick days, as a primary strategy it leads to erratic control, with alternating hyper- and hypoglycemia and often insulin overdosage.

TABLE 11  Use of a Correction Bolus (Alternative to Sliding-Scale Insulin for Short-Term Correction of Hyperglycemia)

Patient with poor short-term control (not a rebound)
Rule of 1800 (lispro/aspart)[a]
1800/TDD = mg/dl drop of glucose expected

*Clinical example*: A 39-year-old man with 12-year history of type 1 diabetes is using 12 units of Ultralente insulin at breakfast and dinner. He takes an average of 5 units of lispro insulin at breakfast, 3 units of lispro at lunch, and 8 units of lispro with his main meal (dinner). You calculate his total daily dose (TDD) to be 40 units for all insulins. Thus, using the 1800 rule predicts that the administration of 1 additional unit of lispro should reduce glucose by 45 mg/dl (1800/40 = 45).

Important caveats
    Do not use at bedtime generally (may risk nighttime hypoglycemia)
    Do not use if you recently took short-acting insulin (additive effect may risk hypoglycemia)
    Use rule of 1500 for regular insulin-based regimens (less peak effect than lispro or aspart)
    Best worked out for leaner patients and those with type 1 diabetes mellitus

TDD = total daily dose of insulin (all types).
[a] Presumably, similar strategies for insulin aspart and lispro will be used.

sponse (SMBG values) over several days or longer. One or two changes in insulin administration aimed at the most consistently abnormal values to bring them into better control are selected, followed by a period of observation to see whether an improved pattern emerges.

Four things are required to make pattern management work in insulin-treated patients. First, pattern management needs *sufficient monitoring* frequency to be able to determine a pattern. Second, it requires clear *communication of appropriate glycemic goals* and their adjustment upward in patients at high risk of hypoglycemia. Third, it requires a *time interval* (typically either 3 or 7 days) after which patterns of glycemia are re-evaluated and changes made if glycemic targets are not met. Fourth, it requires an *increment or decrement size* (commonly 10–20% of the dose) for the dosage adjustment.

## New Monitoring Strategies

Recent innovations in monitoring may soon permit safer attainment of excellent glycemia. The use of subcutaneous glucose sensors (as are available from Mini-

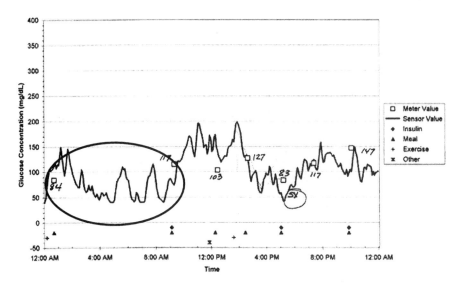

**FIGURE 4** Detection of unsuspected hypoglycemia in a type 1 diabetes mellitus patient using a subcutaneous glucose sensor. The circled area on the left side of the chart illustrates a period of unsuspected and asymptomatic nocturnal hypoglycemia in someone with type 1 diabetes, found by using a subcutaneous continuous glucose-monitoring sensor (MiniMed CGMS system). Because this type of sensing of glucose values still has some errors (sensor decay), its use is currently limited to physicians and not patients.

Med) holds promise in this regard (57). Figure 4 shows an example of unsuspected hypoglycemia that was detected by using a 72-hour subcutaneous glucose sensor in a patient. Another possibility is the use of a Glucowatch Biographer, a wristwatch-like device recently approved for adults by the FDA that detects subcutaneous interstitial fluid glucose by reverse iontophoresis and has a readout similar to that of a large LCD watch (58). These devices are fairly new but seem promising for selected patients.

## INSULIN THERAPY AND HYPOGLYCEMIA

Initially, insulin therapy was available only as Regular insulin from animal pancreas glands. The result was multiple injections and frequent hyper- and hypoglycemia, reflecting difficulty in providing adequate basal insulin replacement. The addition of protamine to insulin, first as PZI (protamine zinc insulin, no longer used) and later as NPH (neutral protamine Hagedorn, after the physician who introduced it), reduced the rate of absorption of insulin and provided the first attempts at a basal insulin strategy. Human insulins have now replaced animal insulins. Despite some initial concern, human insulin does not carry any additional risk for hypoglycemia over animal insulins (59).

## Insulin Analogs and Physiological Insulin Replacement

Regular insulin starts to work within ~30 minutes, has its peak action by ~3 hours, and, although reputed to last only 4–6 hours, has a long tail (see Figure 5) that creates a risk of late postprandial hypoglycemia in many patients. The time-action curve of Regular is also frequently variable in its onset and peak action in different people, and in particular is typically delayed in obese, insulin-resistant type 2 diabetes mellitus patients. In contrast, the insulin analogs lispro and aspart are quicker in onset (~15 minutes) and shorter in duration (3–4 hours), and have a more reliable time of peak action—typically a little less than 2 hours after the injection—which closely mimics the timing of peripheral venous insulin

$$N/R - 0/0 - 0/R - N/0 \ (B\text{-}L\text{-}D\text{-}Hs)$$
$$2{:}1 - 0{:}0 - 0{:}1 - 2{:}0 \ (sum = 6 \ parts)$$

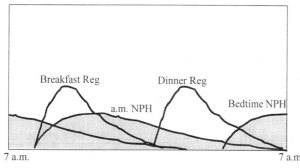

**Pattern management**
**Assess with SMBG**
Bedtime NPH with FBG
a.m. NPH with pre-dinner BG
Dinner Reg with bedtime BG
Morn Reg with pre-lunch BG

Breakfast Reg    Dinner Reg

a.m. NPH    Bedtime NPH

7 a.m.                                    7 a.m.

FIGURE 5  Suggested distribution of insulins in combination of NPH (or Lente) and Regular insulin. NPH and Regular insulin are best distributed throughout the day in the above-depicted manner for those with type 1 or late type 2 diabetes. NPH and Regular can be taken together about 30 minutes before breakfast, usually in a 2:1 ratio. About 30 minutes before dinner the second dose of Regular insulin is given, and the final injection of NPH is given within an hour of bedtime. The best times to sample the self-monitoring of blood glucose (SMBG) pattern of therapy response, to gauge the need for therapy adjustment for the individual doses of NPH, are before breakfast and dinner for the bedtime and morning NPH, respectively. For breakfast Regular and dinner Regular insulin, the therapy response pattern is best gauged by SMBG values before lunch and at bedtime, respectively.

levels with meals in nondiabetic subjects. As shown in Figure 6, Regular insulin needs to be taken 30 minutes or more before meals to act in time to prevent hyperglycemia from food absorption.

## NPH-Based Regimens

Most primary-care providers prescribe NPH and Regular insulin, typically given together as a pre-breakfast and pre-dinner strategy (often referred to as split-mixed insulin). Fixed-insulin-ratio preparations, e.g., 70/30 insulin, are also popular because of their convenience and presumed greater dosing accuracy. NPH insulin given at dinnertime works reasonably well for some patients with type 2 diabetes mellitus, especially the more obese patients (60). However, the use of dinnertime NPH insulin in leaner type 2 diabetes mellitus (BMI $\leq$ 28) patients and those with insulin deficiency from type 1 diabetes mellitus or pancreatic diabetes often causes nocturnal hypoglycemia because the expected peak effect of NPH insulin (maximum glucose lowering) occurs within 8 hours of administration, sometimes earlier. For example, if dinnertime is 6 P.M., then the NPH peak effect occurs between midnight and 6 A.M., when patients are asleep and less able to recognize and effectively treat hypoglycemia. SMBG at 2–3 A.M. may be needed to detect this problem.

### Preventing Nocturnal Hypoglycemia on NPH Regimens

The remedy for nocturnal hypoglycemia from dinnertime NPH is to move the NPH (but not the short-acting meal insulin) to near bedtime. If the patient is on a fixed-insulin-ratio preparation (such as 70/30), this means determining the dose of Regular and NPH from the total 70/30 administered and dosing them separately. For example, to determine the correct starting dose of someone who is on 50 units of 70/30 insulin, multiply the total dose by 0.7 to determine NPH amount (35 units) and by 0.3 to determine the Regular insulin dose (15 units). The Regular insulin would then be given around 30 minutes prior to dinner and the NPH would be given at bedtime (see Figure 5). Most type 1 diabetes mellitus patients and leaner type 2 diabetes mellitus patients (see Table 8) need to separate evening NPH and Regular and use a three-shot regimen to avoid middle-of-the-night hypoglycemia.

### Hypoglycemia with Fixed-Ratio Insulins

Patients on fixed-ratio insulin preparations may have postprandial hypoglycemia because the few available ratios in the United States (70/30 and 50/50 NPH and Regular, 75/25 lispro and NPL) limit the chance of having a ratio that is exactly right for that patient. Further flexible dosing of Regular insulin to match the carbohydrates for different meals is not possible. As illustrated above, the remedy to this kind of problem is the separate dosing and proper timing of the insulins.

Individual dosing for NPH and short-acting insulin allows more precise matching of insulin effects to the glucose peak, leading to improved control of postprandial glucose excursions.

## Erratic Schedules, Missed Meals, and Intermediate Insulins

NPH and Lente insulin have similar (but not identical) delayed peak hypoglycemic actions (intermediate insulins) that result in a prolonged insulin effect. For example, patients simply cannot skip lunch or delay dinner after morning NPH injections without late-afternoon hypoglycemia. Likewise, when NPH or Lente insulin is given near bedtime, breakfast cannot be delayed or omitted, as morning hypoglycemia may ensue. This commonly happens to patients who come for fasting blood tests. In patients who have an early peak of NPH or Lente action, mid-morning or middle-of-the-night hypoglycemia can occur. An insulin preparation such as insulin glargine may improve this kind of situation.

Patients with erratic schedules that lead to unpredictable eating and physical activity patterns often do poorly on NPH- or Lente-based insulin regimens. Peaking of the insulin effect at unwanted times results in frequent hypoglycemia and/or poor glycemic control. Switching to a different basal insulin combined with a bolus of quick-acting insulin with meals (i.e., a basal-bolus regimen) may remedy this kind of problem with hypoglycemia. Recent studies suggest that use of insulin glargine, a newly manufactured long-acting "designer" insulin, may help some patients reduce the frequency of hypoglycemia especially at night (61,62), and may be a superior basal insulin strategy, owing in part to greater reproducibility. Some tradeoffs exist, however, because glargine cannot be mixed with other insulins and there is occasionally more discomfort with its injection because this insulin is constituted in an acidic pH 4.0 solution.

## The Dawn Phenomenon

The "dawn phenomenon" represents a challenge for patients on insulin therapy. The term describes the normal early-morning fall of tissue insulin sensitivity that is counteracted by increased insulin secretion in nondiabetic individuals but is manifest as rising glycemia in persons with diabetes. The physiology is believed to be due to the delayed effect of growth hormone during deep sleep, creating a later temporary period of insulin resistance in the early morning (63). The dawn phenomenon is typically more intense in younger patients and tends to wane with increasing age. Worse glycemic control predicts a greater dawn phenomenon (64). Bedtime intermediate insulin (NPH or Lente) may be advantageous in some patients with a marked dawn phenomenon, with the peak effect of the insulin countering the rise in morning glucose. Often a problem with the dawn phenomenon is the increased risk of hypoglycemia either just before or just afterward (that is, in either the middle of the night or mid-morning). In people with an extreme dawn phenomenon, a basal-bolus approach to insulin therapy may fail to control morning hyperglycemia without unacceptable hypoglycemia at other times of day. Such a problem often leads to selection of insulin-pump therapy, which allows programmed changing of the basal infusion rates during the night.

## Basal Insulin Strategies

For most patients with erratic schedules or who have problematic hypoglycemia when on NPH (or Lente) and Regular or another short-acting insulin, a switch to a better basal insulin may reduce hypoglycemia frequency and severity. Basal insulin normally comprises about half of the total daily insulin dose. This insulin controls hyperglycemia between meals, which is due to hepatic glucose production. Overreliance on basal insulin, however, risks delayed hypoglycemia; this may be seen when basal insulin far exceeds 50% of total daily dosage. Until recently, a basal-bolus strategy for most patients meant a switch to Ultralente insulin, usually given as two injections a day of roughly equal doses before breakfast and dinner. Bolus insulin in the form of quicker-acting insulin would also be given for meal coverage. The bolus of quicker-acting insulin could be Regular, lispro or aspart (see Figure 3). This combination has been shown to be effective and flexible, although most diabetes specialists recognize that Ultralente insulin has some peak action and its peaks are somewhat unpredictable. In outpatient practice, long-acting bolus insulin doses are usually adjusted once a week to minimize risk of overinsulinization as doses are adjusted upward.

## Bolus Insulin Strategies

Matching bolus insulin to meals is an ongoing challenge for many patients with diabetes mellitus, particularly those who are markedly insulin-deficient. Important variables that are often not attended to include the factors mentioned in Table 8. In particular, it is clear from older studies that the timing of insulin can be as important as the dose (see Figure 6).

### *Manipulation of the "Lag Time" to Avoid Hypoglycemia from Bolus Insulin*

As Figure 6 illustrates, altering the lag time—the time between insulin injection and meal ingestion—is a successful strategy to achieve postprandial glycemic control without hypoglycemia. For example, patients may be concerned about using quick-acting insulin preparations when they have hypoglycemia. Omission or reduction of bolus insulin, however, produces marked hyperglycemia. Attempting to correct the postprandial hyperglycemia with later supplemental insulin may risk later hypoglycemia due to overcorrection. A safe approach to bolus dosing in the face of before-meal hypoglycemia is to reduce the lag time (for Regular insulin) or to take quick-acting insulins (lispro or aspart) after the meal

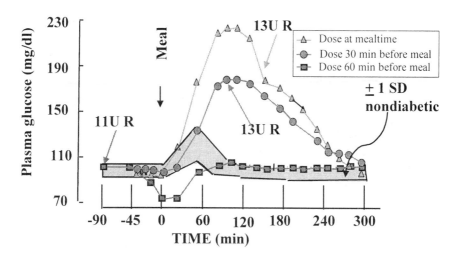

FIGURE 6 Importance of timing of subcutaneous insulin. In this study, the authors examined the glycemic response to mealtime Regular (R) insulin (doses from 11 to 13 units) in well-controlled type 1 diabetes mellitus patients at varying lag times: 0 minutes (triangles), 30 minutes (circles), and 60 minutes (square) before a mixed meal (10 kCal/kg, 45% carbohydrate, 35% fat, and 20% protein). One may conclude from this study that timing of insulin may be as important as dose in determining postprandial hypoglycemia or hyperglycemia. (From Ref. 67.)

to minimize hypoglycemia. This avoids hypoglycemia before the food is absorbed and minimizes the hyperglycemic rebound that insulin omission would foster. Conversely, when pre-meal hyperglycemia is marked, increasing the time between giving the insulin and beginning the meal instead of increasing the dose of insulin (see Table 11) may be helpful. In practice, the lag time for Regular may be from 1 hour before to a half hour after meals (the latter usually in patients with gastroparesis) and with lispro or aspart from one half hour before to one half hour or more after meals.

### Bolus Timing Inconsistency

It is important to inquire specifically about the timing and consistency of the interval between insulin administration and meals. Many patients do not time their insulin properly or consistently at meals. The recommended lag time for Regular insulin is 30–45 minutes; however, patients often take it 5–10 minutes before meals, resulting in hyperglycemia (see Figure 6) due to the lack of correlation between the insulin peak effect and the postprandial glucose peak. If the dose is increased to compensate, late postprandial hypoglycemia may ensue. Timing of insulin injections may need to be changed when patients eat out. Because restaurant meals are often high in fat, which slows food absorption, use of Regular rather than lispro or aspart may be preferred.

### Quick-Acting Insulins and Carbohydrate Counting

The total carbohydrate content of a meal is probably the best guide to the amount of insulin needed as a bolus to "cover" the meal. Insulin/carbohydrate ratios can be estimated in most patients based on standard ranges (1:10–1:20, i.e., 1 unit of bolus insulin for every 10–20 grams of total carbohydrate in the meal) and then adjusted with a skilled dietitian's advice. However, successful use of this technique requires skill in the correct counting of the grams of carbohydrate in a meal, which is initially difficult for some patients to learn. A simple strategy is to ask patients to perform SMBG 2 or 4 hours after common meals (if using lispro/aspart or Regular, respectively) to observe glycemic responses. Where hypoglycemia or hyperglycemia occurs, the patient can adjust the standard bolus doses accordingly.

Strategies for carbohydrate counting come to a large degree from insulin-pump therapy. Learning "carb counting" requires motivation and attention to detail. Several visits with a registered dietitian skilled in dealing with bolus insulin adjustments are usually required. The individual range for insulin/carbohydrate ratios is wide, however; accurate ratio determination involves working closely with a skilled dietitian or certified diabetes educator. Although relative consistency is observed in individuals, insulin/carbohydrate ratios can also change according to circumstances. For example, they may be markedly reduced after exercise (e.g., 1:10 → 1:20) or may be increased as a result of the dawn phenomenon. Some patients carry books listing the carbohydrate content of common foods or use electronic tools such as Palm programs to calculate meal carbohydrate content.

### Postprandial Insulin–Food Absorption Mismatch

Gastroparesis is a challenge to the achievement of stable glycemic control and avoidance of hypoglycemia. It is important to remember that absorption of liquids is much less affected than that of solids. Administration of Regular insulin either with no lag time or after meals may be required to avoid early postprandial hypoglycemia. Unfortunately, hyperglycemia itself tends to worsen gastroparesis. A trial of metoclopramide (10 mg p.o. q.i.d.) or erythromycin (250 mg b.i.d.) may be warranted in some patients with very erratic control and problematic hypoglycemia to see whether improved gastric emptying can stabilize glycemic control. Use of thickened liquid diets may be required. Lispro or aspart may raise the risk of early postprandial hypoglycemia in gastroparesis patients, requiring caution if they are used when gastroparesis is suspected.

Ultimately, for some patients with severe hypoglycemia, insulin-pump therapy will be the only solution with sufficient power and flexibility to achieve stable glycemic control. In appropriately motivated patients, willing to monitor frequently and learn carbohydrate counting and its variations, it will be the best solution for the avoidance of severe hypoglycemia. Implementation of pump therapy requires a team approach and is best done in centers with expertise in pump therapy.

## Combination of Pills and Insulin as Therapy

When combining insulin with oral hypoglycemic pills, it is important to recognize that different pills result in different hypoglycemia patterns. Sulfonylureas, such as glyburide, appear to have a high propensity for causing hypoglycemia in the daytime (65). Metformin appears to have a lesser tendency to do so in combination with insulin, but certainly may require downward insulin-dosage adjustment to avoid hypoglycemia. Thiazolidinediones often cause hypoglycemia if doses of insulin are not reduced because of the improvement in insulin sensitivity. How-

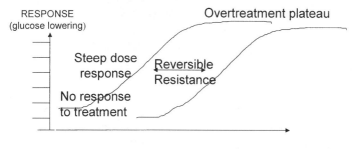

FIGURE 7 Insulin dose-response curve: therapy implications. The dose-response curve is S-shaped, not linear. This means that: 1) undertreatment produces little therapeutic response (glucose lowering), 2) achieving moderate glycemic control improves insulin sensitivity and small changes in dose show significant glycemic alterations, and 3) the glycemic pattern of patients overtreated with insulin is similar whether slightly or severely overtreated; that is, they have both hypoglycemia and hyperglycemia. It is therefore difficult to know how much to reduce the dose to avoid hypoglycemia; several reductions may be needed. Also, overtreated patients become more insulin-resistant, and this gradually reverses as insulin doses are reduced. With greater insulin sensitivity returning, hyperglycemia is followed by recurrent hypoglycemia in some overtreated patients as insulin doses are reduced.

ever, one study suggests that they may also improve counterregulatory hormone defenses. Because hypoglycemia may take from 1 to 6 months to become clinically manifest given the slow time to maximal effect for these drugs, some patients find the hypoglycemia unexpected. Insulin-dose reductions of 25% or more may be required. Figure 7 illustrates how the insulin dose-response curve influences the reoccurrence of hypoglycemia despite dose reductions in such situations.

## SUMMARY

Hypoglycemia is the biggest obstacle to excellent control of diabetes with insulin. The physiological defects that create most of the risk—hypoglycemia unawareness and defective insulin counterregulation—appear in many patients to be largely reversible simply by avoiding hypoglycemia. Identifying those at increased risk is very important since their goals may be adjusted for safety. Full treatment of hypoglycemia is crucial for the safety of patients. Modern insulin therapy is tailored toward avoidance of hypoglycemia. It avoids insulin peaks at times of known susceptibility to hypoglycemia, such as during sleep, and anticipates needs for therapy rather than simply reacting to high and low blood sugars. Increasingly, insulin-therapy strategies are recommended that mimic physiological insulin secretion using a basal-bolus approach. This is accomplished partly through use of insulin preparations that more accurately mimic the way $\beta$ cells secrete insulin.

## REFERENCES

1. American Diabetes Association Position Statement. Standards of medical care for patients with diabetes mellitus. Diabetes Care 24(suppl 1):S33–S43, 2001.
2. The Diabetes Control and Complications Trial Research Group. The effect of intensive treatment of diabetes on the development and progression of long-term complications in insulin-dependent diabetes mellitus. N Engl J Med 329:977–986, 1993.
3. UK Prospective Diabetes Study (UKPDS) Group. Intensive blood-glucose control with sulphonylureas or insulin compared with conventional treatment and risk of complications in patients with type 2 diabetes. Lancet 352(9131):837–853, 1998.
4. UK Prospective Diabetes Study (UKPDS) Group. Effect of intensive blood-glucose control with metformin on complications in overweight patients with type 2 diabetes (UKPDS 34). Lancet 352(9131):854–865, 1998.
5. Frier BM, Fisher BM, editors. Hypoglycemia and Diabetes. London: Edward Arnold, 1993.
6. Cryer PE. Hypoglycemia: Pathophysiology, Diagnosis and Treatment. New York: Oxford, 1997.
7. Purnell JQ, Hokanson JE, Marcovina SM, Steffes MW, Cleary PA, Brunzell JD.

Effect of excessive weight gain with intensive therapy of type 1 diabetes on lipid levels and blood pressure: results from the DCCT. JAMA 280(2):140–146, 1998.

8. The Diabetes Control and Complications Trial Research Group. Hypoglycemia in the Diabetes Control and Complications Trial. Diabetes 46(2):271–286, 1997.

9. Reichard P, Nilsson BY, Rosenqvist U. The effect of long-term intensified insulin treatment on the development of microvascular complications of diabetes mellitus. N Engl J Med 329:304–309, 1993.

10. Reichard P, Pihl M. Mortality and treatment side-effects during long-term intensified conventional insulin treatment in the Stockholm Diabetes Intervention Study. Diabetes 43(2):313–317, 1994.

11. Cox DJ, Gonder-Frederick LA, Kovatchev BP, Young-Hyman DL, Donner TW, Julian DM, Clarke WL. Biopsychobehavioral model of severe hypoglycemia. II. Understanding the risk of severe hypoglycemia. Diabetes Care 22(12):2018–2025, 1999.

12. Kinsley BT, Weinger K, Bajaj M, Levy CJ, Simonson DC, Quigley M, Cox DJ, Jacobson AM. Blood glucose awareness training and epinephrine responses to hypoglycemia during intensive treatment in type 1 diabetes. Diabetes Care 22(7):1022–1028, 1999.

13. Deary IJ, Crawford JR, Hepburn DA, Langan SJ, Blackmore LM, Frier BM. Severe hypoglycemia and intelligence in adult patients with insulin-treated diabetes. Diabetes 42(2):341–344, 1993.

14. Perros P, Deary IJ, Sellar RJ, Best JJ, Frier BM. Brain abnormalities demonstrated by magnetic resonance imaging in adult IDDM patients with and without a history of recurrent severe hypoglycemia. Diabetes Care 20(6):1013–1018, 1997.

15. Fujioka M, Okuchi K, Hiramatsu KI, Sakaki T, Sakaguchi S, Ishii Y. Specific changes in human brain after hypoglycemic injury. Stroke 28(3):584–587, 1997.

16. Kaufman FR, Epport K, Engilman R, Halvorson M. Neurocognitive functioning in children diagnosed with diabetes before age 10 years. J Diabetes Complications 13(1):31–38, 1999.

17. Rovet JF, Ehrlich RM. The effect of hypoglycemic seizures on cognitive function in children with diabetes: a 7-year prospective study. J Pediatr 134(4):503–506, 1999.

18. Rovet JF, Ehrlich RM, Czuchta D. Intellectual characteristics of diabetic children at diagnosis and one year later. J Pediatr Psychol 15: 775–788, 1990.

19. Strachan MW, Deary IJ, Ewing FM, Frier BM. Recovery of cognitive function and mood after severe hypoglycemia in adults with insulin-treated diabetes. Diabetes Care 23(3):305–312, 2000.

20. Gold AE, MacLeod KM, Deary IJ, Frier BM. Hypoglycemia-induced cognitive dysfunction in diabetes mellitus: effect of hypoglycemia unawareness. Physiol Behav 58(3):501–511, 1995.

21. Marques JL, George E, Peacey SR, Harris ND, Macdonald IA, Cochrane T, Heller SR. Altered ventricular repolarization during hypoglycaemia in patients with diabetes. Diabet Med 14(8):648–654, 1997.

22. Trovati M, Anfossi G, Cavalot F, Vitali S, Massucco P, Mularoni E, Schinco P, Tamponi G, Emanuelli G. Studies on mechanisms involved in hypoglycemia-induced platelet activation. Diabetes 35(7):818–825, 1986.

23. Duh E, Feinglos M. Hypoglycemia-induced angina pectoris in a patient with diabetes mellitus. Ann Intern Med 44(7):751–755, 1996.
24. Kamijo Y, Soma K, Aoyama N, Fukuda M, Ohwada T. Myocardial infarction with acute insulin poisoning—a case report. Angiology 51(8):689–693, 2000.
25. Sovik O, Thordarson H. Dead-in-bed syndrome in young diabetic patients. Diabetes Care 22(suppl. 2):B40–B42, 1999.
26. Heller SR. Diabetic hypoglycaemia. Best Pract Res Clin Endocrinol Metab 13(2): 279–294, 1999.
27. Spyer G, Hattersley AT, Macdonald IA, Amiel SA, MacLeod KM. Hypoglycaemic counter-regulation at normal blood glucose concentrations in patients with well controlled type-2 diabetes. Lancet 356: 1970–1974, 2000.
28. Ohkubo Y, Kishikawa H, Araki E, Miyata T, Isami S, Motoyoshi S, Kojima Y, Furuyoshi N, Shichiri M. Intensive insulin therapy prevents the progression of diabetic microvascular complications in Japanese patients with non-insulin-dependent diabetes mellitus: a randomized prospective 6-year study. Diabetes Res Clin Pract 28(2):103–117, 1995.
29. Matyka K, Evans M, Lomas J, Cranston I, Macdonald I, Amiel SA. Altered hierarchy of protective responses against severe hypoglycemia in normal aging in healthy men. Diabetes Care 20(2):135–141, 1997.
30. Shorr RI, Ray WA, Daugherty JR, Griffin MR. Incidence and risk factors for serious hypoglycemia in older persons using insulin or sulfonylureas. Arch Intern Med 157(15):1681–1686, 1997.
31. Veneman TF, Erkelens DW. Clinical review: hypoglycemia unawareness in noninsulin-dependent diabetes mellitus. J Clin Endocrinol Metab 82(6):1682–1684, 1997.
32. Bolli GB, Tsalikian E, Haymond MW, Cryer PE, Gerich JE. Defective glucose counterregulation after subcutaneous insulin in noninsulin-dependent diabetes mellitus: paradoxical suppression of glucose utilization and lack of compensatory increase in glucose production, roles of insulin resistance, abnormal neuroendocrine responses, and islet paracrine interactions. J Clin Invest 73:1532–1541, 1984.
33. Shamoon H, Friedman S, Canton C, Zacharowicz L, Hu M, Rossetti L. Increased epinephrine and skeletal muscle responses to hypoglycemia in non-insulin-dependent diabetes mellitus. J Clin Invest 93(6):2562–2571, 1994.
34. Ohno T, Toyama T, Hoshizaki H, Okamoto E, Naito S, Nogami A, Kamiyama H, Ohshima S, Yuasa K, Taniguchi K, et al. Evaluation of cardiac sympathetic nervous function by 123I-metaiodobenzylguanidine scintigraphy in insulin-treated non-insulin dependent diabetics with hypoglycemia unawareness. Intern Med 35(2):94–99, 1996.
35. Hepburn DA, MacLeod KM, Pell AC, Scougal IJ, Frier BM. Frequency and symptoms of hypoglycaemia experienced by patients with type 2 diabetes treated with insulin. Diabet Med 10(3):231–237, 1993.
36. Fanelli CG, Epifano L, Rambotti AM, Pampanelli S, Di Vincenzo A, Modarelli F, Lepore M, Annibale B, Ciofetta M, Bottini P, et al. Meticulous prevention of hypoglycemia normalizes the glycemic thresholds and magnitude of most of neuroendocrine responses to, symptoms of, and cognitive function during hypoglycemia in intensively treated patients with short-term IDDM. Diabetes 42(11):1683–1689, 1993.

37. Cryer PE. Iatrogenic hypoglycemia as a cause of hypoglycemia-associated autonomic failure in IDDM: a vicious cycle. Diabetes 41(3):255–260, 1992.
38. McCall AL. IDDM, counterregulation, and the brain. Diabetes Care 20(8):1228–1230, 1997.
39. Boyle PJ, Nagy RJ, O'Connor AM, Kempers SF, Yeo RA, Qualls C. Adaptation in brain glucose uptake following recurrent hypoglycemia. Proc Natl Acad Sci USA 91(20):9352–9356, 1994.
40. Boyle PJ, Kempers SF, O'Connor AM, Nagy RJ. Brain glucose uptake and unawareness of hypoglycemia in patients with insulin-dependent diabetes mellitus. N Engl J Med 333(26):1726–1731, 1995.
41. Davis SN, Shavers C, Davis B, Costa F. Prevention of an increase in plasma cortisol during hypoglycemia preserves subsequent counterregulatory responses. J Clin Invest 100(2):429–438, 1997.
42. Davis SN, Shavers C, Costa F, Mosqueda-Garcia R. Role of cortisol in the pathogenesis of deficient counterregulation after antecedent hypoglycemia in normal humans. J Clin Invest 98(3):680–691, 1996.
43. Fritsche A, Stumvoll M, Haring HU, Gerich JE. Reversal of hypoglycemia unawareness in a long-term type 1 diabetic patient by improvement of beta-adrenergic sensitivity after prevention of hypoglycemia. J Clin Endocrinol Metab 85(2):523–525, 2000.
44. Fritsche A, Stumvoll M, Grub M, Sieslack S, Renn W, Schmulling RM, Haring HU, Gerich JE. Effect of hypoglycemia on beta-adrenergic sensitivity in normal and type 1 diabetic subjects. Diabetes Care 21(9):1505–1510, 1998.
45. George E, Marques JL, Harris ND, Macdonald IA, Hardisty CA, Heller SR. Preservation of physiological responses to hypoglycemia 2 days after antecedent hypoglycemia in patients with IDDM. Diabetes Care 20(8):1293–1298, 1997.
46. Bolli GB. How to ameliorate the problem of hypoglycemia in intensive as well as nonintensive treatment of type 1 diabetes. Diabetes Care 22 (suppl 2): B43–52, 1999.
47. Fanelli C, Pampanelli S, Lalli C, Del Sindaco P, Ciofetta M, Lepore M, Porcellati F, Bottini P, Di Vincenzo A, Brunetti P, et al. Long-term intensive therapy of IDDM patients with clinically overt autonomic neuropathy: effects on hypoglycemia awareness and counterregulation. Diabetes 46(7):1172–1181, 1997.
48. Veneman T, Mitrakou A, Mokan M, Cryer P, Gerich J. Induction of hypoglycemia unawareness by asymptomatic nocturnal hypoglycemia. Diabetes 42(9):1233–1237, 1993.
49. Saleh TY, Cryer PE. Alanine and terbutaline in the prevention of nocturnal hypoglycemia in IDDM. Diabetes Care 20(8):1231–1236, 1997.
50. Kaufman FR, Devgan S. Use of uncooked cornstarch to avert nocturnal hypoglycemia in children and adolescents with type I diabetes. J Diabetes Complications 10(2): 84–87, 1996.
51. Beregszaszi M, Tubiana-Rufi N, Benali K, Noel M, Bloch J, Czernichow P. Nocturnal hypoglycemia in children and adolescents with insulin-dependent diabetes mellitus: prevalence and risk factors. J Pediatrics 131(1):27–33, 1997.
52. Matyka KA, Crowne, Havel PJ, Macdonald IA, Matthews D, Dunger DB. Counterregulation during spontaneous nocturnal hypoglycemia in prepubertal children with type 1 diabetes. Diabetes Care 22(7):1144–1150, 1999.

53. Rabasa-Lhoret R, Ducros F, Bourque J, Chiasson JL. Guidelines for premeal insulin dose reduction for postprandial exercise of different intensities and durations in type 1 diabetic subjects treated intensively with a basal-bolus insulin regimen (Ultralente-Lispro). Diabetes Care 24: 625–630, 2001.

54. Gearhart JG, Duncan JL 3rd, Replogle JH, Forbes RC, Walley EJ. Efficacy of sliding-scale insulin therapy: a comparison with prospective regimens. Fam Pract Res J 14(4):313–322, 1994.

55. Sawin CT. Action without benefit: the sliding scale of insulin use. Arch Intern Med 157(5):489, 1997.

56. Guthrie DW, Guthrie RA. Approach to management. Diabetes Educator 16(5):401–406, 1990.

57. Silverstein JH, Rosenbloom AL. New developments in type 1 (insulin-dependent) diabetes. Clin Pediatr 39(5):257–266, 2000.

58. Garg SK, Potts RO, Ackerman NR, Fermi SJ, Tamada JA, Chase HP. Correlation of fingerstick blood glucose measurements with GlucoWatch biographer glucose results in young subjects with type 1 diabetes. Diabetes Care 22(10):1708–1714, 1999.

59. Jones TW, Caprio S, Diamond MP, Hallarman L, Boulware SD, Sherwin RS, Tamborlane WV. Does insulin species modify counterregulatory hormone response to hypoglycemia? Diabetes Care 14(8):728–731, 1991.

60. Riddle MC, Schneider J. Glimepiride Combination Group. Beginning insulin treatment of obese patients with evening 70/30 insulin plus glimepiride versus insulin alone. Diabetes Care 21(7):1052–1057, 1998.

61. Pieber TR, Eugene-Jolchine I, Derobert E. The European Study Group of HOE 901 in Type 1 Diabetes: efficacy and safety of HOE 901 versus NPH insulin in patients with type 1 diabetes. Diabetes Care 23(2):157–162, 2000.

62. Ratner RE, Hirsch IB, Neifing JL, Garg SK, Mecca TE, Wilson CA. U.S. Study Group of Insulin Glargine in Type 1 Diabetes. Less hypoglycemia with insulin glargine in intensive insulin therapy for type 1 diabetes. Diabetes Care 23(5):639–643, 2000.

63. Campbell PJ, Bolli GB, Gerich JE. Prevention of the dawn phenomenon (early morning hyperglycemia) in insulin-dependent diabetes mellitus by bedtime intranasal administration of a long-acting somatostatin analog. Metabolism: Clin Exp 37(1):34–37, 1988.

64. Bolli GB, Perriello G, Fanelli CG, De Feo P. Nocturnal blood glucose control in type I diabetes mellitus. Diabetes Care 16(suppl 3):71–89, 1993.

65. Yki-Jarvinen H, Ryysy L, Nikkila K, Tulokas T, Vanamo R, Heikkila M. Comparison of bedtime insulin regimens in patients with type 2 diabetes mellitus: a randomized, controlled trial. Ann Intern Med 130(5):389–396, 1999.

66. Polonsky KS, Sturis J, Bell GI. Seminars in Medicine of the Beth Israel Hospital, Boston. Non-insulin-dependent diabetes mellitus: a genetically programmed failure of the beta cell to compensate for insulin resistance. N Engl J Med 334(12):777–783, 1996.

67. Dimitriadis GD, Gerich JE. Importance of timing of prandial subcutaneous insulin administration in the management of diabetes mellitus. Diabetes Care 6:374–377, 1983.

# 14

## The Art and Science of Insulin-Pump Therapy

**Alan O. Marcus**

University of Southern California Medical School, Los Angeles, and
Saddleback Memorial Medical Center, Laguna Hills, California

### INTRODUCTION

The appropriate delivery of insulin for achieving euglycemia has been the goal of diabetes therapies in cases of both absolute and relative insulin deficiency. The fact that insulin is the most effective therapeutic choice for lowering blood sugars to normal or near-normal levels was established almost 80 years ago. All people with diabetes mellitus need to achieve the well-known goal of glucose control, set around the world at an $HbA_{1c}$ of 6.5%. The fact that achieving this target results in prevention, stabilization, and reversal of complications associated with diabetes is equally well known as a result of multiple landmark interventional studies. These studies all met the most rigorous of scientific criteria and have set the standards of glucose control to be achieved. The causes of failure to achieve both euglycemia and improvements in the adverse outcomes of patients with diabetes need to be examined, and these factors require rectification.

Investigators and clinicians currently view insulin pumps as the "gold standard" by which all alternative methods of insulin delivery are gauged. What has given rise to this opinion that insulin pumps provide the best method of achieving normal blood sugars is the publication of multiple studies documenting improved control, as measured by reduction in $HbA_{1c}$ levels across all population groups, ages, genders, and socioeconomic backgrounds, in both research and practice settings (Figure 1). This lowering of glucose levels, the accepted goal of all, is tempered only by the associated increasing iatrogenic rate of the most severe of the acute events associated with diabetes: hypoglycemia. In the Diabetes Control and Complications Trial (DCCT), every 10% reduction of HbA1c was associated not only with the well-publicized 43% reduced risk of retinopathy progression but also with an 18% increased risk of severe hypoglycemia associated with coma and seizure (1). Hypoglycemia truly is 'the "rate-limiting step of diabetes," as Phil Cryer stated in 1994. Insulin-pump therapy has demonstrated a reduction not only in blood sugars but also in the number of hypoglycemic events that occur at the same time that blood sugars improve (Figures 2 and 3).

It is estimated that greater than 127,000 people in the United States utilized continuous subcutaneous insulin infusion (CSII)—insulin pumps—to deliver insulin in 2001. Of diabetes health-care professionals who identify themselves as having type 1 diabetes and who belong to the professional sections of the American Diabetes Association or the American Association of Diabetes Educators, 52% and 60%, respectively, use insulin-pump therapy to treat their diabetes. The number of current pump users is growing every year, and this growth is expected to continue. These numbers of professionals using pumps were and still are in sharp contrast to the only 6% of the population of the United States identified as having type 1 diabetes who were on pump therapy at the time of this study, a figure that is now estimated at 12% (2). The acceptance and validation of this technology are due to improvements in all parts of the pumps and advances in

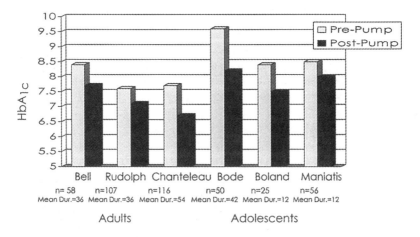

**FIGURE 1** CSII reduces $HbA_{1c}$. (Adapted from Refs. 16, 46–49.)

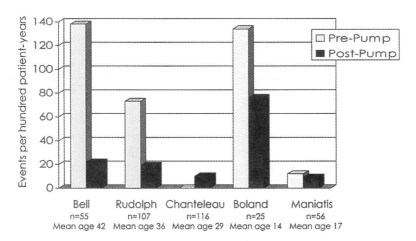

**FIGURE 2** CSII reduces hypoglycemia. (Adapted from Refs. 16, 46–49.)

the formulation of insulins. This has happened at the same time as an explosion in knowledge of patients' real-time, retrospective, and average glucose levels, giving impetus to improve the glucocentric environment of the patient.

Improvement in the technology of the pump itself is easily recognized by the reduction in its size from the impractical but seminal idea of a pump the size of a backpack (proposed by Arnold Kadish of Los Angeles) to the current pumps that weigh as little as 3.5 ounces, or less than 100 grams (the MiniMed 508).

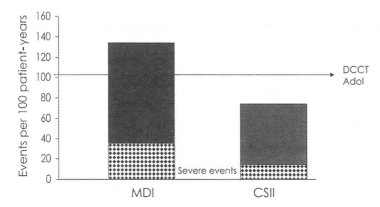

**FIGURE 3** Hypoglycemia reduction in children. $p < 0.01$. (Adapted from Ref. 47.)

Despite this remarkable evolution, the goal is the same: to deliver insulin in a physiological way. The concept of the earliest pumps was to deliver insulin intravenously, but this was modified in subsequent pumps to subcutaneous insulin delivery, which made access—and therefore usage—more feasible, but there were still significant limitations due to their weight and size (400 g and approximately $18 \times 7 \times 6$ cm). These primitive pumps were big and bulky, limited to one infusion rate (insulin rates were adjusted by dilution of insulin), and required a large expenditure of not only battery power but the energy of the patient and the clinicians to maintain its function. The earliest studies on CSII were done with such pumps, and successes were reported in achieving near euglycemia in both adults and adolescents (3,4).

It should be noted that these successes were possible only through the introduction of technology that allowed for the determination of blood sugars rapidly and accurately by the patient. Self-monitoring of blood glucose (SMBG) allows for the evaluation and correction of insulin delivery in terms of basal rate, bolus, and correction bolus and adjustments to these that result in improved glucose due to precise and effective insulin usage.

As described earlier, the pumps themselves have become lighter and smaller and now have the ability to deliver insulin in varying amounts over various time blocks of the day, repetitively or according to the type or characteristics of a given day (e.g., work day, holiday, exercise, travel, premenstrual, or sick). The bolus delivery of insulin can be programmed to match the requirements or challenge presented by every type of meal (its composition or duration) and to accommodate the individual absorptive and gastrointestinal activity of the patient. The bolus can be initiated by remote control, alleviating the fear that "button pushing" by younger patients will result in inappropriate insulin delivery.

The software that accompanies the actual delivery mechanism of the pump allows for added safety features and the accumulation of information on pump performance and patient usage that can be viewed directly or downloaded. This offers additional possibilities for improvement of outcomes as a result of a heightened understanding of what factors resulted in either normal or abnormal glucose levels. Safety alarms on pumps are now standard and provide the added assurance that the insulin pump is doing and will continue to do its primary job of delivering insulin. These features, together with improvements in education and more continuous glucose monitoring, have resulted in a lower incidence of diabetic ketoacidosis (DKA) than with syringe delivery of insulin (5). Additional improvements in the catheters, also called infusion sets, that nonsurgically connect the pump reservoir to the patient and serve as the conduit for the delivery of insulin to the subcutaneous space have also increased the overall acceptance and viability of pump usage. Catheters no longer have the compatibility problems with insulin that in earlier years resulted in catheter binding of insulin and variable delivery; the catheters can be painlessly and effectively inserted by devices such as the Sofserter, specifically designed for this purpose. Multiple options available among catheters allow for variations in subcutaneous fat, individual patient preference, and appropriateness. The ability since 1995 to disconnect from the pump for swimming, taking saunas, and other pursuits in which a pump is not desired was made possible by advances in infusion sets, specifically, by incorporating a quick-release feature into their design. Needles—bent or straight—as part of the catheter have been supplemented by catheters of varying dimension and shape to improve comfort and allow for individual choice of the ideal infusion set. An additional advance has been the development by pharmaceutical companies of insulin analogs. These insulins are designed to have specific desired performance characteristics.

The rapid-acting insulins commercially available and in use (lispro and aspart) possess the ideal characteristics for success with pump therapy. They realize the rapidity of insulin action that was the goal of the original intravenous pump delivery systems while retaining the advantages of subcutaneous delivery. Rapidity of action allows for better matching of insulin to meal requirements temporally as well as limitation of the undesirable "tail effect" of injected insulin that results in increased late postprandial hypoglycemia. These insulins have been proven to reduce hypoglycemia, improve $HbA_{1c}$ levels, and, after 3 months of CSII usage, improve hepatic glucose output in response to glucagon (6–9). Reduction in the "tail effect" of these insulins has not been associated with an increase in the occurrence of DKA. The newer technology of the continuous glucose monitoring system and its usage will provide even more information, pinpointing times and events requiring more or less insulin delivery (10) to achieve a reduction in both hyper- and hypoglycemia. Reduction of events, which will result in optimal glycemic control, is dependent on the individual metabolic characteristics of a given patient and the pharmacodynamics and route of delivery of the insulin (11). When one compares the intrapatient variability of different insulins, it is clear that day-to-day fluctuations in glucose levels are frequently attributable to the insulin formulation utilized and the variability in its glucose-lowering effect in the same person on subsequent days even when all other controllable variables are equal (12). Regular by injection would differ from Regular by CSII in that intrapatient variability is lowest for Regular insulin administered by CSII, greater for glargine and NPH (considered equal in this respect), and still greater for Lente and Ultralente, which has the greatest intrapatient variability whether measured by time of onset, duration of action, or glucose-lowering efficacy (13). The effective use of insulin is dependent on the reproducibility of its effect.

If we accept the premise that all patients need to be considered candidates for intensive therapy and that CSII is the most physiological way to administer insulin and to practice intensive therapy, we need to examine the methods which result in successful insulin pump usage. Some points apply to all groups, but an attempt is made to focus on the individual needs of each patient population and guide the clinician in a practical manner to achieve a positive outcome. The most important guidelines for successful pump use in clinical practice begin with giving the patient—and those involved with the patient—a clear understanding of what a pump is and is not. The pump is a device that enables more precise control over the amounts of insulin delivered and therefore how much insulin will be available at the cell receptor over time. It is not a cure for diabetes. Use of an insulin pump does not in and of itself constitute intensive therapy, which is defined by the targets and goals set for the levels of glucose. The pump itself does not demand more time and effort from the patient or the health-care team; it is the goal of achieving normal or improved glucose levels that calls for a commitment of time and effort from all involved. Pumps are a useful tool for insulin delivery when the goal is near-normal glycemia or ameliorating hypoglycemic events, in the treatment of hypoglycemic unawareness. There is no age limit for pump usage—they have been used in people from 3 days old to over 80 years old. Pumps do allow for more choices and their success depends on the motivation, education, and involvement of all involved.

## ADULT PATIENTS WITH TYPE 1 DIABETES MELLITUS

The key to success with insulin pump therapy can be found in the words of the Chinese philosopher Lao Tsu, first spoken in 500 B.C.:

> Tell me—I'll forget.
> Show me—I may remember.
> Involve me—and I will understand.

All patients with type 1 diabetes mellitus have a complete lack of insulin and therefore require the replacement of both basal (non-food related) insulin and bolus insulin (food-related or necessary for a correction of elevated blood glucose). Patients with type 1 diabetes mellitus who are starting on pump therapy will therefore already be on a regimen intended to deliver insulin for both of these general requirements. Type 1 diabetes mellitus patients can generally be thought to need 40 to 50% of their total daily insulin requirement in the form of basal insulin. To achieve near-euglycemia, the total daily insulin requirement for these patients (basal and bolus) under normal conditions, and if they are within 20% of their ideal body weight, is 0.5 to 1.0 U per kilogram of body weight per day. If stress factors—biological, psychological, or social—are present, the requirement for insulin is frequently greater. This increase may be temporary (e.g., related to events such as menstrual periods or activities such as work and leisure) or permanent (in response to concurrent illness, medications, obesity, and/or insulin resistance). Insulin requirement is also greater in diabetes patients whose BMI (body mass index) is greater than 27, as was true in 33% of the intensive and 19% of the standard treatment groups of the DCCT (14). Any determination of bolus or basal rates before glucose measurement and assessment of insulin-delivery requirements is extremely arbitrary; it should serve only as a place from which to start and then be further refined to match the needs of an individual person as those needs are discovered by observation and interpretation. Commonly, patients going on CSII or pump therapy require 20 to 25% less insulin than they did on injections (15–17).

Targets for glucose levels need to be set (Table 1). The most commonly used targets are those adopted by the American Diabetes Association and utilized in the DCCT (18): preprandial blood sugars of 70–140 mg/dl, 2-hour postprandial blood sugars of less than 180 mg/dl (with the clock starting when chewing begins), bedtime blood sugars of 100–140 mg/dl, and 3 A.M. blood sugars of greater than 90 mg/dl. Additional goals of glucose control recently set by the AACE consensus conference would seem to be appropriate. According to these, blood sugar levels would be a maximum of 110 mg/dl preprandial and 140 mg/dl or less 2 hours postprandial (19). These targets are for patients who are not pregnant and who do not have hypoglycemic unawareness. Those conditions require different targets, which are discussed below.

Starting the pump is an outpatient procedure for the vast majority of patients. A certified pump trainer instructs the patient as to the various features and settings, which need to be in place before using the pump to deliver insulin. A method adopted successfully by most centers and offices is as follows. The patient takes his nighttime insulin the night before beginning to use the pump, and then begins pump therapy that morning prior to any meals. The initiation occurs in the office setting with the patient, others involved with the patient's care, and the physician or health-care provider all being present. The patient inserts the infusion set and is familiarized with such topics as basal rates and targets (Table

**TABLE 1** Target Glucose Ranges (mg/dl; individually set for each patient)

| "Average Joe" adult | |
|---|---|
| Preprandial | 70–110 |
| 2 hr postprandial | <140 |
| Bedtime | 100–140 |
| 3 A.M. | >90 |
| Hypoglycemic unawareness | |
| Preprandial | 100–160 |
| Pregnant | |
| Preprandial | 60–90 |
| 1 hr postprandial | <130 |
| 2 hr postprandial | <120 |

*Source*: Adapted from Refs. 1, 18, 19, 45, 50.

TABLE 2 Calculations of Adult Dosage

---

Basal rate
    50% of pump total daily dose
    Divide total basal by 24 hours to decide on hourly basal
    Start with only one basal rate
    See how it goes before adding additional basals

Basal rate adjustment overnight
    Check BG
    Bedtime
        12 A.M.
        3 A.M.
        6 A.M.
    Adjust overnight basal if readings vary >30 mg/dl

Correction bolus—rule of 1500[a]
    Insulin sensitivity factor
    Determines the estimated BG drop per unit of insulin

Estimating an insulin-to-carbohydrate ratio—rule of 500 (500 divided by
    TDD)
    Example: 500/50 = 10
    = 1 unit of insulin per 10 g carbohydrate

---

[a] *Source*: Ref. 21.

2). Written guidelines are provided on these as well as for the administration of insulin as pre-meal, correction boluses, and basals, with instructions for adapting these initial calculations as necessary. Follow-up is usually scheduled for the next day, once again the following week, and then as often as deemed appropriate.

Initially only one basal rate is set for a 24-hour period. This rate is verified by the patient's checking at 2- or 3-hour intervals for a total of 6 hours, without food or food boluses being taken during this time. If the blood sugar level does not change by more than 30 mg/dl from beginning to end, the basal rate is confirmed as correct. When the glucose level changes in excess of 30 mg/dl, differing basal rates can be added. The newer and original basal rates are changed to accommodate the varying physiological need for insulin during these time periods (e.g., if at 10:00 A.M. blood sugar is 90 and at 12:00, 2 hours later, it is 140, the basal rate is increased over this period by 0.1 or 0.2 units per hour). Any change in insulin should be reconfirmed the following day. The "dawn phenomenon," a sudden increase in glucose prior to awakening, requires an increase in the amount of insulin being pumped or delivered at the time the glucose level is rising; in such cases, blood sugar readings should be taken at midnight, 3 A.M., and 6 A.M. Again, changes in blood sugar by more than 30 mg/dl from the beginning to the end of any of these periods call for a change in the amount of insulin infused. The fact that these infusion rates can be changed, and in micro-amounts, is one of the benefits of pump therapy that are not available to those using syringes to administer insulin.

The pre-meal to post-meal change in blood sugar level should be approximately 50 mg/dl. If the change is greater, an error has been made either in calculating the amount of insulin needed for the meal or in quantification of the meal's carbohydrate content. Most patients can determine the amount of insulin they need to take to balance the amount of food they are going to ingest by practicing carbohydrate counting and assessing how much insulin is necessary to maintain a normal blood sugar. Use of this technique in the DCCT to determine insulin requirements for meals resulted in a reduction in HbA$_{1c}$ of 0.75 (20). The range for this number is large and can vary with each individual, the time of day, and the type of carbohydrate eaten, and with what. Most patients learn by trial and error or—as it is scientifically called—experimentation and observation. An approximate amount of insulin necessary to balance the grams of carbohydrate eaten can be determined initially by calculating the total daily dosage (TDD) of insulin and dividing the number 500 by that amount. The result is the number of grams of carbohydrate that one unit of insulin will be able to balance (e.g., a total daily insulin dosage of 50 units divided into 500 means that every 10 grams of carbohydrate eaten requires one unit of insulin). This number, as in all calculations for insulin requirements, is arbitrary, and adjustments are the rule and not the exception. To make successful adjustments, patients need to frequently monitor glucose levels and other variables and have the skills and training to make changes on an ongoing basis. This "empowerment" of the patient is an essential component for success whatever the method of insulin delivery. For patients who cannot count carbohydrates, remembering the amount of insulin necessary for given foods and amounts is equally adequate and often very successful.

Corrective action is also needed when blood sugars taken other than at mealtimes are out of the predetermined target range. When the blood sugar is too high, the action required is called a correction bolus. The amount of insulin to be taken can be calculated by using the familiar rule of 1500 (21). This aids in determining the insulin sensitivity factor or the estimated drop in blood glucose per unit of insulin. The starting point—the TDD—is divided into 1500 and the result is how much glucose should empirically be lowered following the administration of one unit of insulin (e.g., A TDD of 50 units of insulin divided into 1500 is 30: in this case, one unit of insulin will lower blood sugar by 30 mg/dl. If a patient's blood sugar is 220 and his target is 130, he needs to take 3 additional units to reach that level. The results of some studies using rapid-acting insulin analogs suggest that this rule of 1500 should be corrected to the rule of 1800 or even 2000. Only individual assessment will determine which of these will bring about the correct adjustment for an individual patient.

The infusion site should be checked at least once a day, and pump manufacturers recommend that the infusion site be changed every 48 hours. Because erythema, pain, or irritation at the insertion site may indicate a local anatomical problem that could interfere with insulin delivery, they signal the need for an earlier change of the catheter. If this local irritation is a recurrent or chronic problem attributed to the tape, then a different tape can be used. Rarely, the patient's skin may be irritated by the catheter itself, in which case the "sandwich technique"—placing the catheter between two layers of tape, one on the skin and the other above the catheter to hold it in place—is a suitable remedy. The catheter or infusion set is always inserted subcutaneously, and is inserted using aseptic technique after the skin has been cleansed with a solvent such as i.v. prep. The locations for insertion are wherever the patient feels comfortable; most patients choose the abdomen, sides, or back, but other locations are viable. Special circumstances may affect site selection. For example, in the last trimester of pregnancy, the abdomen, because of its enlargement and stretched skin, is avoided and the upper arms or other locations are chosen.

Tape is used to hold the infusion set in place to prevent hyperglycemia and possibly diabetic ketoacidosis as well as accidental removal. Many tapes are available for this purpose, and most manufacturers will supply a selection of tapes for first-time pumpers to try before deciding on the one best suited for their needs. Some patients have a problem with skin stickiness, most often due to perspiration; specially designed tape such as Skin-Tac or Mastisol liquid adhesive with Detachol to remove it may be useful.

When blood sugar levels are greater than 250 mg/dl, it must be determined whether this state represents simple hyperglycemia or hyperglycemia with diabetic ketoacidosis before a decision can be made on the appropriate therapeutic course. The simplest way to make this determination is through the use of Ketostix, which change color in the presence of ketones in the urine. If no ketones are present, than the patient can take a correction bolus using the insulin pump and recheck his blood sugar level after 1 hour. If the blood glucose has not decreased, then the patient, according to the instructions he should have been given, administers the correction bolus, via syringe and then attempts to determine why the pump-administered insulin was ineffective. The problem is found in greatest to least frequency from "the skin to the pump." The most common mechanical causes involve the catheter (e.g., removal, kinking, partial obstruction). Less often the problem is a faulty connection of the catheter to the pump, absence of insulin, failure of battery supply to the pump, or failure of the pump to deliver insulin because of pump damage. Nontechnological causes include inflammation at the insertion site and insulin decay resulting from physical or chemical alteration to the insulin itself (usually from temperature alterations or incorrect handling).

Prevention of diabetic ketoacidosis is a primary objective of the treatment of type 1 diabetes, whether the patient is on pump or syringe therapy. Special vigilance is required with patients using CSII, even though studies demonstrate that with adequate education and involvement of the patient there is no increased incidence of DKA with pumps. Because pumps use only short-acting forms of insulin, if delivery is interrupted there is no safety net of intermediate- or long-lasting insulin to prevent the breakdown of fat and muscle to prevent the conversion of these substrates into ketone bodies (22,23). If a patient has nausea or vomiting or any other symptoms related to DKA, an immediate check of blood sugars and ketones is warranted. If the patient is unable to drink liquids and replenish fluids, a physician should be called immediately and the patient must go to the hospital for administration of intravenous insulin, replacement of lost fluids and electrolytes, and treatment of the underlying cause of inadequate insulin. If ketones are positive but the patient is able to take liquids orally, then aggressive fluid ingestion is begun and insulin is administered on a schedule determined by the physician and guided by frequent (hourly) self-monitoring of blood glucose levels and recurrent evaluation of the degree of ketosis present or its resolution. Until the ketosis clears, additional insulin is best initiated by syringe injection with a routine change of infusion site and by troubleshooting the pump, insulin, and delivery system prior to resuming pump therapy. As in all cases of ketoacidosis, the cause needs to be determined and corrected to avoid its recurrence.

The other acute event of insulin therapy is hypoglycemia, and its prevention or limitation is of utmost importance in the prevention of premature mortality (24) and the achievement of euglycemia. In type 1 diabetes patients, the adequacy of prevention of hypoglycemia is based on detection, which in turn is dependent on the frequency and regularity of self-monitoring of blood glucoses. Patients on insulin should monitor blood sugar levels four to six times daily and be familiar with the actions necessary to treat an acute event and prevent future episodes.

When hypoglycemia occurs, the most appropriate treatment is to ingest known quantities of glucose to effect a predictable rise in serum glucose levels. The DCCT based the guidelines for treatment on the knowledge that 15 g of glucose will raise blood sugars 15 mg/dl in 15 minutes. If the current level is 40 mg/dl and the target is 100 mg/dl, then 60 g of glucose will achieve that. Patients often overtreat hypoglycemia by taking copious amounts of glucose, for example, in the form of candies or juices, resulting in an exaggerated rise in blood sugars to hyperglycemic ranges.

The occurrence of hypoglycemia is greatest during the overnight or sleep period, when 60% of hypoglycemic events occur (25). Maintaining bedtime and 3 A.M. glucose levels at at least 100 mg/dl diminishes this event rate. Similarly, minimum glucose levels of 100 mg/dl are preferable before engaging in activities such as driving, exercise, drinking, or others that might result in an increased risk or consequence from hypoglycemia. Blood sugars should be checked at the beginning of any such activity that can cause wide swings in plasma glucose and periodically (every hour or two hours) during the activity, to detect and prevent severe hypoglycemia. The knowledge accumulated from monitoring blood glucose levels and their changes should be used as the basis for changing the basal dose of insulin delivered during similar activities in the future. These rates modified for activities, known as temporary basal rates, may vary in size and duration according to the level of activity and its time of occurrence. As with all insulin-administration regimens, these are decided on an individual basis and may need to be adjusted as the patient and health-care team deem appropriate. Before, during, or after any activity that can lower blood glucose, bolus dosages should be reduced to prevent hypoglycemia and then glucose should be measured to determine the correct reduction for future boluses at these times.

For patients with hypoglycemic unawareness, targets appropriate for this condition need to be set. The occurrence of frequent hypoglycemic events (more than three per month) is known to result in a decrease in the catecholamine response to hypoglycemia and a decrease in awareness of these events (26).

The frequency of hypoglycemic unawareness is much greater than previously thought. Only now is it being documented and recognized in studies utilizing systems that continuously monitor interstitial blood glucoses and accumulate these data for later interpretation. Use of this technology prompts adjustment of basal and bolus rates that consistently address the issue of patient under-bolusing at meals and over-basaling at other times. Appropriate targets for patients with hypoglycemic unawareness are 130 mg/dl before meals, bed, and driving, and at 3 A.M. Prevention of hypoglycemia in these patients results in partial correction of hypoglycemic awareness and is one of the goals of and reasons for initiating insulin-pump therapy. Generally the family or other care-givers of the patient with diabetes should be instructed in the recognition of hypoglycemia and the appropriate administration of glucose and/or glucagon if necessary. Patients should wear or carry medical identification bracelets or cards indicating that they have diabetes so hypoglycemia can be recognized and treated. All patients using pump therapy can minimize their exposure to unwanted insulin by setting the auto-off safety alarm so that if they don't actively do something with their pump to tell it that they are alert it will automatically stop delivering insulin at a patient-determined time and prevent hypoglycemia from being prolonged by continued delivery of insulin. Lastly, no insulin pump is waterproof. Putting the pump in water has resulted in hypoglycemia in patients who thought otherwise and unexpectedly received an overdelivery of insulin.

## PEDIATRIC PATIENTS

If the growth in insulin-pump use among adult type 1 diabetes patients has been extraordinary, it has been explosive among pediatric patients with type 1 diabetes. In 1997 the number of young people using pump therapy was less than 500, but by 1999 that number had grown to more than 5000. The reason for this is the realization by the general population of pediatric type 1 patients and their physicians that insulin-pump therapy offers an alternative with more choices and less restriction of behavior and activity than with syringes while also achieving an improved blood sugar environment and an associated lowering of hypoglycemia event rates (27–32). In the study authored by White et al., the rate of severe hypoglycemia in children age 2–16 years in one review was approximately 60 per 100 patient-years whether undergoing usual (two injections per day) or intensive-care regimens; CSII lowered this rate to less than 10 both in and outside the study group. Another study found that the only characteristic predictive of failure to achieve metabolic control with pumps is the fear of needles. Children or adolescents may simply want a pump; have busy, changing schedules; seek more flexibility in activities; or have nocturnal hypoglycemia or many wide swings in their blood sugars with conventional treatment. It is necessary that the child being considered be either performing or willing to perform three or four self-monitored blood glucose measurements per day. Obviously either the patient—or his family, in the case of a very young patient—should be interested in pump therapy and must be reliable. ''Reliable'' can be defined simply as coming in for follow-up visits.

## Starting Dosages for Pediatric Patients

Guidelines for initial starting dosages in children are different from those for adults (Table 3). It is usual to start with the total daily dose for injection therapy and divide it into two parts—basal and bolus—rather than reducing the total dosage by 20% as is done in adults. The basal amount is 50% of the total prepump dosage and is administered as a single rate for the entire 24-hour period. The other 50% is given in evenly divided amounts constituting the boluses for each meal. Insulin needs vary as aging and growth occur. In prepubertal children, the highest basal rate (sometimes as much as twice the normal basal) is usually required between 9 P.M. and 12 A.M. The lowest rate in this age group is often between 3 A.M. and 7 A.M. As a child enters puberty, the most frequent scenario is for the highest basal rates to be between 3 A.M. and 9 A.M. and between 9 P.M. and 12 A.M. (33). As with adults, it is simplest and best to begin pump therapy

TABLE 3 Calculations of Starting Pediatric Dosage

| |
| --- |
| TDD based on injection total daily dose for 3 days averaged per day. |
| Using average per day delivery via pump, 50% basal, 50% bolus. |

*Source*: Adapted from Ref. 51.

with a single basal rate and make changes as indicated by information obtained from SMBG or continuous glucose monitoring. The basic rule of medicine—"Keep it simple"—is applicable to determining bolus requirements. Meal requirements are determined by calculating carbohydrate requirements. The two methods of doing this are to count either grams or servings of carbohydrates. The clinician should devise a meal plan with foods that the child will actually be eating, not an idealized, unrealistic diet program. If neither grams nor servings of carbohydrates can be quantified, patients and their families can be instructed to give appropriate boluses for low-, medium-, and high-carbohydrate meals or foods. The easiest method is to start with a preset amount of carbohydrate at each meal and then determine the amount of insulin required to balance the meal's carbohydrate load. The ratio will frequently vary according to the time of day. If bolus administration is not feasible, an increase in basal rates can minimize blood glucose elevation after snacks or meals. Both the patient and the family should have correction doses written down for them, and, depending on the patient's age and type of insulin, it may be necessary to amend the rule of 1500 to match individual needs and insulin sensitivities.

## Preventing DKA and Treatment of Hyperglycemia in Pediatric Patients

Patients and families should always have available an alternative to pump therapy. This means that pens and/or needles need to be mastered and used when necessary. If the patient has any symptoms of DKA, including but not limited to nausea or abdominal pain, the blood sugar should be checked. If it is above 200 mg/dl and ketones are present in the urine or blood, a correction bolus should be administered by injection and the infusion site should be changed. The pump should be scrutinized for problems (low battery, no insulin, etc.), and these need to be corrected. The blood sugar should be rechecked in 1 hour; if it is not lower or if nausea is present, the health-care team needs to be contacted immediately. If the blood sugar is greater that 200 mg/dl but no ketones or symptoms of DKA are present, the correction bolus can be administered by pump. The blood sugar should be rechecked in an hour. If it is falling, the pump need not be removed. If the blood sugar is not coming down, the patient needs to take the correction bolus by injection and the site must be changed.

In the morning, the blood sugar should be checked at least 1 hour prior to setting off for school. This is enough time so that, as recommended by the Yale Pediatric Pump Program, if the blood sugar is greater than 250 mg/dl the patient will be able to change the site before leaving for school. If the blood sugar is greater than 200 mg/dl while at school, the patient should take a bolus via pump and recheck the blood sugar an hour later. If the blood sugar is not coming down, the child should take the appropriate, predetermined correction bolus by pen or needle and the site can be changed when the child returns home. One of the most common causes of hyperglycemia in this age bracket is the omission of food boluses; this is easily prevented through education.

## Hypoglycemia Prevention in Pediatric Patients

The key to prevention of hypoglycemia is frequent measurements of blood sugar, enabling detection and correction. Often hypoglycemia in children is not associated with classic hypoglycemic symptoms, as documented by studies using continuous glucose measurements (34–36). All these studies highlighted the importance of obtaining 3 A.M. blood sugar measurements intermittently because of the prolonged asymptomatic occurrences of nocturnal hypoglycemia. If the patient has hypoglycemic unawareness, then a review and adjustment of the targets for glycemic control may be needed. Hypoglycemia is frequently due to over-bolusing. Some pumps come with software that allows for downloading and examination of the frequency and amount of boluses. This tool is extremely useful in detecting and correcting errors.

## GETTING STARTED

Pump therapy should not be made unnecessarily complicated for the patient or the family. In most centers, the patient's use of CSII begins after the insulin pump has been delivered, with a visit to the home by the pump trainer. The trainer reviews the features of the pump and techniques for insertion and care of the site. Later, the trainer provides the physician with a checklist of all the activities taught, understood, and mastered.

On the morning of the first visit to the office or clinic for the purpose of starting the pump, the patient, family member, or trainer inserts the infusion set. The decision as to who does the insertion is up to the patient; children should never be forced to do it themselves. Selection of the site is somewhat age-dependent because of the amount of subcutaneous tissue in various anatomical locations. Older children do well with the microinfusion set in the hip area, but many children under 6 are very slender and as a result do best with a silhouette infusion set in the buttocks. To minimize discomfort, "toeing in" is recommended, as is the use of products such as xylocaine spray or EMLA.

The patient has taken insulin the evening before the first session and begins that morning with insulin in the pump. That initial visit includes education about the choice of insulin to be given as boluses and when blood sugars should be checked (before meals and at 3 P.M., bedtime, 12 A.M., and 3 A.M.). Basic instructions are provided on how to suspend the delivery of insulin by the pump, how to disconnect, and how to avoid problems, and numbers to call for help and assistance are given. The next day the patient or a family member calls the center and reports the blood sugar levels, actions taken, and food eaten; in response to these, the nurse explains any changes that are needed. Patients are encouraged to call if they encounter problems or have concerns. On day 3, in another session at the office or clinic, the patient or caregiver fills the reservoir with insulin, attaches the tubing, and demonstrates the ability to insert the infusion set. Whoever is responsible needs to show during this visit how he or she changes basal rates and suspends the pump. Adjustments in basal rates, correction doses, and boluses based on redetermining the carbohydrate sensitivity are made during this session. The need to disconnect for exercise is emphasized, and, as in all sessions, questions are encouraged and answered. If the pump has the remote feature, it is taught at either the first visit or this one. For the next 6 weeks, the patient continues to monitor blood sugars and report levels that are out of range; any other problems are dealt with over the phone. A routine follow-up visit is scheduled at 6 weeks poststart to obtain an $HbA_{1c}$ level, to instruct in the advanced features of the pump, to troubleshoot, and to assess competence and comfort with the pump and its use.

## TYPE 2 DIABETES

It is estimated that 40% of all type 2 diabetes patients are using insulin to control their blood sugar levels. Pancreatic insulin production decreases, and typically continues to decline over time. In some of these patients, the dosages required are in excess of 100 units per day. The greater the dosage given of a long-lasting insulin, the greater the intrapatient variability, resulting in a wide variation in blood sugar levels from day to day. The reproducibility of glucose response to Regular short-acting insulins should make insulin pumps ideal for type 2 diabetes patients who require insulin. Unfortunately, the very few studies that have examined this hypothesis have been short-term or the results have been anecdotal. In one recent study, type 2 diabetes patients were effectively treated with insulin-pump therapy and a short-acting insulin analog. In the pump group, a smaller percentage of patients (5%) experienced hyperglycemia (>350 mg/dl) than in the multiple-daily-injection (MDI) group (18%) (37). It is reasonable to apply the same criteria and guidelines to this group when pump therapy is chosen and to follow the same guidelines for determining insulin dosage rates for delivery by pump as those used in the adult type 1 diabetes population. A useful tool is the recognition that for patients requiring very high insulin dosages (>200 units/day) the use of U500 Regular insulin can result in both improved battery life for the pump and an increased responsiveness to insulin, as reported by clinicians. Insurance coverage for intensive therapy in non-Medicare patients using insulin is frequently available for both pumps and supplies and should be investigated on an individual basis.

## PREGNANCY

Pregnancy offers the clinician the unique opportunity to reap immediate rewards for good glucose control. In a science in which adverse long-term events frequently take 15 years to occur, normoglycemia during pregnancy and preconception results in healthy pregnancies and reduced complications for both the mother and the child. The targets for blood glucose are constant during preconception and pregnancy. Fasting blood sugars should be in the range of 60–90 mg/dl. This is the same level that should be aimed for in the overnight, 3 A.M., and preprandial periods. One-hour postprandial blood sugars should be 120–140 mg/dl (38–40). The challenge of adhering to this is made somewhat easier by the use of insulin pumps.

In terms of insulin sensitivity, pregnancy can be divided into four distinct periods of time determined by the gestational age and the resulting milieu for glucose production, uptake, and utilization. This progressive, diminished insulin sensitivity is caused in large part by the hormones being produced to maintain the pregnancy as it progresses. Weeks 6–18 require the least insulin, estimated at 0.7 U/kg current body weight. The requirement from 18 to 26 weeks' gestation rises, on average, to 0.8 U/kg current body weight and then to 0.9 U/kg for weeks 26–36. In the final stage of pregnancy—week 36 till delivery—the estimated total insulin daily requirement is 1.0 U/kg (41). As with all dosage guidelines, individual determinations on a patient-by-patient basis must be done because requirements can vary widely.

Special considerations during pregnancy include the avoidance of diabetic ketoacidosis, which can have a fetal death rate as great as 50% (42). Emphasis is on early detection: frequent monitoring of blood sugars to detect an increase in these values at the earliest signal of diminished insulin delivery, prompt action by giving correction bolus by injection for any blood sugar greater than 160 mg/dl if the glucose does not respond to one given by pump, and conscientiously checking urine for ketones every morning and whenever the blood sugar is higher than target. In our practice, use of a combination of long-lasting insulin given by injection at bedtime together with pump therapy has prevented any events of nocturnal DKA.

The sites used for the infusion set are different than in the nonpregnant state only in the last trimester and during the actual delivery. The abdomen is to be avoided because of the stretching and the increased risk of cellulitis. This also prevents having to remove the pump during delivery in the event of a caesarian section. The infusion rate during delivery may need to be reduced dramatically and can even be put on suspend. Although not specifically approved for use either in pumps or during pregnancy, the fast-acting insulin analogs are commonly used.

Insulin pumps enable meeting the challenges presented by pregnancy, which may include dramatic decreases in food intake because of morning sickness as well as demands for rigid control while limiting hypoglycemia and its adverse effects. The most important part of intensive therapy during pregnancy is the frequent monitoring of blood sugars—usually before and after meals, at bedtime, and periodically during the middle of the night. It is essential to thus continuously verify the appropriate basal and bolus amounts as the pregnancy proceeds. There is no contraindication for starting insulin pumps during pregnancy, and no special risks.

## SPECIAL CONSIDERATIONS

### Hypoglycemic Unawareness

Even the nonintensively controlled group in the DCCT was not spared hypoglycemic events. In patients with impaired awareness, the number of events has been estimated at 160 per year (43,44). This rate is six times that in people with type 1 diabetes with unimpaired awareness. Analysis of meter downloads demonstrated that even at $HbA_{1c}$ levels of 8.5%, 12% of all readings were below the targets set by the DCCT. When euglycemia is attempted, iatrogenic hypoglycemia is common, especially compared with that reported by standard blood glucose measurement. Analysis of continuous glucose monitoring revealed that 87% of all subjects had hypoglycemic events and 62% had nocturnal hypoglycemia that was not accompanied by symptoms and therefore would be unrecognized. For an average of 2.4 hours per day, blood sugar levels were in the the range considered hypoglycemic; there were 1.8 distinct hypoglycemic episodes per 24 hours, and each of these episodes lasted an average of 72 minutes. It is known that brain metabolism is severely impaired at blood glucose levels under 55 mg/dl; this is linked to the decrease in counterregulatory hormone release. Diabetes of longer duration typically results in repetitive hypoglycemia and unawareness. In these patients, careful avoidance of low blood sugars can result in partial restoration of awareness, indicating that targets for glucose should be set higher with the goal being to prevent low blood sugars. The recommended preprandial, bedtime, and overnight targets in this population are 100–160 mg/dl, and postprandial targets should be approximately 50 mg/dl higher than the preprandial targets (45).

### Renal Disease and Neuropathies Such as Gastroparesis

When there is a decrease in either glucose absorption or its predictability, as in gastroparesis, judicious raising of blood sugar targets to those that will result in prevention of hypoglycemia is a justifiable strategy of therapy.

This is also applicable when insulin action and its disappearance from the blood are affected by renal function. In both of these special clinical states, the fact that there is no long-lasting insulin in the patient is a tremendous benefit in terms of prevention of unexpected hypoglycemia and its adverse results.

Maintenance of long-term euglycemia is achievable in most, if not all, patients with diabetes. Intensive therapy should achieve two goals: the lowering of blood sugars to levels that have a positive impact on microvascular complications of diabetes and the avoidance of hypoglycemia and its short- and long-term damaging effects. Both of these goals need to be accomplished while allowing the patient to enjoy a normal lifestyle. These targets are attainable only if insulin is delivered in a physiological way. This means inclusion of the patient in the decision-making process of determining insulin requirements based on current glucose levels and expected insulin need for meals and activity. It is the patient's knowledge of glucose levels and their response to administered insulin that makes all this possible. The most physiological mode of delivering insulin is by use of insulin pumps. Patients must be willing to take part in the glucose testing and the quantification of insulin needs for the multiple events that make a day eventful in terms of glucose excursions and insulin requirements. Pumps are a way to ''decriminalize'' diabetes and allow people with this disease to once again actively participate in the many aspects of a normal life.

## REFERENCES

1. Diabetes Control and Complications Trial Research Group. The effect of intensive treatment of diabetes on the development and progression of long-term complications in insulin-dependent diabetes mellitus. N Engl J Med 329:977–986, 1993.
2. Graff MR, Rubin RR, Walker EA. How diabetes specialists treat their own diabetes: findings from a study of the AADE and ADA membership. Diabetes Educ 26:460–467, 2000.
3. Pickup JC, Keen H, Parsons JA, Alberti KGMM. Continuous subcutaneous insulin infusion: an approach to achieving normoglycemia. Br Med J 1:204–207, 1978.
4. Tamborlane WV, Sherwin RS, Genel M, Felig, P. Reduction to normal of plasma glucose in juvenile diabetes by subcutaneous administration of insulin with a portable infusion pump. N Engl J Med 300:573–578, 1979.
5. Haardt MJ, Berne C, Dorange C, Slama G, Selam JL. Efficacy and indications of CSII revisited: the Hotel-Dieu cohort. Diabet Med 14(5):407–408, 1997.
6. Tsui EY, Chiasson JL, Tildesley H, Barnie A, Simkins S, Strack T, Zinman B. Counterregulatory hormone responses after long-term continuous subcutaneous insulin infusion with lispro insulin. Diabetes Care 21(1):93–96, 1998.
7. Bruttomesso D, Pianta A, Mari A, Valerio A, Marescotti MC, Avogaro A, Tiengo A, Del Prato S. Restoration of early rise in plasma insulin levels improves the glucose tolerance of type 2 diabetic patients. Diabetes 48:99–105, 1999.
8. Launay B, Zinman B, Tildesley HD, Strack T, Chiasson JL. Effect of continuous subcutaneous insulin infusion with lispro on hepatic responsiveness to glucagon in type 1 diabetes. Diabetes Care 21(10):1627–1631, 1998.

9. Zinman B, Tildesley H, Chiasson JL, Tsui E, Strack TR. Insulin lispro in CSII: results of a double-blind crossover study. Diabetes 46:440–443, 1997.

10. Gross TM, Mastrototaro J. Efficacy and reliability of the continuous glucose monitoring system. Diabetes Technol Therapeutics 2:(1):S19-S26, 2000.

11. Fischer U, Freyse EJ, Salzsieder E, Rebrin K. Artificial connection between glucose sensing and insulin delivery: implications of peritoneal administration. Artif Organs 16(2):151–162, 1992.

12. Scholtz HE, et al. Diabetologia 42(suppl):A235, 1999.

13. Lauritzen T, Pramming S, Deckert T, Binder C. Pharmacokinetics of continuous subcutaneous insulin infusion. Diabetologia 24:326–329, 1983.

14. Hirsh RF, ed. Intensive Diabetes Management. Alexandria, VA: American Diabetes Association, 1995.

15. Bode BW, et al. Diabetes 48(1), 1999.

16. Bell DS, Ovalle F. Improved glycemic control with use of continuous subcutaneous insulin infusion compared with multiple insulin injection therapy. Endocrine Pract 6:357–360, 2000.

17. Crawford LM, Sinha RN, Odell RM, Comi RJ. Efficacy of insulin pump therapy; mealtime delivery is the key factor. Endocr Pract 6:239–243, 2000.

18. Diabetes Control and Complications Trial Research Group. The effect of intensive treatment of diabetes on the development and progression of long-term complications in insulin-dependent diabetes mellitus. N Engl J Med 329:977–986, 1993.

19. ACE Diabetes Consensus Conference on Guidelines for Glycemic Control White Paper Review Consensus Panel, 2001.

20. Bode BW, et al. Diabetes 46(suppl 1):143, 1997.

21. Davidson PC. The Insulin Pump Therapy Book: Insights from the Experts, pp 59–71, 1995.

22. Marcus AO, Bode B, Drexler A, et al. Patient reported experience with velosulin human insulin in continuous subcutaneous insulin infusion. Clin Ther 17(2):204–213, 1995.

23. Shipp JC. Practical problems with insulin pumps. N Engl J Med 306:1369–1370, 1982.

24. Sovik O, Thordarson H. Dead-in-bed syndrome in young diabetic patients. Diabetes Care 22(suppl 2):B40–42, 1999.

25. Gross TM, Mastrototaro JJ, et al. Efficacy and reliability of the continuous glucose monitoring system. Diabetes Technol Ther 2(suppl 1):S19–26, 2000.

26. Polonsky K, Bergenstal R, Pons G, Schneider M, Jaspan J, Rubenstein A. Relation of counterregulatory responses to hypoglycemia in type 1 diabetics. N Engl J Med 307(18):1106, 1982.

27. White N, Hollander AS, Sadler M, Daniels L. Risks and benefits of continuous subcutaneous insulin infusion (CSII) in children. Diabetes 50(suppl 2):267, 2001.

28. Ahern J, Tamborlane WV. Pumps in kids: safe and successful. Diabetes 50(suppl 2):268, 2001.

29. Laffel L, Loughlin C, Ramchandani N, Butler D, Laffel N, Levine BS, Anderson B. Glycemic challenges of pump therapy (CSII) in youth with type 1 diabetes (T1DM). Diabetes 50(suppl 2):269, 2001.

30. Siegel L, Schachner H, Vargas I, Goland R. Continuous subcutaneous insulin infusion therapy in young children with type 1 diabetes. Diabetes 50(suppl 2):271, 2001.

31. Maniatis AK, Toig SR, Klingensmith GJ, Fay-Itzkowitz E, Chase HP. Life with continuous subcutaneous insulin infusion (CSII) therapy: child and parental perspectives and predictors of metabolic control. Pediatric Diabetes 2:51–57, 2001.

32. White NH. Endocrinol Metab Clin North Am Dec;29(4):657–682, 2000.

33. Conrad SC, McGrath MT, Adi S, Greenspan LC, Lee J, Rosenthal M, Gitelman SE. Transition from multiple daily injections (MDI) to continuous subcutaneous insulin infusion (CSII): characteristics of a pediatric population. Diabetes 49(suppl 1):409, 2000.

34. Boland EA, et al. Diabetes 49(suppl 1):397, 2000.

35. Gibson LC, et al. Diabetes 49(suppl 1):438, 2000.

36. Chase HP, Kim LM, Owen SL, MacKenzie TA, Klingensmith GJ, Murtfeldt R, Garg SK. Continuous subcutaneous glucose monitoring in children with type 1 diabetes. Pediatrics 107(2):222–226.

37. Raskin P, Bode B, Marks J, et al. Insulin Aspart (Asp) is as effective in continuous subcutaneous insulin infusion as in multiple daily injections for patients with type 2 diabetes. Diabetes 50(suppl 1):515, 2001.

38. Santiago JV, ed. Pregnancy. In: Medical Management of Insulin Dependent Type 1 Diabetes. 2nd ed. Alexandria, VA: American Diabetes Association, pp 90–98, 1994.

39. Jovanovic L, Druzin M, Peterson CM. Effect of euglycemia on the outcome of pregnancy in insulin-dependent diabetic women as compared with normal control subjects. Am J Med 71:921–927, 1981.

40. Jovanovic L, Peterson CM, Saxena BB, Dawood MY, Saudek CD. Feasibility of maintaining normal glucose profiles in insulin-dependent diabetic women. Am J Med 68:105–112, 1980.

41. Steel JM, Johnstone FD, Hume R, Mao J-H, Insulin requirements during pregnancy in women with type 1 diabetes. Obstet Gynecol 83:253–258, 1994.

42. Kitzmiller JL. Diabetic ketoacidosis and pregnancy. In: Queenan JT, ed. Managing Ob-Gyn Emergencies. 2nd ed. Oradell, NJ: Medical Economics, pp 44–55, 1983.

43. Gold AF, MacLeod KM, Frier BM. Frequency of severe hypoglycemia in patients with type 1 diabetes with impaired awareness of hypoglycemia. Diabetes Care 17: 697–703, 1994.

44. Orskov L, et al. Diabetologia Jul;34(7):521–526.

45. Fanelli CG, Pampanelli S, Epifano L, Rambotti AM, et al. Long-term recovery from unawareness, deficient counterregulation and lack of cognitive dysfunction during hypoglycemia, following institution of rational, intensive insulin therapy in IDDM. Diabetologia 37:1265–1276, 1994.

46. Bode BW, Steed RD, Davidson PC. Reduction in severe hypoglycemia with long-term continuous subcutaneous insulin infusion in type I diabetes. Diabetes Care 19: 324–327, 1996.

47. Boland EA, Grey M, Oesterle A, Fredrickson L, Tamborlane WV. Continuous subcutaneous insulin infusion: a new way to lower risk of severe hypopglycemia, improve metabolic control, and enhance coping in adolescents with type 1 diabetes. Diabetes Care 22:1779–1784, 1999.

48. Chantelau E, Spraul M, Muhlhauser I, Gause R, Berger M. Long-term safety, efficacy and side-effects of continuous subcutaneous insulin infusion treatment for type

1 (insulin-dependent) diabetes mellitus: a one centre experience. Diabetologia 32: 421–426, 1989.
49. Maniatis AK, Klingensmith GJ, Slover RH, Mowry CJ, Chase HP. Continuous subcutaneous insulin infusion therapy for children and adolescents: an option for routine diabetes care. Pediatrics 107:351–356, 2001.
50. Jovanovic-Peterson L, Peterson CM, Reed GF, et al. Am J Obstet Gynecol 164: 103–111, 1991.
51. Kaufman FR, Halvorson M, Kim C, Pitukcheewanont P. Use of insulin pump therapy at nighttime only for children 7–10 years of age with type 1 diabetes. Diabetes Care 23:579–582, 2000.

## BIBLIOGRAPHY

Akhter J, Struebing P, Larsen JL, et al. Determination of insulin requirements: excessive insulin dosages common in type 1 diabetes mellitus. Endocr Pract 4:133–136, 1998.

American Association of Diabetes Educators. Education for continuous subcutaneous insulin infusion pump users (AADE position statement). Diabetes Educ 23:397–398, 1997.

American Diabetes Association. Continuous subcutaneous insulin infusion (position statement). Diabetes Care 23(suppl 1):S90, 2000.

American Diabetes Association. Standards of medical care for patients with diabetes mellitus (position statement). Diabetes Care 23(suppl 1):S32–S4.2, 2000.

Amiel SA, Tamborlane WV, Simonson DC, Sherwin RS. Defective glucose counterregulation after strict glycemic control of insulin dependent diabetes mellitus. N Engl J Med 316:1376–1383, 1987.

Clarke WL, Cox DJ, Gonder-Frederick LA, Julian D, Schlundt D, Polonsky W. Reduced awareness of hypoglycemia in adults with IDDM. Diabetes Care 18:517–522, 1995.

Cryer PE, Fisher JN, Shamoon H. Hypoglycemia. Diabetes Care 17:734–755, 1994.

Gabbe SG, Holding E, Temple P, Brown ZA. Benefits, risks, costs, and patient satisfaction associated with insulin pump therapy for the pregnancy complicated by type 1 diabetes mellitus. Am J Obstet Gynecol 182:1283–1291, 2000.

Marcus AO, Fernandez MP. Insulin pump therapy: acceptable alternative to injection therapy. Postgrad Med 99:125–132, 142–144, 1996.

Mastrototaro J. The MiniMed Continuous Glucose Monitoring System (CGMS). J Ped Endocrinol Metab 12:751–758, 1999.

Rebrin K, Steil GM, Van Antwerp WP, Mastrototaro J. Subcutaneous glucose predicts plasma glucose independent of insulin: implications for continuous monitoring. Am J Physiol 277:E561–E571, 1999.

Rizvi AA, Petry R, Arnold MB, Chakraborty M. Beneficial effects of continuous subcutaneous insulin infusion in older patients with long-standing type 1 diabetes. Endocr Pract 7:364–369, 2001.

# 15

## Noninvasive Insulin-Delivery Systems
Options and Progress to Date

**William T. Cefalu**

University of Vermont College of Medicine, Burlington, Vermont

## INTRODUCTION

Since its discovery, insulin has been the mainstay of treatment for patients with type 1 diabetes. For patients with type 2 diabetes, we have traditionally relied on the oral agents, and these pharmaceutical agents have served us well. With the various drug classes now available, the oral agents address the pathophysiological abnormalities recognized to be present in the patient with type 2 diabetes. Specifically, oral hypoglycemic agents such as the sulfonylureas depend on insulin production by β cells and can markedly increase meal secretion of insulin. The biguanides, i.e., metformin, and the more recently introduced thiazolidinediones improve glycemic control by decreasing hepatic glucose production and sensitizing the peripheral tissues to insulin. Nevertheless, the mode of action for these two classes of drugs also depends on adequate endogenous insulin production or on exogenous insulin. In addition, the results of long-term prospective studies have demonstrated that the natural history of type 2 diabetes suggests a progressive disease in which multiple therapies may be required to achieve glycemic control. In this regard, the combination of drugs from the various classes has shown additive benefits to improve diabetic control, and combination oral therapy may be considered a routine approach in the management of type 2 diabetes. However, with the progressive nature of the disease, and the failure of combination oral therapy to adequately control the patient, insulin has emerged as a more viable treatment option much earlier in the disease process in patients with type 2 diabetes.

Type 2 diabetes, as discussed in detail in other chapters of this book, can be considered a disease in which a "relative" insulin deficiency exists at any given level of insulin resistance. Essentially, type 2 diabetes presents when the pancreas fails to compensate for the increased insulin demand and this failure to adequately compensate results in hyperglycemia. It has been observed that patients with type 2 diabetes will develop progressive insulin deficiency during the course of their disease. As a result, exogenous insulin may be required to achieve glycemic control for most patients at some point, either as monotherapy or in combination. The European Diabetes Policy Group has suggested guidelines for diabetes care that recommend using insulin in type 2 diabetic patients with $HbA_{1c}$ levels $>7.5\%$. It may be because of these suggested guidelines that the use of insulin in patients with type 2 diabetes appears to be more widely accepted in Europe than in the United States at this time. The National Institutes of Health has estimated, however, that in the United States approximately 40% of patients with type 2 diabetes currently receive exogenous insulin therapy.

The benefits of insulin therapy, although well established for type 1, have also become important in the management of patients with type 2 diabetes when one considers the benefits of improved glycemic control in both types of diabetes (for review, see Chapter 1). The Diabetes Control and Complications Trial demonstrated conclusively that the risk of microvascular complications (e.g., retinopathy, nephropathy, neuropathy) can be reduced significantly in patients with type 1 diabetes with tight glycemic control. Evidence for a benefit of improved glycemic control in type 2 patients was provided by the United Kingdom Prospective Diabetes Study. This study confirmed that in patients with type 2 diabetes, improved glycemic control significantly reduced the number of microvascular complications, as well as offering some indications of a favorable effect on macrovascular disease. Thus, when adequate glycemic control is not achieved in the type 2 diabetic patient, as determined by failure to achieve the target $HbA_{1c}$ level with traditional oral therapies, it is appropriate to consider exogenous insulin administration. In the effort to achieve glycemic control, exogenous insulin therapy can be considered the "gold standard" because the dose can be titrated to achieve the desired glycemic target.

It can be argued that the benefits obtained by achieving good glycemic control with insulin therapy outweigh any theoretical or unsubstantiated risks. However, both physicians and patients have concerns about the safety and adverse effects (e.g., hypoglycemia, weight gain, increased cardiovascular risk) of exogenous insulin therapy. These concerns, whether real or perceived, may serve as major barriers and contribute to the reasons that intensive insulin therapy has not gained widespread clinical acceptance. The inconvenience of having to take multiple daily injections and carry around insulin supplies may contribute to poor compliance. Further, the time required of both the provider and the patient to successfully implement the intensive insulin regimen and the resources required to do so may limit acceptance. There is obviously a psychological component— patients with type 2 diabetes may feel that advancing to insulin therapy is related to a serious progression of their disease state.

Thus, both practical and psychological hurdles contribute to the resistance to advance to insulin and, when insulin is administered, may lead to errors in technique and anxiety, further hindering improvement of metabolic control. Such real concerns are demonstrated in studies that suggest that between 60 and 80% of patients may perform some aspect of insulin administration incorrectly, e.g., timing of administration or taking correct dose. As physicians, we may not recognize the importance of injection-related anxiety in our patients. In 1999, Zambanini and colleagues assessed injection-related anxiety in 115 patients with either type 1 or 2 diabetes. Their findings suggest a cause for concern: 1) 14% of patients admitted avoiding injections because of anxiety; 2) 42% reported concern at the prospect of having to inject more frequently, which may be essential to achieve control; and 3) of the 28% of patients with marked anxiety, 45% had avoided injections and 70% reported concern at the prospect of having to inject more frequently. These concerns will adversely influence compliance and greatly interfere with the clinical goal of achieving glucose control. What, then, is the optimal approach? On one hand, we recognize in patients with type 2 diabetes that glycemic control is required to reduce the complications; on the other, significant concerns exist regarding required therapy. Our traditional means of providing exogenous insulin has therefore been re-evaluated. To understand this re-evaluation, a brief review of the development of insulin may help in the understanding of the current focus on alternative insulin delivery.

## HISTORY OF INSULIN DEVELOPMENT

The insulin era began in 1921, when Frederick Banting and Charles Best excited the medical world by reporting that they had isolated the active ingredient in the pancreas believed to regulate blood glucose. In collaboration with a biochemist named Collip, Banting and Best produced an extract of insulin. The real significance of this work in providing a viable clinical therapy, however, was not realized until January 11, 1922. On this date, a 14-year-old boy named Leonard Thompson was dying of diabetes in the Toronto General Hospital when Banting and Best provided him with injections of pancreatic extract. The injections lowered the boy's blood glucose levels and the treatment allowed him to return home within weeks. The successful treatment of this disease, which had been considered essentially untreatable, was one of the major medical breakthroughs of the 20th century. As a result, the Nobel Prize in 1923 went to Banting and department head John Macleod. Although Best's and Collip's roles were unrecognized by the Nobel committee, the four researchers shared the award.

Shortly after Banting and Best's breakthrough, insulin became widely available. Since that initial treatment over 80 years ago, there have been incredible advances in the development of formulations with different onset of action, duration, and roles in therapy. Advances have also been made in our understanding of the pathophysiology of both type 1 and type 2 diabetes, as well as of the molecular structure of insulin. Subsequently, techniques of recombinant DNA technology have been developed and synthetic human insulin has become a reality. Advances made by manipulating insulin's structure have led to a number of short- and long-acting analogs that provide tremendous options for patients. In particular, the short-acting analogs represent an important therapeutic advance. These analogs, intended for use just prior to ingesting a meal, more closely mimic the pharmacokinetic and pharmacodynamic properties of endogenous insulin and overcome the limitations of injected Regular insulin.

However, despite the remarkable advances made in understanding insulin's structure, activity, and physiological role, a major limitation that exists even today is that the only available route of insulin administration is still by injection. Attempts have been made to develop alternative means of delivery, and significant technological innovations have made self-injection easier. For example, the insulin pen devices use smaller-gauge needles, are convenient, offer more accurate delivery, are less painful to use than conventional needles, and may enhance compliance. Unfortunately, injection with a pen is still an injection, and self-injection is required several times a day to optimize glucose control. In addition to the goal of noninvasive insulin delivery to eliminate the injection, broader and more important aims of alternative insulin delivery should include mimicking the normal physiological insulin time–concentration profile as closely as possible. As discussed in Chapter 1, a 24-hour normal endogenous profile can be divided into basal levels of insulin in postabsorptive states and the postprandial rise after meal ingestion. The physiological insulin profile peaks within 30–60 minutes of eating and returns to baseline within 2–4 hours. Unfortunately, following a subcutaneous injection, Regular human insulin has a slow absorption, meaning that patients may have to inject 30–60 minutes prior to meals and insulin may persist in the circulation for 4–6 hours. Additional concerns for the intermediate- and long-acting human insulin preparations, e.g., NPH and Ultralente, is that they may have an undesirable peak profile after subcutaneous injection while still lacking sufficient duration in action. It is for this reason that the short- and long-acting analogs of human insulin were developed that offer a more physiological insulin pharmacokinetic profile than that achieved with previous formulations. Unfortunately, despite the ability of the new formulations to closely mimic a normal physiological profile, all these preparations still have the drawback that they require an injection.

## THE SEARCH FOR A PRACTICAL NONINVASIVE INSULIN-DELIVERY SYSTEM

The major goals when considering a practical noninvasive insulin-delivery system are to: 1) overcome the major limitation associated with conventional insulin injections and 2) preserve a more physiological insulin profile. Achieving these goals will allow for more intensive insulin delivery, a regimen clinically proven to significantly improve glycemia and reduce complications, while enhancing patient compliance. Such goals are lofty, but they are receiving increased research attention. Current areas of ongoing research are outlined in Table 1.

### Jet Injectors

Jet injectors are devices that administer insulin without needles by delivering a high-pressure stream of insulin into subcutaneous tissue. Even though needles are not used, the discomfort associated with jet injectors is reported to be comparable to that with injections. In subjects with great anxiety about needles, however, these devices can obviously have a benefit. Unfortunately, these devices may negatively impact the pharmacokinetics of long-acting insulin, forc-

---

**TABLE 1**  Current Approaches to Penetrating the Skin Barrier

**Jet injectors**: Devices that administer insulin without needles by delivering a high-pressure stream of insulin into subcutaneous tissue

**Ionotophoresis**: Process using low-level electrical current to speed the delivery of drug ions into the skin and surrounding tissues

**Low-frequency ultrasound**: Process by which ultrasound increases, by several-fold, the permeability of human skin to macromolecules such as insulin

**Transfersomes**: Composites of pharmaceutically accepted ingredients designed to deliver drugs across the skin barrier by opening temporary channels between adjoining cells

**Intranasal administration**: Delivery of insulin to nasal mucosa for absorption; bioavailability is low

**Oral insulin**: Via the buccal mucosa in the mouth or mucosa in the gastrointestinal tract

**Pulmonary delivery**: Takes advantage of favorable pulmonary anatomy (e.g., permeability, increased surface area) for absorption of insulin for rapid systemic effect

---

ing more frequent administration . Although they are not widely used, they have been recommended only for people intolerant of conventional needle injection systems.

## Transdermal Delivery by Iontophoresis

Iontophoresis is a process very similar to that of the passive transdermal medication patches that deliver nicotine for smoking cessation or hormone therapy for postmenopausal women. Iontophoresis uses low-level electrical current to speed the delivery of drug ions into the skin and surrounding tissues. It appears to be an effective and rapid method of delivering medication into the skin. Such a process has been evaluated for insulin in diabetic rats that had been depilated; transdermal delivery of bovine insulin using iontophoresis produced a concentration-dependent reduction in plasma glucose levels. However, the method did not appear to be as effective in rats that had not been depilated, which suggests that either the depilation was effective in reducing the skin's barrier function or the creams used with the iontophoretic device acted as a penetration enhancer. Although this is an area of great interest, the factors critical to transdermal absorption and delivery of insulin will need to be defined in further studies.

## Low-Frequency Ultrasound

The use of low-frequency ultrasound has also been evaluated as a means of noninvasively administering insulin. It has been demonstrated to increase, by several-fold, the permeability of human skin to macromolecules. This technique may augment delivery of drugs such as interferon-gamma and erythropoietin. However, given that a goal of noninvasive delivery is to mimic physiological insulin patterns, this approach provides a rate of delivery of insulin that is too slow to be a viable clinical option.

## Transfersomes

Transfersomes—composite phosphatidylcholine-based vesicles—are composites of pharmaceutically accepted ingredients designed to deliver drugs across the skin barrier. This technology takes advantage of the natural moisture gradient across the skin; the mechanism by which it works is believed to be by opening up temporary channels between adjoining cells. It thus has the potential to deliver macromolecules, e.g., insulin, across the skin barrier. Transfersomes have shown effectiveness in delivering local and systemic steroids, proteins, and other hydrophilic macromolecules. Transfersomes have the property of deformability, which facilitates their rapid penetration through the intercellular lipids of the skin— they are flexible enough to pass through pores smaller than their own size. Indeed, transfersomes pass through pores with an efficacy similar to that of water, despite being some 1000 times larger. With particular regard to insulin, transfersomes coupled with insulin allow insulin to cross intact skin cells with a bioefficiency of approximately 50% of the subcutaneous dose. It has been estimated that, with present technology, a skin surface area of approximately 40 cm$^2$ is sufficient to cover the basal daily insulin requirements of most patients with type 1 diabetes. However, limitations regarding delay in onset, making prandial use problematic, are of concern. Additional studies will be needed to determine the clinical utility of this approach.

## Intranasal Delivery

The use of intranasal insulin as a viable clinical option has received considerable attention. The major problem associated with nasal administration of insulin is poor bioavailability, which is typically observed to be between 8 and 15%. Factors affecting bioavailability include timing of dose and frequency of administration. Nasal formulations have used permeability enhancers to augment bioavailability, but these result in nasal irritation in many patients. Nasal insulin, however, has been shown to have clinical effect. The effectiveness of intranasal insulin in 31 patients was evaluated by Hilsted and colleagues in 1995. They reported that the insulin dose needed to reach given markers of glycemic control by intranasal administration was 20 times higher than that given by subcutaneous injection. Although no difference in the number of hypoglycemic episodes between subcutaneous and nasal delivery was observed, markers of metabolic control worsened slightly but significantly during nasal insulin treatment. Nevertheless, nasal insulin has been shown to reduce postprandial glycemia. The reduction is especially marked following repeated dosing. Therefore, intranasal administration of insulin is promising, and has shown to be effective in lowering glucose. However, further studies to establish long-term safety, patient acceptance, and effectiveness are needed.

## Oral Insulin

Oral administration of insulin can be viewed as having two specific areas of uptake: 1) via the buccal mucosa in the mouth and 2) via mucosa in the gastrointestinal tract. Oral insulin delivery is obviously an attractive concept to both patients and physicians, but this approach has significant hurdles to clear before it is a clinically feasible option. Large polypeptides such as insulin will have limited bioavailability due to two factors. First and foremost, the molecules tend to be too large and hydrophilic to cross the mucosa. Second, such polypeptides undergo extensive enzymatic and chemical degradation within the enzymatic barrier of the gastrointestinal-tract mucosa. In an effort to overcome these anatomical and physiological barriers, several research approaches have been attempted to promote the bioavailability of oral insulin, including: 1) *acyl derivatives*; attachment of caproic acid molecules and coating with chitosan stabilizes degradation and improves permeability, 2) *concurrent administration with protease inhibitors*; experiments in dogs suggest that protease inhibitors may augment the oral bio-availability of insulin, but this has not been tested in humans and the long-term side effects are unknown, 3) *enclosing insulin within microspheres*, protecting against hydrolization or enzymatic degradation by attaching insulin to carrier molecules, and 4) *use of absorption enhancers*, an approach similar to nasal for-mulation to enhance buccal delivery and that avoids reliance on lower gastrointes-tinal absorption.

Of all the suggested approaches, it appears that only buccal delivery has recently advanced to more widespread testing in patients with diabetes, and re-ports suggest clinical benefits.

## Pulmonary Delivery

### Concept and Science

Many of the limitations outlined above that exist for other routes of noninvasive insulin delivery appear to be nicely addressed because of the favorable anatomy of the lung. First, the lung's large surface area is highly permeable, and it is suggested that peptides such as insulin will cross the alveolar cells in a process called transcytosis, although this has not been conclusively proven. The process is believed to occur as follows: 1) the inhaled insulin molecules, once deposited in the alveoli, are believed to be taken up into vesicles; 2) the insulin particles are then transported across the epithelial cells and released into the interstitial fluid between the epithelium and the alveolar capillary endothelium; and 3) the insulin is then taken up into vesicles, transported across the capillary endothe-lium, and released into the bloodstream (Figure 1). This process results in a rapid systemic effect as pulmonary inhalation of insulin results in peak levels after 15–20 minutes. A second major advantage for pulmonary delivery is the large surface area of the lung—the normal human lung may have a surface area of 100 m$^2$. This large surface area, combined with the favorable permeability properties, makes the lung a very attractive route for the administration of insulin.

The feasibility of inhaling insulin is not a new idea; it was first reported three years after Banting and Best's extraction of insulin. In 1925, Gänsslen ob-served a lowering of blood glucose approximately 2 hours after administering pulmonary insulin in five diabetic patients. Despite Gänsslen's finding, this non-invasive approach was not pursued further until Wigley and colleagues revisited pulmonary insulin delivery over 45 years later. They reported increased levels of plasma immunoreactive insulin in both normal volunteers and patients with diabetes after delivering pork–beef insulin using a nebulizer. The observation that hypoglycemia closely followed the rise of plasma insulin confirmed proof of concept for the approach.

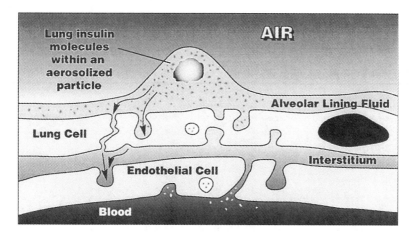

FIGURE 1    Pulmonary transport and uptake mechanism. (From Patton, 1998.)

Once the feasibility of pulmonary delivery had been established, the next step was to design an effective pulmonary delivery system appropriate for patient use. In this regard, the vast experience gained in the management of asthma has greatly aided the development of pulmonary delivery systems for insulin. The asthma drug–delivery devices—e.g., nebulizers, metered-dose inhalers, and dry-powder inhalers—although very useful in the management of local respiratory diseases such as asthma, are not appropriately designed to deliver drugs deep into the alveoli for systemic drug delivery. For inhaled insulin to work effectively, a device would need to allow insulin to reach the alveloli, and to do so in a very reproducible manner. The pulmonary delivery systems currently in clinical development have been designed to deliver both dry-powdered and soluble insulin to the alveoli (for reviews, see Klonoff, 1999, and Greener, 2000).

### Factors Influencing Pulmonary Insulin Delivery

In addition to the requirement that the device be able to administer insulin to the deep reaches of the lung, a number of other potential limitations must be overcome for effective pulmonary drug delivery (Table 2). One factor is particle size—it has been suggested that the lungs very effectively filter particles with the exception of very small (mean aerodynamic diameter <5 μm) particles. These observations established that particle size is a main determinant of efficient pulmonary insulin delivery. Studies have established that particles should have low velocity and an aerodynamic diameter of 1–3 μm. Larger particles are observed to deposit in the bronchial tubes and smaller particles are exhaled. Thus, the early attempts to develop pulmonary delivery systems, by not sufficiently controlling particle size, failed to reliably and sufficiently deliver drug. Only in the recent

**TABLE 2**  Factors Affecting Pulmonary Drug Delivery

Type of propellants utilized
Airflow speed
Losses within the device and the environment
Particle size and velocity
Drug clearance and absorption
Drug deposition into the throat and bronchial tubes
Patient compliance
Potential impact of concomitant diseases

past have technological advances in manufacturing, by now having the ability to control particle size, enabled the development of a range of inhaled formulations and delivery systems including the dry-powder insulin inhalation systems and aqueous insulin aerosol. These systems are undergoing extensive clinical evaluations, but, as described, the dry-powder formulations may have several advantages over conventional liquid formulations, including product and formulation stability, and high-drug-volume delivery.

Once the aerosolized drug reaches the alveloi, its bioavailability must be high enough to make the delivery system feasible. This was the apparent problem with the earlier studies. Despite the successful demonstration of the principle of insulin inhalation for the treatment of diabetes in 1925, the bioavailability was low (<3%). However, more recent inhalation studies that have compared insulin administration by inhalation devices with subcutaneous injection for reproducibility of dosing have shown that the variability in glucose response to the two methods was equivalent. Recent observations suggest that the bioavailability with aerosol insulin is approximately 20%, supporting the use of pulmonary delivery as a method of insulin administration.

Although studies have not evaluated pulmonary delivery in pulmonary diseases such as emphysema or COPD, it has been suggested that active smoking greatly influences the pharmacokinetic profile. It appears that smoking, while not altering the time of peak effect (approximately 15 minutes), can greatly elevate the concentrations obtained.

### Pharmacokinetics of Inhaled Insulin

One of the major advantages of inhaled insulin is that its pharmacokinetics appear to be similar to those of the new insulin analogs and may be closer to a physiological profile. In support of such observations is the evidence suggesting that the time–concentration profile of inhaled human insulin in blood is similar to that of physiological insulin secretion in healthy volunteers. Several studies have evaluated intravenous, subcutaneous (both Regular and fast-acting), and inhaled insulin. Heinemann et al. demonstrated in 1997 that the relative effectiveness of inhaled insulin was approximately 10% with regard to intravenous insulin administration and 8% with regard to subcutaneous insulin administration. In addition, Heise et al. reported that the onset of action of inhaled insulin appears to be more rapid than that of subcutaneous insulin. Inhaled insulin demonstrated a faster onset of action than subcutaneous Regular insulin and even insulin lispro (early $t_{50\%}$: 32, 48, and 40 minutes, respectively). The maximal metabolic action (based on glucose infusion rates) was comparable with that of Regular insulin and lower than that of lispro. The duration of action of inhaled insulin (late $t_{50\%}$) was between that of lispro and Regular insulin (382, 309, and 413 minutes, respectively) (Figure 2). In addition to the above, it appears from several other evaluations that the pharmacokinetic and pharmacodynamic profiles of pulmonary delivery of insulin mimic those of the normal physiological response.

## Clinical Results with Inhaled Insulin

On a clinical level, however, studies have suggested that inhaled insulin may be effective in both type 1 and type 2 subjects who are taking insulin and is effective in type 2 diabetic patients failing on oral agents. In 1999, Weiss et al. examined the effect of adding inhaled insulin (using a dry-powder formulation) to oral

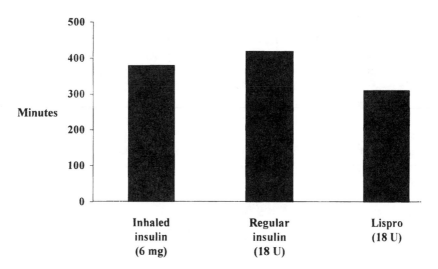

FIGURE 2   Duration of action (late $t_{50\%}$) for inhaled insulin, Regular insulin, and insulin lispro.

agents in a study in 69 patients with poorly controlled type 2 diabetes (HbA$_{1c}$ 8.1–11.9% despite receiving therapeutic doses of a sulfonylurea and/or metformin). Patients were randomized to either continue with their current oral agent alone or take the oral agent in combination with inhaled insulin (one or two inhalations three times daily, i.e., before meals). Inhaled insulin treatment was observed to significantly improve HbA$_{1c}$ in subjects receiving inhaled insulin compared with the level in those receiving an oral agent alone ($-2.28$ vs. $-0.06\%$, respectively; $p < 0.001$). Inhaled insulin therapy was well tolerated, with only one report of severe hypoglycemia. In addition, pulmonary function tests remained stable over the 3-month study period.

Two phase 2 studies have been reported on clinical use of the dry-powder formulation for treatment of type 1 and 2 diabetic subjects who were on insulin injections. Skyler et al. recently evaluated 73 patients with type 1 diabetes who received either their usual insulin regimen of two or three injections daily or pre-meal inhaled insulin plus an injection of Ultralente insulin at bedtime, for 12 weeks. At 12 weeks, there was no significant difference in HbA$_{1c}$ or fasting or postprandial glucose concentrations between those randomized to inhaled insulin versus those taking subcutaneous insulin. In a study of 26 patients with type 2 diabetes who were receiving insulin therapy prior to study, patients were administered one or two inhalations of the dry-powder insulin formulation (between 3 and 18 units, according to the glucose response) before each meal plus bedtime Ultralente insulin. Insulin doses were adjusted at weekly intervals to achieve the target preprandial glucose of 100–160 mg/dl. Mean HbA$_{1c}$ levels were observed to significantly decrease by 0.71% when compared with the baseline value. The limitation of both the type 1 and 2 studies of inhaled insulin versus subcutaneous insulin is that they were of open-label design. Nevertheless, these studies strongly suggested that inhaled insulin may be a viable option for patients with either type 1 or type 2 diabetes currently on insulin therapy.

An important component of the early inhaled-insulin protocols is that patients appeared to be very satisfied with inhaled-insulin treatment. Patient-satisfaction surveys have confirmed that, after 1 year of treatment, patients receiving inhaled dry-powder insulin maintained their satisfaction with significantly greater improvements than those using conventional insulin injections, in global satisfaction and convenience/ease of use. Gerber et al. found that patients who switched from subcutaneous insulin to inhaled insulin showed a significant improvement ($p < 0.05$) in global satisfaction (20% improvement), convenience/ease of use (28% improvement), and social stigma (16% improvement). In contrast, patients who switched from inhaled to subcutaneous insulin showed a trend toward worsening satisfaction. Thus, adherence to treatment with inhaled insulin may be better than that observed with injection regimens, although this must await confirmation by long-term studies.

## SUMMARY

It is now unquestioned that glycemic control is required to prevent progression of diabetic complications. This has been firmly established not only for type 1 diabetes but also for type 2 diabetes. Insulin is the only treatment for type 1, and the natural history of type 2 diabetes suggests that insulin may be required for it too, given the progressive nature of the disease. Thus, regardless of the type of diabetes, multiple injection therapy may be required to adequately control glucose levels. Unfortunately, a number of barriers exist at both the patient and physician levels that may prevent the advancement to intensive insulin therapy. In addition to other relevant concerns, one obstacle is that injection remains the only viable means of administering insulin. However, numerous approaches have been evaluated to administer insulin noninvasively. Although the research is still very active in this area, pulmonary delivery, at this date, appears to have the most potential to become a clinically viable alternative to insulin injections. The clinical evidence shows that inhaled insulin is effective and well tolerated. It has a more physiological insulin profile than conventional subcutaneous insulin making it ideal for preprandial administration. Inhaled insulin, in the early studies, has met with increased patient satisfaction. The additional studies needed to confirm long-term efficacy and long-term pulmonary safety are underway. However, the evidence to date suggests that pulmonary insulin delivery may offer the potential to improve compliance and thereby help reduce the number of complications associated with diabetes.

## BIBLIOGRAPHY

Berger M, Jorgens V, Muhlhauser I. Rationale for the use of insulin therapy alone as the pharmacological treatment of type 2 diabetes. Diabetes Care 22(suppl 3):C71–C75, 1999.

Birkeland KI. Improving glycaemic control with current therapies. Diabet Med 15:S13–S19, 1998.

Bohannon NJ. Insulin delivery using pen devices: simple-to-use tools may help young and old alike. Postgrad Med 106:57–58, 1999.

Boyne MS, Saudek CD. Effect of insulin therapy on macrovascular risk factors in type 2 diabetes. Diabetes Care 22(suppl 3):C45–C53, 1999.

Cefalu WT, Balagtas CC, Landschulz WH, Gelfand RA. Sustained efficacy and pulmonary safety of inhaled insulin during 2 years of outpatient therapy. Diabetes Res Clin Pract 50(suppl 1):S73, 2000.

Cefalu WT, Skyler JS, Kourides IA, Landschulz WH, Balagtas CC, Cheng SL, et al. Inhaled human insulin treatment of patients with type 2 diabetes mellitus. Ann Intern Med 134:203–207, 2001.

Cevc G, Gebauer D, Stieber J, Schatzlein A, Blume G. Ultraflexible vesicles, transfersomes, have an extremely low pore penetration resistance and transport therapeutic amounts of insulin across the intact mammalian skin. Biochim Biophys Acta 1368:201–215, 1998.

Chetty DJ, Chien YW. Novel methods of insulin delivery: an update. Crit Rev Ther Drug Carrier Syst 15:629–670, 1998.

Coates PA, Ismail IS, Luzio SD, Griffiths I, Ollerton RL, Volund A, et al. Intranasal insulin: the effects of three dose regimens on postprandial glycaemic profiles in type II diabetic subjects. Diabet Med 12:235–239, 1995.

Davis SS. Overcoming barriers to the oral administration of peptide drugs. Trends Pharmacol Sci 11:353–355, 1990.

Diabetes Control and Complications Trial (DCCT) Research Group. The effect of intensive treatment of diabetes on the development and progression of long-term complications in insulin-dependent diabetes mellitus. N Engl J Med 329:977–986, 1993.

Dimitriadis GD, Gerich JE. Importance of timing of preprandial subcutaneous insulin administration in the management of diabetes mellitus. Diabetes Care 6:374–377, 1983.

European Diabetes Policy Group. Guidelines for Diabetes Care: A Desktop Guide to Type 2 Diabetes Mellitus. Brussels: International Diabetes Federation (Europe), 1999.

Frauman AG, Jerums G, Louis WJ. Effects of intranasal insulin in non-obese type II diabetics. Diabetes Res Clin Pract 3:197–202, 1987.

Galloway JA, Spradlin CT, Nelson RL, Wentworth SM, Davidson JA, Swarner JL. Factors influencing the absorption, serum insulin concentration, and blood glucose responses after injections of regular insulin and various insulin mixtures. Diabetes Care 4:366–376, 1981.

Gänsslen M. Über Inhalation von Insulin. Klin Wochenschr 4:71, 1925.

Gelfand RA, Schwartz SL, Horton M, Law GG, Pun EF, et al. Pharmacological reproducibility of pre-meal inhaled insulin is comparable to injected insulin in patients with type 2 diabetes. Diabetes 47(suppl 1):A99, 1998.

Gerber RA, Cappelleri JC, Bell-Farrow AD, English JS, Agramante RF, Gelfand EA, et al. Improved patient satisfaction with inhaled insulin in subjects with type 1 diabetes mellitus after one year: results from a multicenter extension trial. Diabetes 49(suppl 1):A108, 2000.

Gizurason S, Bechgaard E. Intranasal administration of insulin to humans. Diabetes Res Clin Pract 12:71–84, 1991.

Golden MP, Haymond M, Hinnen DA, Kruger DF, Schumacher OP. Position statement on jet injections. Diabetes Care 11:600–601, 1988.

Graff MR, McClanahan MA. Assessment by patients with diabetes mellitus of two insulin pen delivery systems versus a vial and syringe. Clin Ther 20:486–496, 1988.

Greener MJ. Leading applications of inhaled delivery systems for systemically active drugs. Spectrum Drug Deliv Reform Tech 2:1–16, 2000.

Heinemann L, Traut T, Heise T. Time–action profile of inhaled insulin. Diabetic Med 14: 63–72, 1997.

Heise T, Rave K, Bott S, Sha S, Willavize SA, Carroll RS, et al. Time–action profile of an inhaled insulin preparation in comparison to insulin lispro and regular insulin. Diabetes 49(suppl 1):A10, 2000.

Heller SR. Diabetic hypoglycaemia. Baillieres Best Pract Res Clin Endocrinol Metab 13: 279–294, 1999.

Hilsted J, Madsbad S, Hvidberg A, Ramussen MH, Krarup T, Ipsen H, et al. Intranasal insulin therapy: the clinical realities. Diabetologia 38:680–684, 1995.

Hirata Y, Kohama T, Ooi K. Nasal administration of insulin in healthy subjects and diabetic patients. In: Sakamoto N, Alberti KGMM, eds. Current and Future Therapies with Insulin. Amsterdam: Excerpta Medica, pp 263–271, 1982.

Hoffman A, Ziv E. Pharmacokinetic considerations of new insulin formulations and routes of administration. Clin Pharmacokinet 33:285–301, 1997.

Hunt LM, Valenzuela MA, Puch JA. NIDDM patients' fears and hopes about insulin therapy: the basis of patient reluctance. Diabetes Care 20(3):292–298, 1997.

Jacobs MAJM, Schreuder RH, Jap-A-Joe K, Nanta JJ, Andersen PM, Heine RJ, et al. The pharmacodynamics and activity of intranasal administered insulin in healthy male volunteers. Diabetes 42:1649–1655, 1993.

Kanikkannan N, Singh J, Ramarao P. Transdermal iontophoretic delivery of bovine insulin and monomeric human insulin analogue. J Controlled Release 59:99–105, 1999.

Klonoff DC. Inhaled insulin. Diabetes Tech Ther 1:307–313, 1999.

Köhler D, Schlüter KJ, Kerp L, Matthys H. [Non-radioactive method to measure lung permeability: inhalation of insulin.] Atemw Lungenkrh 13:230–232, 1987.

Laube BL, Benedict GW, Dobs AS. The lung as an alternative route of delivery for insulin in controlling postprandial glucose levels in patients with diabetes. Chest 114: 1734–1739, 1998.

Laube BL, Benedict GW, Dobs AS. Time to peak insulin level, relative bioavailibility, and effect of site of deposition of nebulized insulin in patients with noninsulin-dependent diabetes mellitus. J Aerosol Med 11:153–173, 1998.

Laube BL, Georgopoulus A, Adams GK III. Aerosolized insulin delivered through the lungs is effective in normalizing plasma glucose levels in non-insulin dependent diabetic subjects (NIDD). J Biopharm Sci 3:163–169, 1993.

Mitragotri S, Blankschtein D, Langer R. Ultrasound-mediated transdermal protein delivery. Science 269:850–853, 1995.

Moses AC, Gordon GS, Carey MC, Flier JS. Insulin administered intranasally as an insulin-bile salt aerosol: effectiveness and reproducibility in normal and diabetic subjects. Diabetes 32:1040–1047, 1983.

National Institute of Diabetes and Digestive and Kidney Diseases. Diabetes Statistics. NIH Publication 99–3892: Bethesda, MD: National Institutes of Health, 1999.

Patton J. Nature Biotechnol, 1998.

Pattrick AW, Cullen A, Matthews DM, Macintyre CCA, Clark BF. The importance of the time interval between injection and breakfast in determining postprandial glycemic control: a comparison between human and porcine insulin. Diabetes Med 5:32–35, 1988.

Pontiroli AE, Alberetto M, Secchi A, Dossi G, Bosi I, Pozza G, et al. Insulin given intranasally induces hypoglycaemia in normal and diabetic subjects. Br Med J 294:303–306, 1982.

Ramdas M, Dileep KJ, Anitha Y, Paul W, Sharma CP. Alginate encapsulated bioadhesive chitosan microspheres for intestinal drug delivery. J Biomater Appl 13:290–296, 1999.

Ruige JB, Assendelft WJ, Dekker JM, Kostense PJ, Heine RJ, Bouter LM. Insulin and risk of cardiovascular disease: a meta-analysis. Circulation 97:996–1001, 1998.

Saudek CD. Novel forms of insulin delivery. Endocrinol Metab Clin North Am 26:599–610, 1997.

Schilling RJ, Mitra AK. Degradation of insulin by trypsin and alpha-chymotrypsin. Pharm Res 8:721–727, 1991.

Schlüter KJ, Köhler D, Enzmann F, Kerp L. Pulmonary administration of human insulin in volunteers and type 1 diabetes. Diabetes 33(suppl):298, 1984.

Silverstein JH, Rosenbloom AL. New developments in type 1 (insulin-dependent) diabetes. Clin Pediatr (Phila) 39:257–266, 2000.

Skyler JS, Cefalu WT, Kourides IA, Landschulz WH, Balagtas CC, Cheng S-L, et al. on behalf of the Inhaled Insulin Phase II Study Group. Efficacy of inhaled insulin in type 1 diabetes mellitus: a randomised proof-of-concept study. Lancet 357:331–335, 2001.

Taylor R, Home PD, Alberti KGMM. Plasma free insulin profiles after administration of insulin by jet and conventional syringe injection. Diabetes Care 4:377–379, 1981.

UK Prospective Diabetes Study (UKPDS) Group. Intensive blood-glucose control with sulphonylureas or insulin compared with conventional treatment and risk of complications in patients with type 2 diabetes. Lancet 352:837–853, 1998.

Wallace TM, Matthews DR. Poor glycemic control in type 2 diabetes: a conspiracy of disease, suboptimal therapy and attitude. Q J Med 93:369–374, 2000.

Weiss SR, Berger S, Cheng S-L, Kourides IA, Landschulz WH, Gelfand RA, et al. Adjunctive therapy with inhaled insulin in type 2 diabetic patients failing oral agents: a multicenter phase II trial. Diabetes 48(suppl 1):A12, 1999.

Wigley GM, Londono JH, Wood SH, Shipp JC, Waldman RH, et al. Insulin across respiratory mucosae by aerosol delivery. Diabetes 20:552–556, 1971.

Winter LB. On the absorption of insulin from the stomach. J Physiol 58:18–21, 1923.

Zambanini A, Newson RB, Maisey M, Feher MD. Injection related anxiety in insulin-treated diabetes. Diabetes Res Clin Pract 46:239–246, 1999.

Ziel FH, Davidson MB, Harris MD, Rosenberg CS. The variability in regular insulin action is more dependent on changes in tissue sensitivity than absorption. Clin Res 35:160–166, 1987.

# Index

Absorption of insulin and factors that affect, 33, 75, 95

Algorithms (*see* Dosing adjustments)

American Diabetes Association (ADA) standards of diabetes care, 14

Analogs (*see* Insulin analogs)

Aspart insulin (*see* Insulin analogs)

Aspirin use for primary and secondary prevention of macrovascular complications, 19

Basal-bolus intensive insulin therapy (*see* Insulin therapy, intensive basal-bolus)

Bedtime insulin in type 2 diabetes, protocol for, 123

Benefits of insulin therapy, 117–118

BIDS, bedtime insulin, daytime sulfonylurea, 118–119

Blood pressure guidelines in diabetes, 17
ACE inhibitors for treatment of, 17
National High Blood Pressure Education program, 17

Carbohydrate counting, 56–57, 134, 216

Cardiovascular complications in diabetes (*see* Macrovascular complications in diabetes)

Certified diabetes educator (CDE), 21

Children with diabetes, 127–138
blood pressure guidelines in, 17
cholesterol guidelines in, 17
diet in, 134
exercise in, 134–135
glargine insulin use in, 132
goals of treatment in, 128, 133
hemoglobin $A_{1c}$ goal in, 133
honeymoon effect on insulin requirements in, 129–130
hypoglycemia in, 135–136
insulin pump therapy in, 130–131, 234–238
insulin regimens in, 128–131
microalbuminuria screening in, 18
outpatient care in, 135
retinopathy screening in, 18

[Children with diabetes]
  self-blood glucose monitoring in, 133
    meter selection in, 37
  sick-day rules in, 136–137
Cholesterol guidelines in diabetes, 2, 16–17
Combination insulin and oral hypoglyce-
    mic pills, 217–218
  bedtime insulin in type 2 diabetes,
    protocol for, 123
  BIDS, bedtime insulin, daytime sul-
    fonylurea, 118–119
  treatment with, 120–123
  weight gain with, 116–117
Concerns over insulin use, 116–117
  hypoglycemia, 116
  cardiovascular disease, 116
  weight gain, 116
CSII (*see* Insulin pump)

Dawn phenomenon, 90, 213–214
DCCT study (*see* Diabetes control and
    complications trial)
DECODE study, 9
Detemir insulin, 82
Diabetes education, 21–45
  factors that affect insulin absorption,
    33, 75, 95
  injection aids, 33–34
  for injection anxiety, 117, 247
  injection difficulties, 31–33, 117
  injection technique, 29–30
  insulin absorption, 33, 75, 95
  insulin pens, 25–28
  insulin storage, 28–29
  for insulin therapy, 23–24, 95, 117
  mixing insulins, 30–31
    microprecipitation changing absorp-
      tion from, 30, 79
  painful injections, 31
  rotating sites, 32–33
  self-blood glucose monitoring, 34–43
    meter accuracy and troubleshoot-
      ing, 42–43
    record keeping, 41–42
    technique for, 41
  sick-day rules, 43–44

[Diabetes education]
  survival skills, 22
  syringes, 24–25
    reuse and disposal, 25
  urine ketone testing, 44
Diabetes control and complications trial
    (DCCT) in type 1 diabetes, 2–3,
    92–94, 195–196
  incidence of hypoglycemia in, 195–196
Diabetes Epidemiology: Collaborative
    Analysis of Diagnostic Criteria
    in Europe (DECODE), 9
Diabetic ketoacidosis, 173–192
  clinical features of, 177–179
  diagnosis and initial evaluation of,
    179–182
  differential diagnosis versus non-
    ketotic hyperosmolar syndrome,
    183
  general management of, 188–190
    with insulin pump use, 233
  incidence and mortality of, 174
  ketone measurement in, 181–182
  pathogenesis of, 175–177
  protocol for treatment of, 190–191
  treatment of, 183–190
    bicarbonate, 187–188
    general management, 188–190
    hydration, 183–185
    insulin, 185–186
    phosphorus, 188
    potassium, 186–187
    protocol for, 190–191
Diabetes Mellitus Insulin Glucose
    Infusion in Acute Myocardial
    Infarction study (*see* DIGAMI
    study)
Diagnosis of diabetes, impaired glucose
    tolerance and impaired fasting
    glucose, 14–15
Diet therapy of diabetes, 47–59
  ADA recommendations for, 48–49
  carbohydrate counting, 56–57, 216
  in children, 134
  exchange lists, 56
  gastroparesis and, 216

[Diet therapy of diabetes]
hypoglycemia and treatment of, 57–58, 203–205
insulin programs for inpatients receiving:
enteral nutrition, 164–166
meals, 161–163
parenteral nutrition, 166
meal planning strategies, 54–57
nutrition needs in inpatients, 155–156
in pregnancy, 145–146
USDA food pyramid, 55
DIGAMI study, 157, 170
DKA (*see* Diabetic ketoacidosis)
Dosing adjustments, 107–109, 208–210
bedtime insulin in type 2 diabetes, protocol, 123
in insulin pumps, 230–231
rule of 1500 or 1800, 108–109, 209, 230–231
sliding scales and problems with:
in hospitalized patients, 158–160
in outpatients, 107–109, 208

Education (*see* Diabetes education)
Elderly and hypoglycemia risk, 199
Exchange list for meal planning, 56
Exercise and insulin therapy, 95
in children, 134
reducing insulin to avoid hypoglycemia, 207

Fasting glucose level, 61–63, 65–68
hepatic glucose production in the control of, 7, 61–62
Foot care, 19
Fructosamine test to assess glycemic control, 7

Glargine insulin, 80–81
cannot mix with other insulins, 30, 81, 101
intensive insulin program with mealtime short-acting insulin analog, 100–102
not proven for use in pregnancy, 144
use in children, 132

Glucose homeostasis (*see* Physiology of blood glucose level)
Glucotoxicity and reversal by insulin therapy, 118
Glycated hemoglobin (*see* Hemoglobin A$_{1c}$)
Glycemic control:
assessment of, 6–7
by fructosamine, 7
by hemoglobin A$_{1c}$ (HbA$_{1c}$), 5–6, 15–16, 114
blood glucose guidelines for, 15, 92, 229
contribution of fasting and postprandial glucose level to, 7–10
insulin pump success in achieving, 224
postprandial glucose levels contribution to, 8–10
rationale and strategies for achieving, 1–11
in pregnancy, 140–142
to prevent macrovascular complications, 6, 113
to prevent microvascular complications, 2–6
in type 1 diabetes, 2–3
in type 2 diabetes, 3–6
relationship to diabetes complications, 1–11
studies showing benefit of:
Diabetes Control and Complications Trial (DCCT) in type 1 diabetes, 2–3, 92–94, 195, 196
Kumamoto Study in type 2 diabetes, 3–4
Stockholm Diabetes Intervention Study in type 1 diabetes, 3
United Kingdom Prospective Diabetes Study (UKPDS) in type 2 diabetes, 4–6
tests to assess, 6–7
Goals of treatment (*see* Treatment guidelines)
Guidelines of treatment (*see* Treatment guidelines)

HAAF syndrome (*see* Hypoglycemia-associated autonomic failure *and* Hypoglycemia unawareness)

Hemoglobin $A_{1c}$ (Hb$A_{1c}$)
  to assess glycemic control, 5–6, 15–16, 114
  in children, 133
  in pregnancy, 148
  contribution of fasting and postprandial glucose level to, 7–10
  guideline for optimal glycemic control, 5–6, 15–16, 114
  lack of use for the diagnosis of diabetes, 15
  methods to measure, 7

Honeymoon effect on insulin requirements, 129–130

Honolulu heart study, 9

Hospitalized patients with diabetes, 153–171
  blood glucose monitoring in, 156–157
  dosing adjustment of insulin by algorithm, 160–161
    lack of effectiveness of sliding scales, 158–160
  guidelines for glucose control in, 157–158
  insulin infusion, 160–161, 163–164
  insulin programs for, 161–169
    acute myocardial infarction (DIGAMI protocol), 170
    glargine use in, 162
    intravenous infusion, 160–161, 163–164
    lispro use in, 162
    patient who is eating, 161–163
    patient receiving enteral nutrition, 164–166
    patient receiving parenteral nutrition, 166
    preoperative patient, 166–169
  nutrition needs in, 155–156
  preoperative diabetes management, 166–169
  sliding scales and lack of effectiveness in, 158–160

Humalog (*see* Insulin analogs, lispro)

Hyperglycemic emergencies (*see* Diabetic ketoacidosis *and* Nonketotic hyperosmolar syndrome)

Hypertension (*see* Blood pressure guidelines in diabetes)

Hypoglycemia and insulin therapy, 57–58, 92–94, 193–222
  avoidance strategies of, 214–217, 234
  in children with diabetes, 135–136
  in combination insulin and oral hypoglycemic pills, 217–218
  counterregulation in type 2 diabetes, 199–200
  and dawn phenomenon, 213–214
  in elderly, 19
  with exercise, 207
  factors that impair hypoglycemia defenses, 202
  and gastroparesis, 216
  hypoglycemia unawareness, 92–94
    HAAF syndrome, 200–201
    insulin pump therapy in, 240
    management of, 201, 202–203
    reversibility of, 200–202
    self-blood glucose monitoring in, 208
  incidence of:
    in Diabetes Control and Complications Trial (DCCT), 195–196
    in type 1 and type 2 diabetes, 116, 193–195, 198–200
    with insulin pump therapy, 224, 233
    lispro versus Regular insulin, 77–78, 98–100
  in insulin pump therapy, 224, 233
    prevention and treatment in adults, 233–234
    prevention and treatment in children, 236–237
  neurological dysfunction from, 197–198
  nocturnal hypoglycemia, 201
    with commercial premixed insulin, 212
    with insulin pump therapy, 233
    with NPH insulin, 212
    with Ultralente insulin, 99
  risk factors for severe, 195, 199

[Hypoglycemia and insulin therapy]
risk with intensive insulin therapy, 92–94
role in causing hypoglycemia unawareness, 200–202
and sudden death, 198
symptoms of, 196–197
treatment of, 57–58, 203–205
Hypoglycemia-associated autonomic failure (HAAF syndrome), 200-202
Hypoglycemia unawareness, 92–94
factors that impair hypoglycemia defenses, 202
insulin pump therapy in, 240
management of, 201, 202–203
reversibility of, 200–202
self-blood glucose monitoring in, 208

Inhaled insulin, 252–256
in children, 132
Inpatient insulin use (*see* Hospitalized
patients with diabetes)
Insulin analogs, 75, 211–212
aspart, 77–78
in insulin pump, 77–78, 227
detemir, 82
glargine, 80–81
cannot be mixed with other insulins, 30, 81, 101
in children, 132
in hospitalized patients, 162
intensive insulin program with pre-
meal short-acting insulin analog,
100–102
not proven for use in pregnancy, 144
lispro, 76–78
caution with gastroparesis, 216
in hospitalized patients, 162
in insulin pump, 77–78, 227
less hypoglycemia than Regular insulin, 77–78, 98–100
in pregnancy, 142–145
premixed commercial insulin preparations, 80
Insulin injection technique, 29–30
assistance devices, 33–34
difficulties with, 31–33

Insulin infusions (*see* Intravenous insulin infusion)
Insulin pens, 25–28
manufacturer phone numbers, 26
Insulin pharmacokinetics, 73–85, 91
intermediate-acting insulins, 78–80
long-acting insulins, 80–81
short-acting insulins, 76–78
variable day-to-day profiles, 75
Insulin programs, 96–106
bedtime insulin in type 2 diabetes,
protocol for, 123
bedtime NPH and pre-meal Regular,
102–103
daytime NPH, 103–106, 212
glargine with pre-meal short-acting analog, 100–102
premixed commercial preparations,
79–80, 212–213
Ultralente with pre-meal short-acting
analog, 98–100
Insulin pump therapy, 223–244
blood glucose guidelines with, 229
hypoglycemia unawareness, 234
in children, 130–131, 234–238
diabetic ketoacidosis and prevention
of, 233
dosing adjustments with, 230–231
effectiveness at achieving glycemic
control with, 224
in gastroparesis, 240–241
and hypoglycemia:
lowered incidence with, 224
prevention and treatment in adults,
233–234
prevention and treatment in children, 236–237
in hypoglycemia unawareness, 240
in pregnancy, 143–144, 238–240
in renal disease, 240
sandwich technique for skin irritation,
232
troubleshooting high blood glucose
level:
in adults, 232
in children, 236–237

[Insulin pump therapy]
in type 1 diabetes, 228–234
in type 2 diabetes, 238
use of insulin analogs lispro and
aspart, 77–78, 227
Insulin secretion and regulation of the
blood glucose level, 63-65, 88–
91
and dawn phenomenon, 90
Insulin storage, 28–29
Insulin therapy:
absorption of insulins and factors that
affect, 33, 75, 95
in acute myocardial infarction based
on the DIGAMI study, 157,
170
bedtime insulin in type 2 diabetes,
protocol for, 123
benefits of, 117–118
BIDS–bedtime insulin, daytime sulfonylurea, 118–119
concerns over insulin use, 116–117
hypoglycemia, 116
cardiovascular disease, 116
weight gain, 116
dawn phenomenon, 90, 213–214
in diabetic ketoacidosis, 183–190
and diet therapy, 47–59
ADA recommendations, 48–49
dosing adjustments in, 107–109,
208–210
insulin pumps, 230–231
rule of 1500 or 1800, 108–109,
209, 230–231
sliding scales in hospitalized patients, 158–160
sliding scales in outpatients, 107–
109, 208
equipment:
injection aids, 33–34
injection technique, 29–30
insulin storage, 28–29
pens, 25–28
pump, 223–244
syringes, 24–25
syringe reuse and disposal, 25

[Insulin therapy]
glucose metabolism in fasted and fed
state for insulin replacement,
65–69
glucotoxicity and reversal by, 118
in hospitalized patients, 153–171
insulin infusion, 160–161, 163–164
preoperative, 166–169
receiving enteral nutrition, 164–166
receiving meals, 161–163
receiving parenteral nutrition, 166
in hyperglycemic emergencies, 173–
192
and hypoglycemia, 57–58, 193–222
inhaled insulin, 252–256
in children, 132
injection aid devices, 33–34
injection anxiety, 117, 247
injection difficulties, 31–33
injection technique, 29–30
insulin infusion, 160–161, 163–164
insulin storage, 28–29
intensive basal-bolus, 87–112
dosing adjustments in, 107–109
eligibility for, 91–92
goals and risks of, 92–94
how to, 95–102
hypoglycemia with, 92–94
insulin programs, 96–106
normal insulin secretion profile,
63–65, 88–91, 205–206
self-blood glucose monitoring in, 109
24-hour insulin dose calculation, 96
in type 2 diabetes, 119–120
weight gain with, 94
in labor, 148–149
mixing insulins, 30–31
microprecipitation changing insulin
absorption, 30, 79
in nonketotic hyperosmolar syndrome, 173–192
noninvasive insulin delivery, 245–260
inhaled insulin, 252–256
intranasal insulin delivery, 251
jet injectors, 249–250
oral insulin, 251–252

[Insulin therapy]
  patient education in, 23–24, 95, 117
  pens, 25–28
    manufacturer phone numbers, 26
  pharmacokinetics, 73–85, 91
    intermediate-acting insulins, 78–80
    long-acting insulins, 80–81
    short-acting insulins, 76–78
    variable day-to-day profiles, 75
  postpartum, 149
  in pregnancy, 139–151
  premixed commercial insulin prepara-
    tions, 79–80, 212–213
  preoperative, 166–169
  programs, 96–106
    basal insulin strategies, 214
    bedtime insulin in type 2 diabetes,
      protocol, 123
    bedtime NPH and pre-meal Regu-
      lar, 102–103
    bolus insulin strategies, 214–217
    daytime NPH, 103–106, 212
    glargine with pre-meal short-acting
      analog, 100–102
    premixed commercial insulin prepa-
      rations, 79–80, 212–213
    Ultralente with pre-meal short-act-
      ing analog, 98–100
  that do not promote macrovascular dis-
    ease based on results of UKPDS
    in type 2 diabetes, 5, 116
  pump, 223–244
  rotating sites, 32–33
  self-blood glucose monitoring, 34–43
  sick day management, 43–44
  syringes, 24–25
  timing of short-acting insulin to avoid
    hypoglycemia, 214-215
  24-hour insulin dose calculation, 96
  in type 1 diabetes, 87–112 (*see also*
    Insulin therapy, Intensive basal-
    bolus)
  in type 2 diabetes, 113–125
    bedtime insulin, protocol for, 123
    BIDS, bedtime insulin, daytime sul-
      fonylurea, 118–119

[Insulin therapy]
  indications for, 114–115
  intensified insulin regimens, 119–120
  treatment of, 120–123
  urine ketone testing, 44
Intranasal insulin delivery, 251
Intravenous insulin infusion, 160–161,
  163–164

Jet insulin injectors, 249–250

Ketone measurements, 181–182
Kumamoto Study in type 2 diabetes, 3–4

Labor, insulin therapy in, 148–149
Lantus (*see* Insulin analogs, Glargine)
LADA, latent autoimmune diabetes in
  adults, 115, 154–155,
Lente insulin, 78–79
  microprecipitation of Regular insulin
    when mixed with, 30, 79
Lipid guidelines in diabetes, 16–17
  cholesterol guidelines, 2, 16–17
Lipoatrophy, 31–32
Lipohypertrophy, 32–33
Lispro (*see* Insulin analogs)

Macrosomia, 140
Macrovascular complications in diabetes:
  glycemic control for prevention of, 6,
    113
  insulin infusion in acute myocardial in-
    farction, DIGAMI study, 157, 170
  insulin treatment not cause, based on
    results of UKPDS in type 2 dia-
    betes, 5, 116
  prevention of:
    ACE inhibitors, MICRO-HOPE
      study, 17
    aspirin use for primary and second-
      ary prevention of, 19
    cholesterol guidelines, 2, 16–17
    glycemic control in UKPDS study,
      113
    lipid guidelines, 16–17
    smoking, 19

[Macrovascular complications in diabetes]
  risk with insulin therapy, 116
  studies showing importance of post-
      prandial glucose in:
    DECODE, 9
    Honolulu Heart Study, 9
Microalbuminuria screening for nephrop-
    athy, 18
Microvascular complications in dia-
    betes:
  glycemic control for prevention of,
      2–6
Mixing insulins, 30–31
  microprecipitation changing absorp-
      tion, 30, 79

National Cholesterol Education Program
    (NCEP) guidelines, 2, 17
National High Blood Pressure Education
    program guidelines, 17
Natural history and progressive nature
    of type 2 diabetes based on
    UKPDS study, 114
Noninvasive insulin delivery, 245–260
Nonketotic hyperosmolar syndrome,
    173–192
  clinical features of, 177–179
  diagnosis and initial evaluation of,
      182–183
  differential diagnosis versus diabetic
      ketoacidosis, 183
  general management of, 188–190
  incidence and mortality of, 174–175
  pathogenesis of, 175–177
  treatment of, 183–190
    general management, 188–190
    hydration, 184–185
    insulin, 185–186
    potassium, 186–187
    phosphorus, no indication for, 188
Novolog (*see* Insulin analogs, Aspart)
NPH insulin, 79–80, 212
  bedtime NPH and pre-meal Regular,
      102–103
  daytime NPH, 103–106, 212
Nutrition (*see* Diet therapy)

Oral agent failures and insulin therapy
    in type 2 diabetes, 114-115
Oral insulin, 251–252

Painful injections, 31
Pattern management (*see* Dosing adjust-
    ments)
Pens (*see* Insulin pens)
Physiology of blood glucose level, 61–
    71
  dawn phenomenon, 90
  and fasting glucose level, 7, 61–63
  glucose metabolism in fasted and fed
      state for insulin replacement,
      65–69
  insulin secretion, 63–65, 88–91,
      205–206
  and postprandial glucose level, 7
  in pregnancy, 141
  in type 2 diabetes, 7–8
Postpartum insulin requirements, 149
Postprandial glucose level, 68–69
  factors that influence, 7
  in level of hemoglobin $A_{1c}$, 8–10
  role in macrovascular complications, 9
    DECODE study, 9
    Honolulu Heart Study, 9
  role in neonatal macrosomia, 140
Pregnancy and diabetes, 139–151
  diet in, 145–146
  guidelines for:
    glucose control, 146–147
    hemoglobin $A_{1c}$, 148
    screening for complications, 147
  insulin analogs in:
    glargine, 144
    lispro, 142–145
  insulin pump therapy in, 143–144,
      238–240
  insulin requirements:
    during labor, 148–149
    during pregnancy, 142–145
    postpartum, 149
  neonatal care, 149
  normal carbohydrate metabolism in,
      141

[Pregnancy and diabetes]
rationale for glycemic control in,
140–142
self-blood glucose monitoring in,
146–147
urine ketone testing in, 44
Premixed commercial insulin preparations, 79–80, 212–213
Preoperative diabetes management,
166–169
Proteinuria (*see* Microalbuminuria
screening for nephropathy)
Pulmonary insulin (*see* Inhaled insulin)
Pump (*see* Insulin pump)

Rationale for intensive glycemic control
(*see* Glycemic control)
Registered dietician, 49–50
Regular insulin, 76–78
intensive insulin therapy with bedtime
NPH and pre-meal Regular,
102–103
more hypoglycemia than lispro, 77–
78, 98–100
wait 30–45 minutes before eating,
214–216
Risk of macrovascular complications
with insulin therapy, 116
Rule of 1500 or 1800 for dosing adjustments, 108–109, 209, 230-231

Screening for diabetes complications:
American Diabetes Association
(ADA) guidelines, 14
blood pressure, 17
foot exams, 19
lipids, 16–17
nephropathy 17–18
retinopathy, 18
Self-blood glucose monitoring (SBMG),
34–43,
in children, 133
education for, 36–37
frequency of, 40
with hypoglycemia unawareness,
208

[Self-blood glucose monitoring (SBMG)]
guidelines for blood glucose control, 15
in pregnancy, 146–147
inpatient glucose monitoring, 156–
157
with intensive insulin therapy, 109–
110
meters:
accuracy and troubleshooting, 42
manufacturer phone numbers, 38–
39
selection, 37–40
for visually impaired, 37–40
postprandial measurements in hemoglobin $A_{1c}$ level, 9–10
in pregnancy, 146–147
record keeping, 41–42
technique, 41
Sick-day management:
in adults, 43–44
in children, 136–137
Sliding scales (*see* Dosing adjustments)
Stockholm diabetes intervention study
in type 1 diabetes, 3
Syringes, 24–25
reuse and disposal, 25

Total glycosylated hemoglobin (*see* Hemoglobin $A_{1c}$)
Treatment guidelines, 13–20
American Diabetes Association
(ADA) standards, 14
blood glucose, 15, 92, 229
blood pressure, 17
cholesterol, 2, 16–17
foot care, 19
hemoglobin $A_{1c}$ (Hb$A_{1c}$), 5–6, 15–16,
114
immunizations for influenza and pneu-
mococcus, 19
inpatient glycemia goals, 157–158
lipids, 16–17
microalbuminuria screening, 17–18
in pregnancy, 147
retinopathy screening, 18
smoking, 19

Type 1 diabetes, 87–112
    diabetic ketoacidosis, 173–192
    diet therapy in, 51–52
    incidence of hypoglycemia, 193–196
        in Diabetes Control and Complica-
        tions Trial (DCCT) 195-196
        risk factors for, 195
    insulin pump in, 228–234
    LADA, latent autoimmune diabetes in
        adults, 115, 154–155
Type 2 diabetes, 113–125 (*see also*
        United Kingdom Prospective Dia-
        betes Study)
    bedtime insulin, protocol for, 123
    BIDS, bedtime insulin, daytime sul-
        fonylurea, 118–119
    combination insulin and oral hypogly-
        cemic pills, 118–119, 120–123,
        217–218
    diet therapy in, 52–54
    glucotoxicity and reversal by insulin
        therapy, 118
    incidence of hypoglycemia, 193–194,
        198–200
        combination insulin and oral hypo-
          glycemic pills, 217-218
        counterregulation in, 199–200
        risk factors for, 199
    indications for insulin therapy in,
        114–115
    insulin pump in, 238

[Type 2 diabetes]
    intensified insulin regimens in, 119–
        120
    natural history and progressive nature
        based on UKPDS study, 114
    nonketotic hyperosmolar syndrome,
        173–192
    treatment of, 120–123
    24-hour glucose profiles, 7–8

Ultralente insulin, 80
    intensive insulin progam with pre-meal
        short-acting analog, 98–100
    microprecipitation of Regular insulin
        when mixed with, 30, 79
United Kingdom Prospective Diabetes
        Study (UKPDS) in type 2 diabe-
        tes, 4–6
    glycemic control shown to lower mac-
        rovascular disease in, 6, 113
    insulin therapy does not promote mac-
        rovascular disease, 5
    natural history and progressive nature
        of type 2 diabetes from, 114
UKPDS (*see* United Kingdom Prospec-
        tive Diabetes Study)

Weight gain
    with combination insulin and oral hy-
        poglycemic pills, 116-117
    with intensive insulin therapy, 94